Quantitative Methods for Precision Medicine

Modern medicine is undergoing a paradigm shift from a "one-size-fits-all" strategy to a more precise patient-customized therapy and medication plan. While the success of precision medicine relies on the level of pharmacogenomic knowledge, dissecting the genetic mechanisms of drug response in a sufficient detail requires powerful computational tools. *Quantitative Methods for Precision Medicine: Pharmacogenomics in Action* presents the advanced statistical methods for mapping pharmacogenetic control by integrating pharmacokinetic and pharmacodynamic principles of drug–body interactions. Beyond traditional reductionist-based statistical genetic approaches, statistical formulization in this book synthesizes elements of multiple disciplines to infer, visualize, and track how pharmacogenes interact together as an intricate but well-coordinated system to mediate patient-specific drug response.

Features:

- Functional and systems mapping models to characterize the genetic architecture of multiple medication processes
- Statistical methods for analyzing informative missing data in pharmacogenetic association studies
- Functional graph theory of inferring genetic interaction networks from association data
- Leveraging the concept of epistasis to capture its bidirectional, signed, and weighted properties
- Modeling gene-induced cell–cell crosstalk and its impact on drug response
- A graph model of drug–drug interactions in combination therapies
- Critical methodological issues to improve pharmacogenomic research as the cornerstone of precision medicine

This book is suitable for graduate students and researchers in the fields of biology, medicine, bioinformatics, drug design and delivery who are interested in statistical and computational modeling of biological processes and systems. It may also serve as a major reference for applied mathematicians, computer scientists, and statisticians who attempt to develop algorithmic tools for genetic mapping, systems pharmacogenomics, and systems biology. It can be used as both a textbook and research reference. Professionals in pharmaceutical sectors who design drugs and clinical doctors who deliver drugs will also find it useful.

Chapman & Hall/CRC Biostatistics Series

Series Editors

Shein-Chung Chow, *Duke University School of Medicine, USA*
Byron Jones, *Novartis Pharma AG, Switzerland*
Jen-Pei Liu, *National Taiwan University, Taiwan*
Karl E. Peace, *Georgia Southern University, USA*
Bruce W. Turnbull, *Cornell University, USA*

RECENTLY PUBLISHED TITLES

Hybrid Frequentist/Bayesian Power and Bayesian Power in
Planning Clinical Trials
Andrew P. Grieve

Advanced Statistics in Regulatory Critical Clinical Initiatives
Edited By Wei Zhang, Fangrong Yan, Feng Chen, and Shein-Chung Chow

Medical Statistics for Cancer Studies
Trevor F. Cox

Real World Evidence in a Patient-Centric Digital Era
Edited by Kelly H. Zou, Lobna A. Salem, and Amrit Ray

Data Science, AI, and Machine Learning in Pharma
Harry Yang

Model-Assisted Bayesian Designs for Dose Finding and Optimization
Methods and Applications
Ying Yuan, Ruitao Lin, and J. Jack Lee

Digital Therapeutics: Strategic, Scientific, Developmental, and
Regulatory Aspects
Oleksandr Sverdlov and Joris van Dam

Quantitative Methods for Precision Medicine
Pharmacogenomics in Action
Rongling Wu

Drug Development for Rare Diseases
Edited by Bo Yang, Yang Song, and Yijie Zhou

For more information about this series, please visit: https://www.routledge.com/
Chapman--Hall-CRC-Biostatistics-Series/book-series/CHBIOSTATIS

Quantitative Methods for Precision Medicine
Pharmacogenomics in Action

Rongling Wu

With Contributions from
Mengmeng Sang and Li Feng

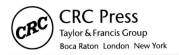

CRC Press
Taylor & Francis Group
Boca Raton London New York

CRC Press is an imprint of the
Taylor & Francis Group, an **informa** business

A CHAPMAN & HALL BOOK

First edition published 2023
by CRC Press
6000 Broken Sound Parkway NW, Suite 300, Boca Raton, FL 33487-2742

and by CRC Press
4 Park Square, Milton Park, Abingdon, Oxon, OX14 4RN

© 2023 Taylor & Francis Group, LLC

CRC Press is an imprint of Taylor & Francis Group, LLC

Library of Congress Cataloging-in-Publication Data
Names: Wu, Rongling, author. | Sang, Mengmeng, contributor. | Li, Feng (Computational biologist), contributor.
Title: Quantitative methods for precision medicine : pharmacogenomics in action / Rongling Wu (the Pennsylvania State University, USA) ; with contributions from Mengmeng Sang (Institute of Reproductive Medicine, Nantong University Medical School, China), Feng Li (Centre for Computational Biology, College of Biological Science and Technologies, Beijing Forestry University, China).
Description: First edition. | Boca Raton : C&H/CRC Press, 2023. | Series: Chapman & Hall/CRC biostatistics series | Includes bibliographical references and index.
Identifiers: LCCN 2022030449 (print) | LCCN 2022030450 (ebook) | ISBN 9781482219456 (hardback) | ISBN 9781032398877 (paperback) | ISBN 9780429171512 (ebook)
Subjects: LCSH: Precision medicine--Statistical methods. | Precision medicine—Mathematical models. | Personalized medicine—Statistical methods. | Personalized medicine--Mathematical models.
Classification: LCC RM301.3.G45 W78 2023 (print) | LCC RM301.3.G45 (ebook) | DDC 615.701/51—dc23/eng/20221013
LC record available at https://lccn.loc.gov/2022030449
LC ebook record available at https://lccn.loc.gov/2022030450

ISBN: 9781482219456 (hbk)
ISBN: 9781032398877 (pbk)
ISBN: 9780429171512 (ebk)

DOI: 10.1201/9780429171512

Typeset in Palatino
by codeMantra

Contents

Part 2   Network Pharmacogenetics

Preface

We are all different in many ways, including susceptibility to a particular disease, biology by which the disease develops, and response to a specific medical treatment. Some people break down drugs more quickly than is needed, resulting in an inadequate amount of the drugs to fight the disease, while for other people, the drugs do not break down rapidly enough so that they accumulate in the body and cause side effects. Because of these differences, catalyzed by the human genome project, modern medicine has made a paradigm shift from a conventional "one-drug-fits-all" strategy to the thinking of precision medicine aimed to tailor and customize therapeutic practices for the best healthcare of individual patients.

The central cause of our discrepancies is the differential action of our genomes and related exposomics and metabolomics as well as their interactions with non-genetic factors, such as lifestyle, living environment, age, and body weight among others. For this reason, pharmacogenetics, also interchangeably called pharmacogenomics, which studies genetic variation associated with drug-body interactions, stands at the core of precision medicine. In recent years, sophisticated technologies have emerged that enable researchers to collect and stream an avalanche of data to omnidirectionally track biological, medical, and health processes of drug response. At the same time, it is very clear that dissecting the molecular mechanisms of interindividual differences at a level of details that are informative enough for the design of precision medicine sorely relies on how these data can be omnidirectionally modeled and analyzed in accord with fundamental principles of biology, biomedicine, biophysics, and engineering. We write this book by focusing on interdisciplinary statistical methodologies that can potentially promote pharmacogenetic and pharmacogenomic research.

The book is organized into ten chapters. In the first chapter, we review the current status of pharmacogenetic mapping and association studies and discuss the challenges of moving pharmacogenomic research from a phenomenological observation to mechanistic understanding. The following eight chapters are divided into two balanced parts. Part 1 – Pharmacokinetic–Pharmacodynamic Pharmacogenetics is comprised of four chapters that present the statistical principle of integrating pharmacokinetic–pharmacodynamic principles into pharmacogenetic mapping and its broader and more effective applications to pharmacogenetic clinical trials. Part 1 is the refinement and expansion of Wu and Lin's (2008) *Statistical and Computational Pharmacogenomics*. Part 2 – Network Pharmacogenetics consists of four chapters that depict the statistical models for coalescing all possible interactive pharmacogenes into pharmacogenetic networks to chart personalized genetic architecture as an essential step toward precision medicine.

Part 2 records our latest conceptual methodological development of how to understand pharmacogenomics from a holistic, systems-oriented thinking. We write the last chapter to provide a prospect on the methodological leverage of pharmacogenomic research in several areas that can make it more tangible to precision medicine.

This book is a systematic collection of statistical models and methods for pharmacogenomic research developed in my program during the past decades. It is intended to provide analytical tools for pharmacogeneticists who are interested to explore the pharmacogenetic mechanisms underlying why some people are more responsive to medications than others, why some people produce significant drug side-effects whereas others do not, and why some people generate drug resistance more rapidly than others from a multidisciplinary perspective. It is also intended to attract the beginners' interest to pursue pharmacogenomic research by providing model derivations, practical examples, and detailed result interpretations. It is our hope that this book can help bring pharmacogeneticists into the cutting-edge frontiers of genetic research that facilitate the translation of precision medicine. Although our examples are from a small-scale pharmacogenetic association study, the concepts and methods described in the book can be appropriately applied to any large-scale association cohorts and consortia.

Writing a book is never an easy job, and it relies on tremendous involvements of many people. Mengmeng Sang and Li Feng performed data analysis, wrote computer code, drew figures for most chapters, and provided their unique insight into computational pharmacogenetics. Their contributions reach a level that deserves recognition on the cover of the book as collaborators. Many other people, including my current and previous students and collaborators, have made substantial contributions to this book in some ways. The following people need to be specially mentioned. Ang Dong helped perform computer simulation for ordinary systems mapping in Chapter 5. A small example of stochastic systems mapping with Euphrates poplar in Chapter 5 is derived from Dr Jingwen Gan's thesis. The main text of Chapter 4 was derived from my previous publications with Dr Hongying Li and Dr Zhong Wang. Some figures are cited and adapted from our early papers, which have been acknowledged. The example of a dobutamine-based pharmacogenetic association study, used in our previous publications and re-used many times in several chapters of this book, was provided by Prof. Julie Johnson at the University of Florida. Special appreciation is given to Dr Libo Jiang whose contribution to my research program has fostered our methodological development in the area.

This work was completed at my home university – Pennsylvania State University College of Medicine. A special gratitude is due to Distinguished Professor Vernon Chinchilli, Chair of the Department of Public Health, for his tireless support of my research program. His leadership creates a free and stimulating academic atmosphere, enabling me to focus on my independent and collaborative research. I wish to thank Professor Christopher Griffin, whose expertise in game theory has enlightened my thinking of introducing this fascinating theory into genetic mapping to open up a new gateway for pharmacogenetic research. I would also like to thank Editor Rob Calver for inviting me to publish an advanced statistical pharmacogenetic book at Chapman Hall/CRC and Vijay Shanker for his editorial and technical assistance in improving the presentation of this book.

Last, not least, I extend my warmest thanks to my family. My wife, Professor Lidan Sun, has always given me her unwavering encouragement, support, and love during my book writing and beyond. My parent-in-laws have helped me take care of my son, letting me write this book without worrying about his daily life and schooling. I am grateful to my two older sisters for caring so much for me that they could not sleep in the nights when the COVID-19 pandemic spread in the United States. My son, Jialu (Barron) Wu, is the best stimulator for me to work hard to achieve my goals in both life and career.

Rongling Wu
Hershey, PA

Biography

Rongling Wu develops a transdisciplinary approach for building up multilayer, multiscale, and multifunctional bridges that link genotype to phenotype. Dr Wu asks, answers, and disseminates biologically meaningful questions in the boundaries of statistics, genetics, ecology, and evolution. He invented a statistical method called functional mapping to reveal the genetic architecture of developmental trajectories and incorporated this approach into the context of eco-evo-devo research aimed to unveil the genetic and ecological mechanisms underpinning evolutionary novelties. More recently, Dr Wu has integrated evolutionary game theory and predator-prey theory through naturally omnipresent allometric scaling law into graph theory to create a new theory – functional game-graph theory. This new theory can unravel the internal workings of complex systems at an unprecedented level of detail by charting and tracing the causal, signed, and weighted roadmap of relationships among any set of variables (including high- or even ultrahigh-dimensional variables) from any data domains. The second part of this book represents the application of this theory to pharmacogenomic research. Dr Wu received his PhD in quantitative genetics at the University of Washington in 1995. He was appointed an Assistant Professor of Statistics at the University of Florida in 2000 and awarded the University Foundation Professorship in 2007. Since 2008, Dr Wu has been Professor of Public Health Sciences and Statistics, promoted to Distinguished Professor in 2015 and served as Director of the Center of Statistical Genetics at The Pennsylvania State University. Dr Wu is a Fellow of the American Statistical Association and a Fellow of the American Association for the Advancement of Science.

Dr Mengmeng Sang and Ms Li Feng are collaborators of this book writing project under the leadership of Dr Wu. Dr Sang received his PhD degree at Beijing Forestry University in 2019 and is currently working as Lecturer of Medical Informatics at Nantong University Medical School, China. Ms Feng is a PhD candidate in computational biology at Beijing Forestry University and will graduate in 2023. The research interest of both Dr Sang and Ms Feng lies in the statistical modeling of computational biology and its applications to a broader area of agriculture, forestry, medicine, and beyond.

1

Methodological Foundation of Precision Medicine

1.1 Interpersonal Variability in Drug Response

Not all patients respond to drug therapy in an effective and efficient way. Interindividual variability in drug response involves a strong genetic component (Weinshilboum 2003; Eichelbaum et al. 2006; Madian et al. 2012; Suarez-Kurtz and Parra 2018). Pharmacogenetics, as a term first proposed in 1959 (Vogel 1959), has already emerged as a discipline, aimed to identify and study single DNA variants that control the response to a drug. With the availability of high-throughput sequencing and genotypic data, pharmacogenetics has been shifted to a higher level of pharmacogenomics at which all of genes throughout the genome for drug response are characterized (Weinshilboum and Wang 2006, 2017; Tse et al. 2011; Primorac et al. 2020). DNA variants influence drug response through mediating protein function. Much of the early pharmacogenetic research focused on non-synonymous DNA variants; i.e., those that alter protein function by changing the encoded amino acids. Contemporary genomics has uncovered a much broader array of genetic variants for drug response. Although they do not encode proteins, non-coding variants can still affect drug response through regulating gene expression (Xie et al. 2019; Park et al. 2020; Cano-Gamez and Trynka 2020). A similar role may also be played by epigenetic changes and small mRNAs that are identified as important mechanisms modulating gene expression and function (Sadée and Dai 2005; Cecil et al. 2016; Hanna et al. 2019; You et al. 2020).

Pharmacogenomics, as an approach to identifying the genomic determinants of drug response, is a catch-all term that fails to characterize a cascade of biological pathways that affect the body's response to drugs. There are two main types of interactions between drugs and the body, known as pharmacokinetics (PK) and pharmacodynamics (PD), both of which are related to drug response (Meibohm and Derendorf 1997; Prantil-Baun et al. 2018; Zou et al. 2020), influenced by genomic factors (de Vries Schultink et al. 2015; Schärfe et al. 2017; Lu et al. 2020). PK interactions determine how a drug is processed by the body, i.e., how it is absorbed, distributed, metabolized, and excreted. An individual genome may determine the bioavailability (the amount of the drug available to the body) at target sites through PK interactions, producing an impact on the appropriate dosing for that individual. For example, the cytokine CYP2D6 is a protein mediating the body's metabolism of many drugs (Davis et al. 2018; Takahashi et al. 2020). Alterations in the *CYP2D6* gene determine the rate of metabolism for certain medications. If the *CYP2D6* variant an individual carries is a fast metabolizer of a CYP2D6-sensitive medication, the drug will be broken down and eliminated from the body more quickly so that it would be less effective. In contrast, for slow metabolizers, the drug concentration would build up in the body, which may be more susceptible to side effects.

PD interactions describe how a drug impacts the body by modulating cellular reactions in space and time, including treatment efficacy and adverse effects (Pirmohamed 2014). This process is also influenced by genomic factors (Lin et al. 2005a, b; Kozyra et al. 2017; Lu et al. 2020). An example is the apolipoprotein E (APOE), a polymorphic protein with three alleles (E2, E3, and E4). Recent studies show that APOE polymorphism is associated with the efficacy of donepezil in treating Alzheimer's disease (Waring et al. 2015; Lu et al. 2020). This association may result in the role of APOE in the transformation and metabolism of lipoproteins (Uddin et al. 2019). It is likely that the body's response to a certain drug is affected by multiple genetic variants, some affecting PD interactions and others PK pathways. Warfarin, known to be affected by variants at multiple locations in the genome, is such an example. Variants in two different genes can influence this drug's administration in different ways. Whereas variations in one gene, *CYP2C9*, affect the metabolism of the drug (through the PK effect), variants in another gene, *VKORC1*, can affect the target of the drug, a protein involved in blood clotting (through the PD effect) (Sangviroon et al. 2010).

Given that the influence of genomic factors on endpoint drug response is expressed through various biochemical and physiological pathways, pharmacogenomics can be better studied by incorporating PK-PD processes into genetic associations. Functional mapping, a dynamic model for mapping complex traits (Ma et al. 2002; Wu et al. 2004a, b, c; Wu and Lin 2006), has been implemented to map the genetic architecture of drug response by incorporating the mathematical aspects of PK and PD interactions (Lin and Wu 2005; Lin et al. 2005a, b, 2007; Wang et al. 2015a). The modified functional pharmacogenetic mapping model, systematically reviewed in Wu and Lin (2008), demonstrates its unique statistical power for detecting drug response genes and its biological and clinical relevance of gene detection. By treating a complex trait as a system, functional mapping has been leveraged to systems mapping by which the genetic control of how interconnected components interact with each other to determine trait phenotype can be mapped (Fu et al. 2011; Wu et al. 2011a; Sun and Wu 2015a, b; Fu et al. 2017). Several attempts have been made to implement systems mapping into pharmacogenomic studies, showing a great promise to reveal the mechanistic genetic signatures of drug response (Liu et al. 2013; Wang et al. 2013d). Systems pharmacogenetic mapping organizes systems biology into pharmacogenomics and can provide knowledge about the delivery of the right drug at the right dose at the right time for the right patient. All this forms the central theme of designing personalized medicine.

In traditional medicine, strategies for treating and preventing diseases are made on the basis of the average person, with little consideration for interindividual variability. As opposed to such a one-size-fits-all approach, precision medicine, also known as personalized medicine, tailors disease treatment and prevention strategies for individual persons by taking into account their genetic, environmental, and lifestyle differences. Because of its more precise targeting of subgroups of disease with new therapies, precision medicine can potentially produce increasing therapeutic efficacies and decreasing side effects. The success of precision medicine critically relies on our profound understanding of pharmacogenomics, a study of how genes affect a person's response to drugs. As the combination of pharmacology (the science of drugs) and genomics (the study of genes and their functions), pharmacogenomics forms a core part of precision medicine. This chapter provides an overview of fundamental quantitative approaches for pharmacogenomic research.

1.2 Mechanistic Modeling of Drug Response

The two past decades have witnessed the tremendous growth of using DNA-based polymorphism markers to identify genes responsible for drug response (Weinshilboum 2003; Evans and McLeod 2013; Watters et al. 2004; Daly 2010; Barrett 2019; Koromina et al. 2020). If the genotype of a marker is detected to be significantly associated with a drug-response phenotype through statistical tests, then this marker is regarded as the genetic variants that affect drug response. This approach, although simple and widely applied in practice, cannot provide a mechanistic explanation about how the genes interact with biochemical pathways to determine the end-point phenotype of drug response.

The mechanistic understanding of pharmacogenetic control can be made from two perspectives. In the first (dynamic) perspective, drug response is viewed as a dynamic process involving drug transport, drug metabolism, and drug targets, mathematically described by PK and PD equations (Meibohm and Derendorf 1997). Integrating these biochemically meaningful equations into the functional mapping framework (Ma et al. 2002; Wu and Lin 2006) produces a dynamic mapping approach (Wu and Lin 2007), which can identify specific PK genes that affect time-varying change patterns of drug concentration and specific PD genes that shape dose-effect curves. This approach founded on biochemical reactions can not only identify how genes interact with each other and with developmental and environmental stimuli in a patient's body (Lin et al. 2007) but also quantify the dynamic effects of individual genes and gene-environment interactions on various biochemical pathways and reactions that contribute to drug response (Figure 1.1a).

In the second (regulatory) perspective, drug response is viewed as a complex phenotype, including regulatory and genetic mechanisms between genotype and phenotype. The "Central Dogma" of biology, DNA → mRNA → enzyme (inactive) → enzyme (active) → metabolites → metabolism → cellular physiology → phenotype, subjected to continuous addendums and modifications in the recent past, is thought to be a fundamental rule to the form and control of every aspect of a phenotype. Regulatory control is exerted to affect virtually all these levels. This mechanistic approach based on regulatory control has been developed (Luizon and Ahituv 2015; Wang et al. 2014; Hanson et al. 2016), aimed to identify the "black box" that lies between genotype and drug response through transcript abundance and other intermediate molecular processes (Wu 2021) (Figure 1.1b).

The mechanistic modeling of drug response from dynamic and regulatory perspectives is based on specific modules that are linked through mathematical models. Below, we show how these modules are modeled from genetic, biochemical, and engineering standpoints.

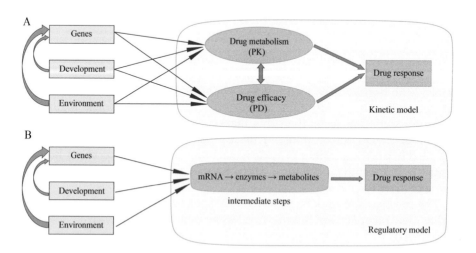

FIGURE 1.1
Kinetic modeling of drug response. (a) Causal effects of genetic, developmental, and environmental factors and their interactions on the outcome of drug response. All these effects operate through PK and PD reactions. (b) Intermediate steps linking signaling, transcriptional and metabolic networks involved in the distribution and action of drugs.

1.2.1 Genetic Architecture Modeling

Genetic architecture, the structure of the mapping from genotype to phenotype, builds and controls a given phenotypic character and its variational properties (Mackay et al. 2009; Rajon and Plotkin 2013). Traditional approaches for linkage and association-based studies have been instrumental in the elucidation of the genetic architecture of complex traits or diseases, such as cardiovascular diseases, metabolic disturbances, diabetes, lipids, inflammation, and cancer. These approaches enable geneticists to address several fundamental questions, i.e., what mode of actions individual genes exert, additive or dominant; whether there are interactions (epistasis) among different genes; what is the pleiotropic effect of genes on different traits; and what is the distribution of allelic effects (Mackay et al. 2009).

Beyond these traditional descriptions, we need to integrate the molecular mechanisms involved in pharmacogenomic effects into drug response. Quantitative genetic theory should be refined to define the molecular effects of genes through mutations, insertions, deletions, copy number variations and, more recently, epigenetic events, such as histone and DNA methylation, and gene expression. To describe the pharmacogenetic control of drug response, the genetic architecture should not be only regarded as a given set of genetic effect parameters, but it should also reflect dynamic trajectories of genetic alteration over time and space and environmental gradients.

1.2.2 Kinetic Models of Drug Reactions

Traditional pharmacogenomics investigates the genetic control of drug response measured as a static state of drug effect. However, when a drug is administered to a patient, it must be absorbed, distributed to its site of action, interact with its targets, undergo metabolism, and finally be excreted (Wang et al. 2008; Tuntland et al. 2014). This so-called PK process influences the concentration of a drug reaching its target, and it interacts with another so-called PD process associated with drug targets to determine drug response (Figure 1.1a). Since functionally important genetic variation also occurs in the drug target itself, or in signaling cascades downstream from the targets, the ability to take into account all of the factors that can influence drug response in the cell would help to better understand the mechanisms involved in the variation of drug response.

As discussed above, the integration of PK and PD equations and functional mapping produces a dynamic mapping approach that can detect genes associated with drug response at varying doses or over a time course. Given that PK and PD are biochemically linked with each other, a more powerful approach to modeling drug response is to treat its formation as a dynamic system in which various biochemical parts are interconnected through a system of ordinary differential equations (ODE) (Sun and Wu 2015a). Thus, by developing and implementing statistical methods for estimating ODE parameters, we can test and quantify the genetic and genomic control of biochemical pathways involved in drug response.

1.2.3 Dynamic Models of Genetic Networks

Current pharmacogenomic studies are based on a direct relationship between genotype and phenotype through simple statistical models that are relatively opaque to biological interpretation. Such "black box" approaches are less helpful in revealing regulatory and genetic mechanisms between genotype and phenotype. As the cost of methods for measuring mRNA, protein, and other indicators continues to fall, it becomes reasonable to design experiments that capture the dynamic processes of phenotypic formation across timescales. With these data, the respective systems disciplines arise from the study of the transcriptome (the set of RNA transcripts) and the metabolome (the entire range of metabolites taking part in a biological process). Other omics (sets) that may also be of interest include: the interactome (complete set of interactions between proteins or between these and other molecules), the localizome (localization of transcripts, proteins, etc.), or even the phenome (complete set of phenotypes) of a given organism (Clayton et al. 2006; Hopkins 2006; Corona et al. 2012; Alarcon-Barrera et al. 2022). New models are needed to reconstruct biological networks by incorporating interactome, localizome, and phenome related to drug response (Busby et al. 2019). Coupling with DNA polymorphism information, these models are capable of mapping quantitative trait loci (QTLs) that control transcriptional (eQTL), proteomic (pQTL), and metabolomic (mQTL) expressions and their interaction networks among these different types of QTLs (Sun et al. 2021; Wu and Jiang 2021; Chen et al. 2022).

1.2.4 Implementing Systems Approaches

Systems biology studies the relationships among elements of a system, aimed to better understand its emergent properties (Wu 2021; Chen et al. 2021). A systems analysis can be applied to molecules, cells, organs, individuals, or even ecosystems. For instance, a system may include just a few protein molecules that together serve a defined task (e.g., fatty acid synthesis), a more complex molecular machine (e.g., a transcription complex), or a cell or group of cells executing a particular function, such as an immune response (Hood and Perlmutter 2004). In each case, a systems analysis describes all of the elements of the system, defines the biological networks that interrelate the elements of a system, and characterizes the flow of information that links these elements to an emergent biological process through their networks. A particular response to medications emerges when the operation of networks is perturbed to some degree. By comparing responsive and non-responsive networks, we can identify critical nodal points (proteins) that, if modulated, are likely to reconfigure the perturbed network structure back toward its non-responsive state (Hopkins 2006). These nodal proteins are likely to represent drug targets.

The detection and identification of nodal proteins in complicated networks is critical in developing the solutions of the models. A system of differential equations can be implemented to model the structure of regulatory networks involved in drug response. Although previous work has utilized ODE to model the change in each gene's expression (Chen et al. 1999; Tegner et al. 2003; Shahrezaei and Swain 2008), these models are structurally too simple to capture the complexity of networks. Also, statistical issues on parameter estimation for differential equations have never been adequately explored. Innovative statistical methods need to be developed for estimating the mathematical parameters defining differential equations with noisy measurements by combining a modified data smoothing method and the generalization of profiled estimation. Also, these statistical methods should be expanded to handle nonlinear differential equations (including stochastic, delay, and partial types) that better describe the complexity of regulatory networks (Kristensen et al. 2005; Fu et al. 2011; Donnet and Samson 2013; Liu et al. 2013; Wang et al. 2013d; Boger and Wigström 2018).

1.3 Statistical Models for Mapping Drug Response

1.3.1 Study Design

The genetic architecture of drug response can better be mapped by integrating its mechanistic foundation into genetic mapping. There are several study designs developed for genome-wide association studies (GWAS) of pharmacogenetic mapping (Guessous et al. 2009; McInnes et al. 2021). One of the most common study designs is the case-control association design in which subjects in the treatment arm of a clinical trial are divided into those with a positive response to the drug and those with a negative or no response (Weiss et al. 2001; Motsinger-Reif et al. 2013; Giacomini et al. 2017). The use of pharmacogenomic GWAS has been instrumental for identifying actionable genetic variants that can inform drug selection and dosage. For example, genetic variants identified in *CYP2C19* have guided the choice of antiplatelet drug and dosage (Scott et al. 2013), whereas variants identified in interleukin-28B has helped determine whether additional drugs should be added to therapeutic regimens of pegylated interferon-α for hepatitis C infections (Muir et al. 2014). The advantage of the case-control design is its capacity to chart a comprehensive picture of pharmacogenetic control without detailed measures of PK and PD processes. Its disadvantage is that it is difficult to integrate the mechanistic processes of drug response into association settings. The second commonest study design is based on population-based association cohorts in which subjects in drug treatment are quantitatively measured for key biochemical and physiological parameters that reflect drug response

(Barrett 2019). In the GWAS of response to methotrexate in rheumatoid arthritis patients, such a parameter was defined as change in disease-activity score from baseline to six months post-administration (Taylor et al. 2018). If these parameters are longitudinally measured at a series of drug doses and time points (Viatte et al. 2015), PK-PD models can be implemented into genetic association studies to explore the mechanistic basis of drug response (Lin et al. 2005a, b; Ahn et al. 2010).

Compared to complex-disease GWAS, pharmacogenetic GWAS may only have a small sample size because of high costs, longitudinal measures at a range of doses or time points, and ethical considerations (Daly 2010; Motsinger-Reif et al. 2013). Small or moderately sized sample sizes lead to overestimated pharmacogenetic effects of a locus and also make it difficult to detect small-size effects (Taylor et al. 2018). To overcome this issue, a family-based design is accommodated, in which both parental and offspring DNA are genotyped and the measurements of drug response are made on offspring. Family-based designs have proven to be powerful for parameter estimation and inference, more informative than population-based designs (Wu and Zeng 2001).

1.3.2 Nonlinear Regression of Drug Response

Consider a population-based cohort, in which subjects differ in age, race, sex, body mass index (BMI), and other demographics, recruited from a natural population to study human response to a particular drug (Wu et al. 2011b). After a drug is administered to these subjects at the same dose, the concentration of the drug reduces with time because of drug absorption, distribution, metabolism, and excretion. Let $\left(y_i(t_{i1}), \ldots, y_i(t_{iT_i})\right)$ denote the concentration value vector of subject i measured at a series of time points $\left(t_{i1}, \ldots, t_{iT_i}\right)$. All these subjects are genome-wide genotyped for polymorphic single nucleotide polymorphisms (SNP), aimed to identify significant genetic variants with drug response. Let us first consider an SNP with three different genotypes AA, Aa, and aa. A nonlinear regression model is used to describe the concentration value of subject i measured at time t_i, affected by the SNP, expressed as

$$y_i(t_i) = \sum_{j=1}^{3} z_{ij} g_j(t_i) + \sum_{r=1}^{R} \alpha_r u_{ir} + \sum_{s=1}^{S}\sum_{l=1}^{L_s} x_{isl} v_{sl} + e_i(t_i) \tag{1.1}$$

where $g_j(t_i)$ is the genotypic value of drug concentration for subject i who carries SNP genotype j ($j=1$ for AA, 2 for Aa, and 3 for aa), z_{ij} is an indicator variable of subject i defined as 1 if this subject carries a genotype considered and 0 otherwise, u_{ir} ($r=1, \ldots, R$) is the value of the rth continuous covariate, such as age and BMI, for subject i, α_r is the effect of the rth continuous covariate, v_{sl} ($l=1, \ldots, L_s$; $s=1, \ldots, S$) is the effect of the lth level for the sth discrete covariate, such as race, gender, and treatment, with $\sum_{l=1}^{L_s} v_{sl} = 0$ where L_s is the number of levels for the sth discrete covariate, x_{isl} is an indicator variable of subject i who receives the lth level of the sth discrete covariate, and $e_i(t_i)$ is a normally distributed random error.

Let $(y_i(c_{i1}),\ldots, y_i(c_{iD_i}))$ denote the drug effect vector of subject i measured at a series of doses $(c_{i1},\ldots, c_{iD_i})$. The phenotype of drug response for subject i at dose c_i be expressed as a function of the SNP, with demographic factors included in covariates, written as

$$y_i(c_i) = \sum_{j=1}^{3} z_{ij} g_j(c_i) + \sum_{r=1}^{R} \alpha_r u_{ir} + \sum_{s=1}^{S}\sum_{l=1}^{L_s} x_{isl} v_{sl} + e_i(c_i) \tag{1.2}$$

where $g_j(c_i)$ is the genotypic value of drug effect at dose c_i for subject i (whose genotype at a given SNP is determined by z_{ij}) and both continuous and discrete covariate effects have the same forms as described in equation (1.1). Similarly, $e_i(c_i)$ is a normally distributed random error.

1.3.3 Mechanistic Mapping

Viewing it as a longitudinal trait, functional mapping dissects drug response into its genetic components by integrating PK and PD models. There are numerous types of mathematical equations describing PK processes, and these equations are used in practice, depending on administration manner and many other factors (Meibohm and Derendorf 1997; Durisová and Dedík 2005; Mager 2006; Lankelma et al. 2013). For example, for the oral administration of a drug by a single dose, the time-varying plasma concentration of the drug can be described by

$$c(t) = \frac{F \cdot d \cdot k_a}{V_d (k_a - k_e)} \left(e^{-k_e t} - e^{-k_a t}\right) \tag{1.3}$$

where F is the fraction of the drug absorbed (bioavailability), d is the dose administered, V_d is the volume of distribution, k_e is the elimination rate constant, and k_a is the absorption rate constant. Given a longitudinal concentration data, we can fit the concentration-time curve by the above PK equation (1.3), from which four parameters $\Phi_K = (F, V_d, k_e, k_a)$ are estimated.

Similarly, a number of PD equations have been derived in the literature, one of which is the Hill equation or the $E_{\max}$ function (Giraldo 2003; Gesztelyi et al. 2012). Let $E(c)$ denote the effect value of a drug at dose c, which is expressed as

$$E(c) = E_0 + \frac{E_{\max} c^H}{EC_{50}^H + c^H} \tag{1.4}$$

where E_0 is the baseline, $E_{\max}$ is the asymptotic drug response, EC_{50} is the drug concentration at which drug effect is the half of $E_{\max}$, and H is the slope of drug response curve (Hill coefficient). Concentration-varying effect data can be fitted by the above PD equation (1.4), with parameters $\Phi_D = (E_0, E_{\max}, EC_{50}, H)$.

Functional mapping, aimed to map PK and PD reactions, integrates the PK and PD equations into the nonlinear regression models of equations (1.1) and (1.2), under which genotype-dependent parameters Φ_{Kj} $(j=1, 2, 3)$ describing concentration-time curves (PK) and genotype-dependent parameters Φ_{Dj} describing effect-concentration curves (PD) are estimated by least-square or maximum likelihood approaches. By comparing and testing these genotype-dependent parameters, functional mapping can determine whether and how a gene affects PK and PD processes and, further, how individual patients respond to drug therapy based on their genotypes. Figure 1.2 diagrams an example of a significant SNP for PK and a significant SNP for PD, in which case, three genotypes at each SNP have different curves.

Drug response is the consequence of interactions among drug, disease, and body (Figure 1.3). The interactions between drug and body can be quantified by PK and PD models. Differential equations and stochastic models, which provide detailed descriptions of dynamic systems that include physically relevant units, can be used to simulate the dynamic behavior of drug response and link the exposure of a drug and the modulation of pharmacological targets, physiological pathways, and ultimately disease systems (Agoram et al. 2007). For example, the PK of a drug with the first-order absorption and Michaelis-Menten elimination following an oral dose is described by a one-compartment model (Jusko 1995; Jusko et al. 1995; Mager et al. 2003; Kristensen et al. 2005; Wang et al. 2008), expressed as

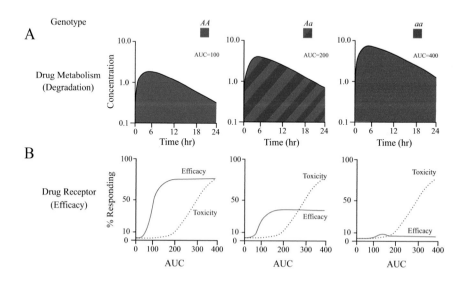

FIGURE 1.2
Three genotypes (*AA*, *Aa*, and *aa*) at a locus each associated with a different curve for drug metabolism (a) and drug receptor (b), showing the pattern of genetic control of drug response through pharmacokinetics and pharmacodynamics. AUC is the area under the concentration-time curve.

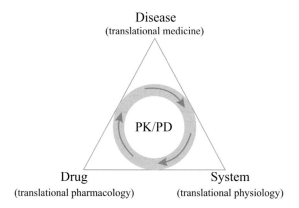

Disease
(translational medicine)

PK/PD

Drug
(translational pharmacology)

System
(translational physiology)

FIGURE 1.3
Drug response as a system with interactions between the drug, disease, and body through PK-PD processes. Thus, translational research in drug discovery and development could be considered to be divided into three broad disciplines – translational physiology, pharmacology, and medicine. Mechanism-based PK-PD modeling, by quantitatively combining system and drug-specific physiological, pharmacological, and pathological properties, has the potential to facilitate translational research.

$$\begin{cases} \dfrac{dQ}{dt} = -\left(\dfrac{V_{max}}{k_m + Q} \right) Q \\[2ex] \dfrac{dc}{dt} = \dfrac{V_{max} Q}{\left(k_m + Q \right) V} - \left(\dfrac{V_{max}}{k_m + c} \right) c \end{cases} \tag{1.5}$$

where t is the time, an independent variable, Q is the amount of drug in the gastrointestinal tract (mg), and c is the plasma drug concentration (mg/l). A Michaelis-Menten equation describes the initial rate of reaction as a function of the substrate concentration, with the reaction reaching a certain maximum rate as the substrate concentration increases, where k_m is the Michaelis-Menten constant and V_{max} is the maximum rate of the reaction. Thus, the PK parameters include k_m, V_{max}, and V, the volume of drug distribution in the plasma.

The PD effect of a drug is described by a one-compartment indirect response model, i.e., an equation specifying the rate of change of the effect (or response) over time in the presence of the drug, expressed as

$$\begin{cases} \dfrac{dc}{dt} = -\left(\dfrac{V_{max}}{k_m + c} \right) c \\[2ex] \dfrac{dR}{dt} = k_{in} \left(1 + \dfrac{E_{max} c^H}{EC_{50}^H + c^H} \right) - k_{out} R \end{cases} \tag{1.6}$$

where t is the time, c is the plasma drug concentration (mg/l), and R is the drug response that can be viewed as blood pressure, body temperature, or other pharmacologic response. The PD parameters include k_{in} and k_{out}, the zero- and first-order rate constant for production and loss of an effect, respectively (Jusko et al. 1995; Mager et al. 2003), and H, E_{max}, and EC_{50} are defined as above.

PK and PD parameters that specify equations (1.4) and (1.5) are genotype-specific. Systems mapping integrates ODEs of equations (1.4) and (1.5) to estimate genotype-specific ODE parameters through regression model (1) or (2) (Liu et al. 2013; Wang et al. 2013d). Testing genotype-dependent differences in these parameters allow us to ask and address new hypotheses about the genetic control of drug response and pleiotropic effects of individual genes on PK and PD processes. If two types of environmental and developmental covariates, those that are discrete (such as gender, race, and smoke/no smoke) and continuous (such as age, nutrient level, and body mass), are incorporated, we will have power to quantify gene-environment interactions and gene-development interactions (Carlsten et al. 2014).

1.4 Network Mapping of Drug Response

Gene regulatory networks play a pivotal role in every process of drug response, including cell differentiation, cell cycle, metabolism, and signal transduction (Nicholson et al. 2004; van der Wijst et al. 2018; Delgado and Gómez-Vela 2019; Lee et al. 2020a). By studying the dynamics of these networks, we can better understand the mechanisms of altering these cellular processes through medications and more precisely predict drug response. With the aid of powerful computational tools, the following specific questions can be addressed: what is the full range of behavior for this system under different conditions? How does the system change when certain parts stop functioning? How robust is the system under extreme conditions?

As a complex trait, drug response is controlled by DNA variants and a cascade of endophenotypes from different spaces that bridge the gap from the genotype to end-point phenotype through multilayer and multispace regulatory networks (Figure 1.4). To show the complexity of this process, we diagram a tridimensional network in which surfaces represent interaction networks of endophenotypes at a single space and vertical edges represent interaction networks of endophenotypes across different spaces. Genes G1–G4 form a surface interaction network at the gene space, whereas transcripts T1–T4 generate a surface interaction network at the transcript space. The genes and transcripts interact across the gene and transcript spaces to form multiple channels of connectivity. By linking the gene space to transcript space, to protein space, to metabolite space, to microbiome space, and finally to PK and PD space, we reconstruct a multiscale tridimensional network from which key nodes and key links can be identified to unveil a roadmap of genotype-phenotype

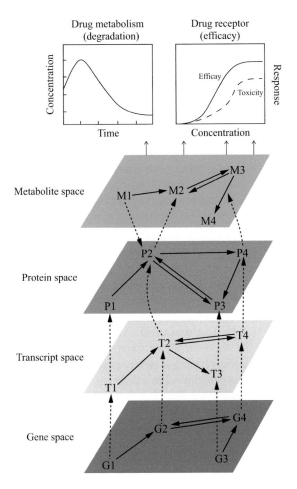

FIGURE 1.4
A multilayer, multispace, multiplex, and multifunctional network that mediates pharmacokinetic and pharmacodynamic processes. The bottom genetic network translates its information into the transcriptional network which transcripts its codes into the protein network that is transmitted to the metabolic network toward drug response. Arrowed lines represent directed interaction between two entities.

relationships. This tridimensional network should be casual, signed, and weighted, uncovering and quantifying the causal relationships of endophenotypes from one space to the other or from the second to first.

In drug discovery, we seek for a targeted perturbation that can typically inhibit or activate function of biomolecules related to a disease (Nelander et al. 2008). We describe the pathways related to drug action as a system characterized by a particular type of cell, its environment, its points of intervention (such as drug targets), time points of observation (such as the phosphorylation state of proteins involved in signaling processes), and a phenotypic change (such as cell death or growth). Mathematical models are used to describe the regulatory network of the system in which nodes denote levels of molecular activity and edges reflect the impact of one node on the time derivative of another. The time evolution of the system can be modeled by a first-order differential equation

$$\frac{dy}{dt} = f(y(t), u(t)) \qquad (1.7)$$

where $y(t)$ represents the activities of the system's components, $u(t)$ represents perturbations of drugs on the components, and f is a linear or nonlinear transfer function. In practice, $y(t)$ can be the abundances of specific mRNAs or proteins, whereas $u(t)$ can be the concentrations of different chemical compounds to which the cells are exposed (Nelander et al. 2008). Equation (1.7) can be linear differential equations for a system, but they can further be modified by a nonlinear transfer function to reflect properties of the system that are not explicitly modeled.

The application of differential equations to the detection of drug targets can be made by inferring functional interactions between pathway components, predicting phenotypic consequences of drug combinations, and controlling the behavior of the system. By incorporating systems modeling of transcriptome, proteome, protein-protein, protein-DNA interactions into a GWAS, we can gain better insight into the genetic architecture of drug response in which specific eQTLs, pQTLs, and mQTLs and their interactions can be identified to better predict the efficacy of drugs. All this constitutes a concrete step toward the active development of network-oriented pharmacology.

Modern medicine has developed to a point at which the paradigm that has dominated drug discovery for decades is shifting to the era of multispecific drugs promised to increase therapeutic efficacy and decrease drug resistance by harnessing the power of biology (Deshaies 2020; Tyers and Wright 2019; Palmer et al. 2019). Many ongoing clinical trials have begun to implement combination therapies for cancer, infectious diseases, and metabolic, cardiovascular, autoimmune, and neurological disorders (Perry et al. 2015; Lai et al. 2018; Ciccolini et al. 2019; Asadzadeh et al. 2020). Unlike conventional therapies, combination therapies are characteristic of drug-drug interactions (DDIs) by which the pharmacological effect of one drug is altered by that of another drug in a combination regimen (Venkatakrishnan and Rostami-Hodjegan 2019; Bain 2019; Meyer et al. 2020). DDIs can be qualitatively classified as synergistic, additive, or antagonistic in nature (Niu et al. 2019; Schafer et al. 2020) and, thus, a systematic characterization of how and how strongly different drugs interact as a whole to modulate drug effects is sorely needed. To better understand the importance of drug regimens, methodologies need to be developed for characterizing the direction, sign, and strength of DDIs and their patient- and context-specific architecture, which enhance the capacity of drug combinations to maximum drug efficacy and minimum drug resistance (Niu et al. 2019; Zhang et al. 2019; Tran and Grillo 2019).

Sang et al. (2022) developed a computational model for coding DDIs into quantitative networks that mediate PK and PD processes. Such DDI networks can help to trace the mechanistic roadmaps of how each drug acts and

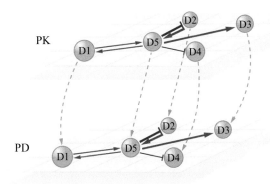

FIGURE 1.5
A tridimensional DDI network among five drugs D1–D5 across PK and PD spaces. The absorption, distribution, metabolism, and erection of a drug are influenced by other drugs, with the degree and sign of this influence used to reconstruct the PK network. Based on the independent and dependent concentration components of each drug estimated by the SEGN model, we use a PD equation, such as the Hill equation, to estimate the corresponding independent and dependent drug effects due to these two concentration components, respectively, which are encapsulated into the PD network. Both PK and PD networks reconstructed by the SEGN model are fully informative, filled by bidirectional, signed, and weighted interactions, equipped with a capacity to characterize various types of DDIs, including synergy, asymmetrical synergy, directional synergy, antagonism, asymmetrical antagonism, directional antagonism, and predation or altruism. Arrowed and T-shaped lines represent the direction by which one drug activates and inhibits the next drug, respectively, with the strength proportional to the thickness of the lines.

interacts with every other drug within the PK-PD context. Sang et al.'s model links DDI networks from two spaces, PK and PD (Figure 1.5). In this example, drug D5 influences the time-varying concentration change of all other four drugs at the PK space, thus regarded as a hub drug that plays a leadership role in mediating the overall PK process of all drugs. D5 tends to block the concentration decrease of drugs D1 and D3 but stimulates the concentration decrease of drugs D2 and D4, although drugs D1 and D4 reciprocally block the concentration decrease of D5. The DDIs at the PK level allow us to portray an interaction network at the PD space (Figure 1.5), from which we can clearly characterize how and how strongly the pharmacological effects of a drug are affected by its interactive drugs.

1.5 Conclusions and Outlook

Precision medicine critically relies on precise analysis and modeling of the ever-growing amounts of complete genome sequences for individual patients and their pharmacological activities, with great potential to provide precise information to engineer new biotechnological solutions to the design and discovery of new drugs. In principle, it is possible to re-engineer new processes by selectively combining otherwise distinct biochemical capabilities, but its success is very much determined by a profound understanding of how the proteins encoded in each individual genome dynamically assemble into biological circuits through their mutual communication and their interactions with the environment. Statistical models and computational tools are central to understand how a simple genetic change or environmental perturbation influences the behavior of an organism at the molecular level and ultimately its phenotype and how we can enable re-engineering of cellular circuits for the system through quantitative alterations. Computational approaches will need to be coordinated and implemented with experimental data to build up a predictive gene regulatory network model for drug response.

The central theme of this book is to introduce computational models for studying the pharmacogenetic architecture of drug response and quantifying drug reactions as a coordinated network of genes, proteins, and biochemical reactions. These models incorporate PK and PD principles into genetic mapping and association studies, which can mechanistically understand how drugs modulate cellular reactions across space and time and how they impact human pathophysiology. The integration of the "omics" data into these models can disentangle the pattern of gene expression (regulation, inhibition, and induction) and systematically screen the pathways that could be involved in drug reactions. The results obtained from these models can facilitate the quantitative prediction of the responses of individual subjects as well as the design of optimal drug treatments that maximize therapeutic efficacy while minimizing the number and severity of adverse drug reactions.

In recent years, precision medicine has developed as an important research focus in medicine, whose ultimate goal is to gain knowledge about the delivery of the right drug at the right dose at the right time for the right patient (Collins and Varmus 2015). This development has been fueled by technological advancement that allows us to collect fundamental data of various genetic elements related to health and disease. The biggest challenge in precision medicine is not data collection but has become how to extract and excavate precise information from these data, used to redefine disease at a higher resolution and design new therapies using knowledge about disease-drug interactions. The computational models introduced in this book may be powerful for unveiling the complexities of particular aspects of drug response. There is a sore need to develop more systematic and sophisticated methods that can capture and chart a more complete picture of pharmacogenetic architecture. It is unlikely that these methods can be developed from a single discipline alone, and multidisciplinary cross-pollination producing $1+1>2$ certainly opens up a new direction of pharmacogenomic research and is a crucial step for shifting traditional medicine to precise, predictive, personalized, and participatory medicine.

Part 1

Pharmacokinetic–
Pharmacodynamic
Pharmacogenetics

2

Pharmacogenetic Dissection by Functional Mapping

2.1 Introduction

The response of patients to a drug is complex in terms of its underlying genetic basis (Weinshilboum 2003; Weinshilboum and Wang 2006; Daly 2010; Bailey and Cheng 2010; Wang et al. 2011). Drug response, either drug efficacy or adverse drug reactions, is usually controlled by a network of genes that operate independently or interactively (Liou et al. 2012; Weigelt and Reis-Filho 2014; Zhang et al. 2020; Lozovsky et al. 2021). Moreover, the genetic effects triggered by the genes rely on the genetic background of a patient, his/her life style, as well as the change in the body's metabolic environment arising from drug administration (Baye and Wilke 2010; Lin et al. 2018; Banerjee et al. 2019). The identification of drug response–related genes and their interactions with each other and with various environmental factors has been a long-standing focus in pharmacogenetic research, aiming at pre-treatment selection and the development of drugs that are effective and safe for individual patients according to their genetic blueprints (Bailey and Cheng 2010; Wang et al. 2011; Lin et al. 2018).

A detailed genetic study of drug response has largely benefitted from the discovery of molecular markers, distinctive segments of DNA that serve as landmarks for a target gene. Since both markers and target genes are distributed through the genome, the latter can be inferred from the former through linkage analysis. The motive force that identifies individual target genes for complex traits, such as drug response, comes from the publication of Lander and Botstein's (1989) seminal paper, which presented a mixture model to map latent quantitative trait loci (QTLs) based on the co-segregation of markers with QTLs. This so-called genetic mapping approach has been widely used to map and identify QTLs for drug response (Watters et al. 2004; Grisel et al. 1997; Choy et al. 2008). In the past decades, the advent of high-throughput sequencing and genotyping techniques has shifted conventional QTL mapping to genome-wide association studies (GWAS) by which a detailed picture of the genetic control of drug response can better be elucidated

DOI: 10.1201/9780429171512-3

(Daly 2010; Bailey and Cheng 2010; Wang et al. 2013a). Through GWAS, significant genetic loci have been detected for interferon-α response (Ge et al. 2009; Suppiah et al. 2009; Tanaka et al. 2009), clopidogrel response (Shuldiner et al. 2009), and anticoagulant dose requirement (Cooper et al. 2008; Takeuchi et al. 2009; Teichert et al. 2009). For adverse drug reactions, GWAS also identified significant associations; for example, those for statin-induced myopathy (Link et al. 2008) and flucloxacillin-induced liver injury (Daly et al. 2009).

In this chapter, we review the basic theory of quantitative genetics used to map the genetic architecture of drug response using a population-based GWAS design. Different from disease mapping, mapping drug response requires an additional dimension of how drug-body interactions mediate and diversify the therapeutic effects of a drug into its efficacy and toxicity. As such, we discuss and describe a more effective and efficient statistical approach for pharmacogenetic mapping – functional mapping. This approach integrates the pharmacokinetic (PK) and pharmacodynamic (PD) processes of drug-body interactions into a mapping setting. In practice, it is highly challenging to collect an adequate number of cases with drug intervention so pharmacogenomics studies are based on small sample sizes, leading to insufficient power to detect small or moderately sized effects (Daly 2010). Functional mapping can at least partially overcome this issue by incorporating physiologically meaningful PK and PD equations into the genetic analysis based on repeated measures of pharmacological parameters at multiple time points or doses (Lin et al. 2005a, b, 2007; Wu and Lin 2008; Wu et al. 2011a; Wang et al. 2015a).

2.2 Quantitative Genetics

The underlying QTLs for variation in drug response can be mapped to the specific regions of the genome. The original model for genetic mapping capitalizes the linkage between the markers and QTLs, derived for a controlled cross between two parents that are segregating at the genetic loci (Wu et al. 2007). For those species, such as humans, in which artificial crosses are not available, genetic mapping has been extended to linkage disequilibrium (LD)-based mapping approaches for natural populations (Wang and Wu 2004; Wang et al. 2005, 2009). While LD mapping has been widely used to study pharmacogenetics in human populations, linkage mapping can also serve as an approach for mapping drug response using model systems, such as the mouse and *Saccharomyces cerevisiae* (Kim and Fay 2009; Button-Simons et al. 2021).

2.2.1 One-Gene Model

Consider a gene, with alleles A and a, which are segregating in a natural human population at Hardy-Weinberg equilibrium (HWE). The two alleles randomly combine to produce three genotypes AA, Aa, and aa, whose genotypic values for a trait of interest are denoted as μ_2, μ_1, and μ_0, respectively. Let p and q ($p+q=1$) denote allele frequencies of A and a, respectively. Under HWE, the genotype frequencies are calculated as p^2 for AA, $2pq$ for Aa, and q^2 for aa. The three genotypes are displayed along a line in the order of aa-Aa-AA:

Genotype	aa	Origin	Aa	AA
Genotypic value	μ_0	$\mu=(\mu_2+\mu_0)/2$	μ_1	μ_2
Net genotypic value	$-a$	0	d	a
Genotype frequency	p^2		$2pq$	q^2
Deviation from population mean	$2pa-2p^2d$		$(q-p)a+2pqd$	$2qa-2q^2d$

$$(2.1)$$

Here, the mean of two homozygotes AA and aa, $\mu=(\mu_2+\mu_0)/2$, is defined as the origin of the line. Thus, the net genotypic values of AA, Aa, and aa are expressed, respectively, as

$$\mu_2 - (\mu_2 + \mu_0)/2 = (\mu_2 - \mu_0)/2 = a$$
$$\mu_1 - (\mu_2 + \mu_0)/2 = d \qquad (2.2)$$
$$(\mu_2 + \mu_9)/2 - \mu_0 = -(\mu_2 - \mu_0)/2 = -a$$

where a is defined as the additive genetic effect of the gene due to a change in the number of a particular allele expressed in a genotype and d is defined as the dominant genetic effect of the gene due to the interaction between two different alleles. Based on equation (2.2), we formulate genotypic values as

$$\mu_2 = \mu + a$$
$$\mu_1 = \mu + d \qquad (2.3)$$
$$\mu_0 = \mu - a$$

We use genotype frequencies and net genotypic values to calculate the weighted population mean as $m = q^2(-a) + 2pqd + p^2a = (p-q)a + 2pqd$. Let $\alpha = a + (q - p)d$, which is defined as the average effect due to the substitution of one allele to the other at the gene. Based on deviations of net genotypic values from the population mean, as shown in display (2.1), we calculate the total genetic variance at the gene as

$$\sigma_g^2 = 2pq\alpha^2 + (2pqd)^2 \qquad (2.4)$$

which is decomposed into additive genetic variance $\sigma_a^2 = 2pq\alpha^2$ and dominant genetic variance $\sigma_d^2 = (2pqd)^2$. The total phenotypic variance of the trait is the sum of genetic variance (σ_g^2) and environmental variance (σ_e^2). Narrow-sense heritability is defined as the ratio of the additive genetic variance to the total phenotypic variance,

$$h^2 = \frac{\sigma_a^2}{\sigma_g^2 + \sigma_e^2} \tag{2.5a}$$

and broad-sense heritability defined as the ratio of the total genetic variance to the total phenotypic variance,

$$H^2 = \frac{\sigma_g^2}{\sigma_g^2 + \sigma_e^2} \tag{2.5b}$$

Both narrow- and broad-sense heritabilities are important genetic parameters that describe the contribution of a specific gene to quantitative genetic variation. The size of the heritability is often used as the criterion for assessing the magnitude of genetic effects for a gene.

2.2.2 Two-Gene Model

Genetic interactions between different genes, coined epistasis, play an important role in contributing to interpersonal variation in drug response (Weigelt and Reis-Filho 2014; Lozovsky et al. 2021). Consider two genes **A** and **B**, with alleles A vs. a and B vs. b, respectively, which are co-segregating to produce nine genotypes. Let a_1 and d_1 denote the additive and dominant genetic effects of gene **A** and a_2 and d_2 denote the additive and dominant effects of gene **B**, respectively. The alleles of two genes interact with each other to form the additive × additive epistatic effect (i_{aa}), additive × dominant epistatic effect (i_{ad}), dominant × additive epistatic effect (i_{da}), and dominant × dominant epistatic effect (i_{dd}). Two-locus genotypic values at genes **A** and **B** are formulated in Table 2.1.

TABLE 2.1

Two-Locus Genotypic Values and Their Decomposition into Additive and Dominant Genetic Effects at Each Locus and Four Types of Epistatic Interactions Between Two Loci

	BB	Bb	bb
AA	$\mu_{22} = \mu + a_1 + a_2 + i_{aa}$	$\mu_{21} = \mu + a_1 + d_2 + i_{ad}$	$\mu_{20} = \mu + a_1 - a_2 - i_{aa}$
Aa	$\mu_{12} = \mu + d_1 + a_2 + i_{da}$	$\mu_{11} = \mu + d_1 + d_2 + i_{dd}$	$\mu_{10} = \mu + d_1 - a_2 - i_{da}$
Aa	$\mu_{02} = \mu - a_1 + a_2 - i_{aa}$	$\mu_{01} = \mu - a_1 + d_2 - i_{ad}$	$\mu_{00} = \mu - a_1 - a_2 + i_{aa}$

By solving the regular equations given in Table 2.1, we can estimate the origin mean as

$$\mu = \frac{1}{4}(\mu_{22} + \mu_{20} + \mu_{02} + \mu_{00})$$

and the genetic effects as

$$a_1 = \frac{1}{4}[(\mu_{22} + \mu_{20}) - (\mu_{02} + \mu_{00})] \tag{2.6a}$$

$$a_2 = \frac{1}{4}[(\mu_{22} + \mu_{02}) - (\mu_{20} + \mu_{00})] \tag{2.6b}$$

$$d_1 = \frac{1}{2}(\mu_{12} + \mu_{10}) - \frac{1}{4}(\mu_{22} + \mu_{20} + \mu_{02} + \mu_{00}) \tag{2.6c}$$

$$d_2 = \frac{1}{2}(\mu_{21} + \mu_{01}) - (\mu_{22} + \mu_{20} + \mu_{02} + \mu_{00}) \tag{2.6d}$$

$$i_{aa} = \frac{1}{4}[(\mu_{22} + \mu_{00}) - (\mu_{20} + \mu_{02})] \tag{2.6e}$$

$$i_{ad} = \frac{1}{2}(\mu_{21} - \mu_{01}) - \frac{1}{4}[(\mu_{22} + \mu_{20}) - (\mu_{02} + \mu_{00})] \tag{2.6f}$$

$$i_{da} = \frac{1}{2}(\mu_{12} - \mu_{10}) - \frac{1}{4}[(\mu_{22} + \mu_{02}) - (\mu_{20} + \mu_{00})] \tag{2.6g}$$

$$i_{dd} = \mu_{11} - \frac{1}{4}(\mu_{22} - \mu_{20} + \mu_{02} + \mu_{11}) - \frac{1}{2}[(\mu_{12} + \mu_{10}) - (\mu_{21} + \mu_{01})] \tag{2.6h}$$

Thus, if genotypic values are estimated from real data, we can use equations (2.6a–h) to estimate each of these genetic effects. Each effect is thought to play a different role in mediating drug response.

Let p_1 and q_1 denote allele frequencies of A and a and p_2 and q_2 denote allele frequencies of B and b. Under random mating and linkage equilibrium, the two-locus genotype frequencies are expressed in Table 2.2. Based on net genotypic values and genotype frequencies, we derive the additive and dominant genetic variances for each gene and the total epistatic genetic variance due to four types of interactions (Cheverud and Routman 1995). The average effects of an allele substitution at genes **A** and **B** are derived as

$$\alpha_1 = a_1 + d_1(q_1 - p_1) + p_1(i_2 - i_1) + q_1(i_1 - i_0) \tag{2.7a}$$

$$\alpha_2 = a_2 + d_2(q_2 - p_2) + p_2(i_2 - i_1) + q_1(i_1 - i_0) \tag{2.7b}$$

TABLE 2.2

Genotype Frequencies Expressed in Terms of Allele
Frequencies in a Panmictic Population

	BB	Bb	bb
AA	$p_1^2 p_2^2$	$2p_1^2 p_2 q_2$	$p_1^2 q_2^2$
Aa	$2p_1 q_1 p_2^2$	$4p_1 q_1 p_2 q_2$	$2p_1 q_1 q_2^2$
Aa	$q_1^2 p_2^2$	$2q_1^2 p_2 q_2$	$q_1^2 q_2^2$

where

$$i_{2.} = p_2^2 \, i_{aa} + 2p_2 q_2 i_{ad} - q_2^2 \, i_{aa} \tag{2.8a}$$

$$i_{1.} = p_2^2 \, i_{da} + 2p_2 q_2 i_{dd} - q_2^2 \, i_{da} \tag{2.8b}$$

$$i_{0.} = - p_2^2 \, i_{aa} - 2p^2 q^2 i_{ad} + q_2^2 \, i_{aa} \tag{2.8c}$$

$$i_{.2} = p_1^2 \, i_{aa} + 2p_1 q_1 i_{da} - q_1^2 \, i_{aa} \tag{2.8d}$$

$$i_{.1} = p_1^2 \, i_{ad} + 2p_1 q_1 i_{dd} - q_1^2 \, i_{ad} \tag{2.8e}$$

$$i_{.0} = - p_1^2 \, i_{aa} - 2p_1 q_1 i_{da} + q_1^2 \, i_{aa} \tag{2.8f}$$

which are the epistatic population means over three genotypes at one gene
for a given genotype at the other. The additive genetic variances at each gene
A or **B** in the two-locus system are derived as

$$\sigma_{a1}^2 = 2p_1 q_1 \alpha_1^2 \tag{2.9a}$$

$$\sigma_{a2}^2 = 2p_2 q_2 \alpha_2^2 \tag{2.9b}$$

The dominant genetic variances at each gene **A** or **B** in the two-locus system
are derived as

$$\sigma_{d1}^2 = \left[2p_1 q_1 d_1 - p_1 q_1 \left(i_{2.} - 2i_{1.} + i_{0.} \right) \right]^2 \tag{2.10a}$$

$$\sigma_{d2}^2 = \left[2p_2 q_2 d_2 - p_2 q_2 \left(i_{.2} - 2i_{.1} + i_{.0} \right) \right]^2 \tag{2.10b}$$

Based on the epistatic values in Table 2.1 and genotypic frequencies in
Table 2.2, we calculate the epistatic population mean over all genotypes as

$$i_{..} = \left(p_1 - q_1 \right)\left(p_2 - q_2 \right) i_{aa} + 2 \left(p_1 - q_1 \right) p_2 q_2 i_{ad} + 2 \, p_1 q_1 \left(p_2 - q_2 \right) i_{da} + 4p_1 p_2 q_2 i_{dd}$$

TABLE 2.3

Epistatic Formulation

	BB	Bb	bb
AA	$i_{aa} - i_{2.} - i_{.2} + i_{..}$	$i_{aa} - i_{2.} - i_{.1} + i_{..}$	$i_{aa} - i_{2.} - i_{.0} + i_{..}$
Aa	$i_{aa} - i_{1.} - i_{.2} + i_{..}$	$i_{aa} - i_{1.} - i_{.1} + i_{..}$	$i_{aa} - i_{1.} - i_{.0} + i_{..}$
aa	$i_{aa} - i_{0.} - i_{.2} + i_{..}$	$i_{aa} - i_{0.} - i_{.1} + i_{..}$	$i_{aa} - i_{0.} - i_{.0} + i_{..}$

from which, in combination with equations (2.8a–f), we derive the epistatic deviations that are given in Table 2.3. Thus, total epistatic variance is calculated as the sum of the squared interaction deviations weighted by the corresponding genotype frequencies given in Table 2.2.

The average effects of alleles and additive genetic variances are contributed by additive, dominant, and epistatic effects, the dominant genetic variances are contributed by dominant and epistatic effects, and the epistatic genetic variance is contributed only by epistatic effects. In other words, epistasis can make contributions to all three component variances, i.e., additive, dominant, and epistatic. This indicates that epistasis plays an important role in trait evolution by influencing additive genetics, i.e., heritable variance.

2.2.3 Haplotype Model

It has well been recognized that genetic polymorphisms can cause the alteration or even loss of activity in drug-metabolizing enzymes, transporters, and receptors (Saito et al. 2007). Numerous studies have pursued to identify these individual polymorphisms for drug response. However, accumulating evidence shows that haplotypes, linear combinations of non-alleles on a chromosomal region, play a more important role in drug response than individual polymorphisms (Snyder et al. 2015; Nkhoma et al. 2021; Ebert et al. 2021; Lim et al. 2022). For example, Saito et al. (2007) found that haplotypes between *CYP2C19*2* or *3* and *CYP2C9*1* and haplotypes between *YP2C9*3* and *CYP2C19*1* are associated with drug metabolism in East Asians. Haplotype mapping using multiple SNPs jointly has been shown to increase power in detecting significant genetic variants (Uemoto et al. 2013; Shirali et al. 2018) and retrieving the missing heritability of complex traits (Shirali et al. 2018).

For a multilocus heterozygote, the discovery of its constituent haplotypes is not straightforward. To detect the association between haplotypes and phenotypes, a series of statistical models based on the Expectation-Maximization (EM) algorithm (Dempster et al. 1977) have been developed (Liu et al. 2004; Lin et al. 2005a, 2007; Wen et al. 2009). More recently, advanced genome sequencing and assembling techniques have been developed and implemented to phase haplotypes from individual whole-genome sequences (Snyder et al. 2015; Ebert et al. 2021). Haplotype-resolved genomes gain insight into the complete picture of structural variants for complex traits.

2.3 A General Framework for Functional Mapping

2.3.1 Why Functional Mapping

Many biological and biomedical traits, such as drug response, are expected to arise as curves. To determine the dynamic changes of genetic effects, we need to measure trait values at a series of discrete time points or states and model how these values for different genotypes at a specific locus change over time or state. In a traditional way, one can extend genetic mapping to accommodate the multivariate nature of time-dependent traits. However, this extension is limited due to the following reasons:

1. This extension estimates the expected means of each genotype at all the points and all variances and covariances, resulting in a substantial computational burden especially when the data dimension is high;

2. The result from this extension is biologically less meaningful because the underlying biological principle for trait dynamics is not incorporated;

3. This extension is not flexible to ask and answer novel biologically or biomedically interesting questions at the interplay of multiple disciplines.

To overcome the above limitations of traditional mapping approaches, a collection of statistical methods implemented with the mathematical aspects of biological processes have been proposed (Ma et al. 2002; Wu et al. 2004a, b, c; Wu and Lin 2006). This method, called *functional mapping*, expresses the genotypic means of a locus at different time points by a mathematical equation with respect to time, e.g., the growth equation. Under this principle, the parameters describing the shape of growth curves, rather than the genotypic means at individual time points, as expected in traditional mapping strategies, are estimated by a maximum likelihood approach or other approaches. Also, functional mapping estimates the parameters that model the covariance structure among multiple time points, which largely reduces the number of parameters being estimated for variances and covariances, especially when the number of time points is large.

2.3.2 The Procedure of Functional Mapping

To demonstrate the utility of functional mapping, we consider a GWAS population in which all subjects are phenotyped for a growth trait at a series of time points and genotyped for a panel of genome-wide SNPs. Growth is the increase of an organism in size or mass over time, which can be explained by the growth equation. Exponential growth, i.e., growth rate increases over time, in proportion to the size of the organism, occurs when there are infinite amounts of resources. However, the organism may not always follow exponential growth because it reaches a particular size at which resources start to be used. Thus, the growth will plateau to form an S-shaped curve. A number of growth equations have been developed to model such an S-shaped curve (Zwietering et al. 1990). As an example, we introduce a three-parameter logistic growth equation, expressed as

$$g(t) = \frac{a}{1 + be^{-rt}} \qquad (2.11)$$

where $g(t)$ is the growth of an organism at time t, a is the asymptotic growth when time tends to be infinite, b is the initial growth, and r is the growth rate or the steepness of the curve. Based on the goodness-of-fit of the growth equation (2.11) to time-dependent observational data, many growth traits can be found to obey the logistic growth law (Zwietering et al. 1990; Ma et al. 2002). This phenomenon has been interpreted from fundamental principles for the allocation balance of metabolic energy between the maintenance of existing tissue and the production of new biomass (West et al. 2001). Functional mapping incorporates the growth equation into a statistical mapping framework to test and identify specific QTLs that govern growth trajectories. Prior to performing functional mapping, we adjust the growth data by removing effects due to covariates involving demographic factors and life style using equation (1.1). Let $\mathbf{y}_i = (y_i(t_{i1}), \ldots, y_i(t_{iT_i}))$ denote a vector of adjusted phenotypic values for subject i measured at T_i time points $(t_{i1}, \ldots, t_{iT_i})$. Consider an SNP with three genotypes AA, Aa, and aa, whose observations are denoted as n_2, n_1, and n_0, respectively. We formulate the likelihood of phenotypic data at this SNP as

$$L(y) = \prod_{i=1}^{n_2} f_2\left(\mathbf{y}_i; \mu_{2|i}, \Sigma_2\right) \prod_{i=1}^{n_1} f_1\left(\mathbf{y}_i; \mu_{1|i}, \Sigma_1\right) \prod_{i=1}^{n_0} f_0\left(\mathbf{y}_i; \mu_{0|i}, \Sigma_0\right) \qquad (2.12)$$

where $f_j(\mathbf{y}_i; \mu_j, \Sigma)$ is the multivariate normal distribution density function with QTL genotype-specific mean vector μ_j ($j = 2$ for AA, 1 for Aa and 0 for aa) and covariance matrix Σ.

Functional mapping models time-dependent means for each genotype by the growth equation, as described in equation (2.11), i.e.,

$$\mu_{j|i} = \left(\mu_j(t_{i1}), \ldots, \mu_j(t_{iT_i})\right)$$

$$= \left(\frac{a_j}{1 + b_j e^{-r_j t_{i1}}}, \ldots, \frac{a_j}{1 + b_j e^{-r_j t_{iT_i}}}\right) \qquad (2.13)$$

where three growth parameters (a_j, b_j, r_j) describe the form of the growth curve for a genotype j. If growth parameters (a_j, b_j, r_j) are different among genotypes, then this suggests that the SNP under consideration is associated with the growth process. As an application of longitudinal data analysis, functional mapping models the longitudinal covariance structure,

$$
\Sigma_j = \begin{pmatrix} \sigma_{t_{i1}}^2 & \cdots & \sigma_{t_{i1}t_{iT_i}} \\ \vdots & \ddots & \vdots \\ \sigma_{t_{iT_i}t_{i1}} & \cdots & \sigma_{t_{iT_i}}^2 \end{pmatrix}
\tag{2.14}
$$

where $\sigma_{t_{i1}}^2, \ldots, \sigma_{t_{iT_i}}^2$ are the variances at different time points, and $\sigma_{tt'} = \sigma_{t't}$ is the covariance between different time points t and t'. Many statistical approaches, such as autoregressive and structured antedependence approaches, nonparametric fitting and semiparametric fitting, have been used to model the covariance structure in functional mapping (Yap et al. 2009).

The first-order autoregressive (AR(1)) model assumes that variances are stable across time points and covariances only depend on the intervals of two time points, regardless of where these two time points come from. Under these two stationarity assumptions, we can model the autocorrelative structure of the matrix by using only two parameters, time-invariant variance (σ^2) and correlation coefficient between two time points distant by a unit of time (ρ). Such an AR(1) model is statistically advantageous because under it the inverse and determinant of the matrix have a closed form (Wu et al. 2002), which facilitates the computation of functional mapping. If these two assumptions are too strong, we introduce the first-order structured antedependence (SAD(1)) model to model the matric structure (Zimmerman and Núñez-Antón 2001, 2009). This model allows variances to change with time and covariances to differ depending on both time interval and the stage of measurements. The advantages of SAD(1) include that (1) it does not need any stationarity assumption and (2) it preserves the advantages of AR(1) (Zhao et al. 2005a, b).

Many computational approaches have been developed to solve the likelihood of functional mapping (Ma et al. 2002; Hou et al. 2005, 2006; Liu and Wu 2009). Zhao et al. (2004) implemented the simplex algorithm into the likelihood (2.11) to estimate genotype-specific parameters that model the mean vectors (2.12) and autoregressive parameters that model the matrix structure (2.14). After these parameters are estimated, we need to confirm whether this SNP is significantly associated with the growth process by testing genotypic differences in growth parameters. Under the null hypothesis, growth parameters have no difference among three genotypes, whereas under the alternative hypothesis, there are genotype-dependent differences in growth parameters. These two hypotheses are formulated as

$$
\mathrm{H_0:}\ \left(a_2, b_2, r_2\right) = \left(a_1, b_1, r_1\right) = \left(a_0, b_0, r_0\right) = \left(a, b, r\right)
$$

$$
\tag{2.15}
$$

$\mathrm{H_1}$: At least one equality does not hold

The null hypothesis only contains a set of growth parameters (a, b, r), which can be estimated from the likelihood

$$L(y) = \prod_{i=1}^{n} f\left(\mathbf{y}_i; \boldsymbol{\mu}_i, \boldsymbol{\Sigma}_i\right) \qquad (2.16)$$

We obtain the maximum likelihood estimates (MLEs) of all parameters under each hypothesis and plug in these MLEs into the likelihoods (2.10) and (2.11), respectively. Let L_0 and L_1 denote the estimated likelihoods under the null and alternative hypotheses. Then, we calculate the likelihood ratio (LR) by

$$LR = -2\left(\log L_0 - \log L_1\right) \qquad (2.17)$$

which serves as a test statistic. To determine the genome-wide critical threshold, we perform permutation tests by shuffling phenotypic data. Each run of shuffling produces an LR value. If this process is repeated 1,000 times or more, we can determine the top 5% quantile as the critical threshold.

2.3.3 Biological Relevance of Functional Mapping

QTLs affect growth trajectories in different ways. One major advantage of functional mapping is that it can discern different types of genetic control over growth. In summary, these types can broadly include:

a. *Early-late QTL:* It affects the time at which the development starts but has no effect on the rate of growth and the pattern and form of developmental processes. As shown in Figure 2.1a, the trait begins developing earlier for one genotype than it does for the other one at an early-late QTL.

b. *Slow-fast QTL:* It triggers an effect on the rate of growth rather than on the starting point of development. In Figure 2.1b, the trait is shown to develop at a higher rate in one genotype than in the other one.

c. *Short-long QTL:* It changes the time at which the development ceases, although it does not alter the developmental trajectory. In Figure 2.1c, the development of the trait considered for one genotype continues beyond the point at which it stopped for the other genotype.

d. *Sequential QTL:* It leads to the change of sequential differentiation in early and late stages. As shown in Figure 2.1d, during the early stage the trait develops at a lower rate for one genotype than for the other one, but this is inverted during the late stage.

Each of these QTL types may play a different role in regulating phenotypic variation and evolution. Integrating these distinct roles into a unified framework can more precisely understand the genetic architecture of complex traits and predict their ecological and evolutionary response to environmental change.

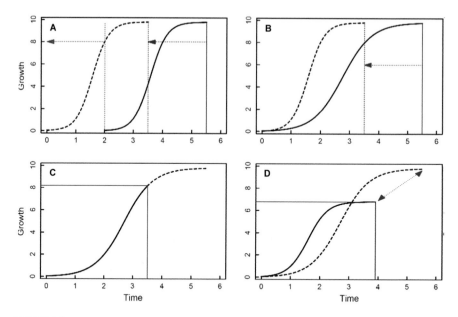

FIGURE 2.1
Four types of genetic control at a QTL detected by functional mapping. (a) Early-late QTL, in which development starts and stops earlier (shown by arrows) for one genotype (solid line) than for the other one (dash line). (b) Slow-fast QTL, in which the rate of growth is accelerated for one genotype (slash line), thus using a shorter time to achieve the maximum growth (shown by an arrow). (c) Short-long QTL, in which growth is prolonged for one genotype (dash line). (d) Sequential QTL, at which one genotype (slash line), relative to the other one (solid line), has decreasing growth in the early stage of development but increasing growth in the late development.

2.3.4 Inferring Casual QTLs

General formulism: If the LR test is significant, then this means that this SNP is significantly associated with growth curves, but this does not imply that this SNP is a causal gene. To infer the casual QTL associated with the significant SNP, we implement a mixture model to distinguish the effect of the casual QTL and the "effect" of the significant SNP due to its LD with the casual QTL. Let p and $1-p$ denote the frequencies of two alternative alleles A vs. a at the SNP, let q and $1-q$ denote the frequencies of two alternative alleles B and b at the QTL, and let D denote the coefficient of LD due to nonrandom association between the marker and QTL in the population. The alleles of the marker and QTL form four possible haplotypes AB, Ab, aB, and ab, with the corresponding frequencies defined as

$$p_{11} = pq + D$$

$$p_{10} = p(1 - q) - D$$

$$p_{01} = (1 - p)q - D \tag{2.18}$$

$$p_{00} = (1 - p)(1 - q) + D$$

where $p_{11}+p_{10}+p_{01}+p_{00}=1$. Haplotypes from the maternal genomes and those from the paternal genomes are randomly combined to produce nine genotypes, with frequencies given in Table 2.4. From these joint genotype frequencies, the conditional probabilities of the QTL genotypes, conditional on the marker genotypes, can be derived according to Bayes' theorem.

Of n subjects, n_1, n_2, and n_3 belong to marker genotypes AA, Aa, and aa, respectively. For a given subject with a particular marker genotype, he or she must carry one and only one of three QTL genotypes with probability depending on the conditional probability provided in Table 2.4 (prior probability) and this subject's phenotypic value. Based on this statement, we reformat the original marker-phenotype data in the form of Table 2.5.

Since the QTL genotypes cannot be directly observed, we construct a mixture-based likelihood to retrieve missing QTL information from observed marker and phenotypic data. Based on Table 2.5, this likelihood is written as

$$L(\mathbf{y}) = \left[\pi_{2|1} f_2\left(\mathbf{y}_1 ; \mu_{2|1}, \Sigma_1\right) + \pi_{1|1} f_1\left(\mathbf{y}_1 ; \mu_{1|1}, \Sigma_1\right) + \pi_{0|1} f_0\left(\mathbf{y}_i ; \mu_{0|i}, \Sigma_1\right) \right]$$
$$\times \left[\pi_{2|2} f_2\left(\mathbf{y}_2 ; \mu_{2|2}, \Sigma_2\right) + \pi_{1|2} f_1\left(\mathbf{y}_1 ; \mu_{1|2}, \Sigma_2\right) + \pi_{0|2} f_0\left(\mathbf{y}_2 ; \mu_{0|2}, \Sigma_2\right) \right]$$
$$\times \dots$$
$$\times \left[\pi_{2|n} f_2\left(\mathbf{y}_n ; \mu_{2|n}, \Sigma_n\right) + \pi_{1|n} f_1\left(\mathbf{y}_n ; \mu_{1|n}, \Sigma_n\right) + \pi_{0|n} f_0\left(\mathbf{y}_n ; \mu_{0|n}, \Sigma_n\right) \right]$$

where $\pi_{j|i}$ is the mixture proportion of QTL genotype j ($j=2$ for QQ, 1 for Qq, and 0 for qq), expressed as the conditional probability of QTL genotype j (Table 2.5), given the marker genotype of subject i and $f_j\left(\mathbf{y}_i ; \mu_{j|i}, \Sigma_i\right)$ is a multivariate normal distribution of phenotypic data $\mathbf{y}_i$ with mean vector represented by genotypic values of the QTL $\mu_{j|i}$ and subject-dependent residual covariance matrix Σ_i.

The unknown parameters involved in the above likelihood are population genetic parameters (p, q, D) and quantitative genetic parameters $(a_j, b_j, r_j, \sigma^2, \rho)$ (because we use the growth equation to model QTL genotypic values and an autoregressive model to fit the covariance structure). To estimate these

TABLE 2.4

Joint Marker-QTL Genotype Frequencies Expressed in Terms of Haplotype Frequencies

	BB	Bb	bb
AA	p_{11}^2	$2p_{11}p_{10}$	p_{10}^2
Aa	$2p_{11}p_{01}$	$2p_{11}p_{00}+2p_{10}p_{01}$	$2p_{10}p_{00}$
aa	p_{01}^2	$2p_{01}p_{00}$	p_{00}^2

TABLE 2.5

Data Structure of Mapping Causal QTL Using Marker Information

Subject	Marker	Conditional (Prior) Probability $(\pi_{j|i})$ Phenotypic Trait (y_i)			Phenotypic Trait (y_i)		
		BB	Bb	bb	t1	t2	t_T
1	AA	p_{11}^2/p^2	$2p_{11}p_{10}/p^2$	p_{10}^2/p^2	$y_1(t_1)$	$y_1(t_1)$	$\cdots$ $y_1(t_T)$
2	AA	$\dfrac{p_{11}^2}{p^2}$	$2p_{11}p_{10}/p^2$	$\dfrac{p_{10}^2}{p^2}$	$y_2(t_1)$	$y_2(t_2)$	$\cdots$ $y_2(t_T)$
$\vdots$							
n_1	AA	$\dfrac{p_{11}^2}{p^2}$	$2p_{11}p_{10}/p^2$	p_{10}^2/p^2	$y_m(t_1)$	$y_m(t_2)$	$\cdots$ $y_m(t_T)$
$n_1{+}1$	Aa	$p_{11}p_{01}/p(1{-}p)$	$(p_{11}p_{00}{+}p_{10}p_{01})/p(1{-}p)$	$p_{11}p_{01}/p(1{-}p)$	$y_{m+1}(t_1)$	$y_{m+1}(t_2)$	$y_{m+1}(t_T)$
$n_1{+}2$	Aa	$p_{11}p_{01}/p(1{-}p)$	$(p_{11}p_{00}{+}p_{10}p_{01})/p(1{-}p)$	$p_{11}p_{01}/p(1{-}p)$	$y_{m+2}(t_1)$	$y_{m+2}(t_2)$	$y_{m+2}(t_T)$
$\vdots$							
$n_1{+}n_2$	Aa	$p_{11}p_{01}/p(1{-}p)$	$(p_{11}p_{00}{+}p_{10}p_{01})/p(1{-}p)$	$p_{11}p_{01}/p(1{-}p)$	$y_{m+n_2}(t_1)$	$y_{m+n_2}(t_2)$	$\cdots$ $y_{m+n_2}(t_T)$
$n_1{+}n_2{+}1$	Aa	$p_{01}^2/(1{-}p)^2$	$2p_{01}p_{00}/(1{-}p)^2$	$p_{00}^2/(1{-}p)^2$	y_{m+n_2+1} (t_1)	y_{m+n_2+1} (t_2)	$\cdots$ y_{m+n_2+1} (t_T)
$n_1{+}n_2{+}2$	Aa	$p_{01}^2/(1{-}p)^2$	$2p_{01}p_{00}/(1{-}p)^2$	$p_{00}^2/(1{-}p)^2$	y_{m+n_2+2} (t_1)	y_{m+n_2+2} (t_2)	$\cdots$ y_{m+n_2+2} (t_T)
$\vdots$							
N	Aa	$p_{01}^2/(1{-}p)^2$	$2p_{01}p_{00}/(1{-}p)^2$	$p_{00}^2/(1{-}p)^2$	$y_n(t_1)$	$y_n(t_2)$	$\cdots$ $y_n(t_T)$

$n = n_{1}{+}n_{2}{+}n_3$

parameters, we implement a hybrid of the EM algorithm and simplex algorithm. In so doing, we rewrite the above mixture likelihood in a general form as

$$L\left(\mathbf{y}\right) = \prod_{i=1}^{n}\left[\pi_{2|i} f_2\left(\mathbf{y}_i;\mu_{2|i},\Sigma_i\right) + \pi_{1|i} f_1\left(\mathbf{y}_i;\mu_{1|i},\Sigma_i\right) + \pi_{0|i} f_0\left(\mathbf{y}_i;\mu_{0|i},\Sigma_i\right)\right] \quad (2.19)$$

Based on these mixtures, we calculate the expected probabilities (posterior probabilities) with which subject i carries a QTL genotype j, given on its marker genotype and phenotypic values, expressed as

$$\Pi_{j|i} = \frac{\pi_{j|i} f_j\left(\mathbf{y}_i;\mu_{j|i},\Sigma_j\right)}{\pi_{2|i} f_2\left(\mathbf{y}_i;\mu_{2|i},\Sigma_2\right) + \pi_{1|i} f_1\left(\mathbf{y}_i;\mu_{1|i},\Sigma_1\right) + \pi_{0|i} f_0\left(\mathbf{y}_i;\mu_{0|i},\Sigma_0\right)} \quad (2.20)$$

Based on these expected probabilities, we calculate haplotype frequencies using the following formulas:

$$p_{11} = \frac{1}{2n}\left[\sum_{i=1}^{n_2}\left(2\Pi_{2|i}+\Pi_{1|i}\right)+\sum_{i=1}^{n_1}\left(\Pi_{2|i}+\phi\Pi_{1|i}\right)\right]$$

$$p_{10} = \frac{1}{2n}\left[\sum_{i=1}^{n_2}\left(2\Pi_{0|i}+\Pi_{1|i}\right)+\sum_{i=1}^{n_1}\left(\Pi_{0|i}+\left(1-\phi\right)\Pi_{1|i}\right)\right]$$

$$p_{01} = \frac{1}{2n}\left[\sum_{i=1}^{n_0}\left(2\Pi_{2|i}+\Pi_{1|i}\right)+\sum_{i=1}^{n_1}\left(\Pi_{2|i}+\left(1-\phi\right)\Pi_{1|i}\right)\right] \tag{2.21}$$

$$p_{00} = \frac{1}{2n}\left[\sum_{i=1}^{n_0}\left(2\Pi_{0|i}+\Pi_{1|i}\right)+\sum_{i=1}^{n_1}\left(\Pi_{0|i}+\phi\Pi_{1|i}\right)\right]$$

and calculate genotype-dependent growth parameters and matrix-structuring parameters using the simplex algorithm. The calculation of the expected probabilities is treated as the E step and the estimation of population and quantitative genetic parameters is treated as the M step. These two steps are repeated until the estimates converge to stable values that are considered the MLEs of model parameters (Table 2.6).

After the MLEs of the model parameters are obtained, we calculate the posterior probabilities of each subject to carry a QTL genotype based on its marker genotype and phenotypic values using equation (2.20). Thus, although three posterior probabilities are calculated for each subject, only

TABLE 2.6

Posterior Probability ($\Pi_{j|i}$) of Each Subject i to Carry a QTL Genotype j

Subject	Marker	v	QTL Genotype	
			Bb	bb
1	AA	$\Pi_{2|1}$	$\Pi_{1|1}$	$\Pi_{0|1}$
2	AA	$\Pi_{2|2}$	$\Pi_{1|1}$	$\Pi_{0|1}$
$\vdots$				
n_1	AA	$\Pi_{2|n_1}$	$\Pi_{1|n_1}$	$\Pi_{0|n_1}$
n_{1+1}	Aa	$\Pi_{2|n_1+1}$	$\Pi_{1|n_1+1}$	$\Pi_{0|n_1+1}$
n_{1+2}	Aa	$\Pi_{2|n_1+2}$	$\Pi_{1|n_1+2}$	$\Pi_{0|n_1+2}$
$\vdots$				
n_1+n_2	Aa	$\Pi_{2|n_1+n_2}$	$\Pi_{1|n_1+n_2}$	$\Pi_{0|n_1+n_2}$
n_1+n_2+1	Aa	$\Pi_{2|n_1+n_2+1}$	$\Pi_{1|n_1+n_2+1}$	$\Pi_{0|n_1+n_2+1}$
n_1+n_2+2	aa	$\Pi_{2|n_1+n_2+2}$	$\Pi_{1|n_1+n_2+2}$	$\Pi_{0|n_1+n_2+2}$
$\vdots$				
$n_1+n_2+n_3=n$	aa	$\Pi_{2|n_1+n_2+n_3}$	$\Pi_{1|n_1+n_2+n_3}$	$\Pi_{0|n_1+n_2+n_3}$

one QTL genotype corresponding to the highest posterior probability is considered the most likely QTL genotype of this subject. For a given marker genotype, we further calculate the proportions of subjects that belong to a QTL genotype, which can be used to determine the degree of the correspondence between QTL and marker genotypes.

Hypothesis test: From the MLEs of haplotype frequencies, we can obtain the MLEs of allele frequencies and LD by solving a group of linear equations (2.18), which are expressed as

$$p = p_{11} + p_{10}$$

$$q = p_{11} + p_{01} \tag{2.22}$$

$$D = p_{11}p_{00} - p_{10}p_{01}$$

Next, we can further test whether the marker is significantly associated with the QTL using the following hypotheses:

$$H_0 : D = 0$$

$$H_1 : D \neq 0 \tag{2.23}$$

Under the null hypothesis, mixture proportions of the mixture likelihood (2.19) are replaced by the conditional probabilities of QTL genotypes given marker genotypes derived from Table 2.2 (assuming no nonrandom association). Note the notation change of allele frequencies from p_1 to p and p_2 to q. We implement the EM algorithm to estimate allele frequencies at the marker and QTL. In the E step, the posterior probabilities are calculated using equation (2.21). In the M step, allele frequencies are estimated using

$$p = \frac{1}{2n} \left[\sum_{i=1}^{n_2} \left(2\Pi_{2|i} + 2\Pi_{1|i} + 2\Pi_{0|i} \right) + \sum_{i=1}^{n_1} \left(\Pi_{2|i} + \Pi_{1|i} + \Pi_{0|i} \right) \right] = \frac{1}{2n} (2n_2 + n_1)$$

$$q = \frac{1}{2n} \left[\sum_{i=1}^{n} \left(2\Pi_{2|i} + \Pi_{1|i} \right) \right] \tag{2.24}$$

where p can be estimated directly from marker observations. Similarly, under the null hypothesis, genotype-dependent growth parameters and matrix-structuring parameters are estimated by the simplex algorithm.

The likelihood values under the null and alternative hypotheses are calculated and used to calculate the LR value using equation (2.17). This LR is thought to follow a chi-square distribution with one degree of freedom. If D is tested to be insignificant, then this means that the significant marker is weakly associated with a causal QTL that is likely to have a large effect. If D is significant, the QTL and marker are either highly linked on a narrow genome interval or evolutionarily have a young age.

2.4 Pharmacogenetic Application of Functional Mapping

2.4.1 A Pharmacogenetic Association Study

Example 2.1

We show how functional mapping can be used to map QTLs for drug response. The example was derived from a published pharmacogenetic study for 163 patients, aimed at investigating the medical effect of dobutamine (Lin et al. 2005a, b, 2007). This drug was designed to improve the heart function of patients who cannot pursue any physical exercise. The association study was conducted to test how patients respond to dobutamine and how drug response is genetically controlled. The study focused on three candidate genes. β-adrenergic receptor (βAR) stimulation occurs in peripheral blood circulation, metabolic regulation, muscle contraction, and central neural activities (Graham et al. 1996). Two subtypes of βAR, $\beta_1 AR$ and $\beta_2 AR$, are found to regulate cardiac structure and function, although they play different even opposite functional roles. The subtype of α_1-adrenergic receptor, $\alpha_1 A$, is an important mediator of sympathetic nervous system responses involved in cardiovascular homeostasis (Woo et al. 2015). Two polymorphisms were genotyped at codons 49 (with two alleles A and G) and 389 (with two alleles C and G) for the $\beta_1 AR$ gene, at codons 16 (with two alleles A and G) and 27 (with two alleles C and G) for the $\beta_2 AR$ gene, and at codon 492 for the $\alpha_1 A$ gene.

The patients studied differ in age, gender, race, body height, and body mass index. As an important pharmacological parameter that assesses drug effect, heart rates were repeatedly measured 5 minutes after the drug was injected at each of increasing dose series, 0 (baseline), 5, 10, 20, 30, and 40 mcg/min. To test how heart rates respond to dose change, we correct heart rate data by removing the baseline effect and plotting the corrected heart rate values against dosage levels (Figure 2.2a). For each patient, dosage-varying change of heart rate can be fitted by the E_{max} equation (Goutelle et al. 2008), expressed as

$$E(c) = \frac{E_{max}c^H}{EC_{50}^H + c^H} \tag{2.25}$$

where E_{max} is the asymptotic (limiting) effect, EC_{50} is the drug concentration that results in 50% of the maximal effect, and H is the slope parameter that determines the slope of the concentration-response curve. Figure 2.2b illustrates the good-of-fitness of the E_{max} equation to heart rates of two randomly chosen subjects, supported by random associations between the fitted values and residuals (Figure 2.2c). Because of their differences in Hill parameters, these two subjects display different forms of dose-response curves.

We draw an LD plot of the five SNPs in the study population (Figure 2.3a) and find that they are generally not associated with each other, except for a moderate association between two SNPs within the $\beta_2 AR$ gene. Because of this, we can perform association

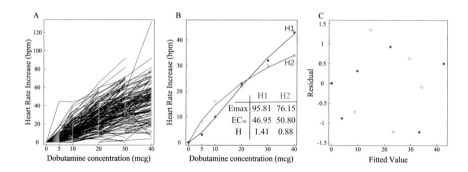

FIGURE 2.2

(a) Changes of heart rate (adjusted for the baselines) for all patients in response to different dosages of dobutamine. (b) Dose-varying heart rates (dot) for two randomly chosen subjects, H1 (blue) and H2 (red), both of which can be fitted by the E_{max} equation. Three Hill parameters estimated for the two subjects are given within the plot. (c) Scatter plots of residuals against the fitted values for the two chosen subjects, H1 (blue) and H2 (red).

studies individually for each SNP without the need to consider possible confound effects due to other SNPs. We incorporate the E_{max} equation into the likelihood of functional mapping to test whether these SNPs are associated with heart rate curves. We calculate the LR values for each SNP. Permutation tests are performed to determine the critical threshold. Only one SNP, codon27 within the $\beta_2 AR$ gene, is significantly associated with response curves to dobutamine (Figure 2.3b). Using the MLEs of the three Hill parameters $(E_{maxj}, EC_{50j}, H_j)$ for different genotypes at codon27, we draw the genotypic curves of drug response (Figure 2.4a), which shows how and how much genotypes differ in the form of the dose-response curve. Genotype CC shows consistently higher heart rates over a window of observed doses (from 0 to 40) than genotypes CG and GG. This difference can be explained by a greater curve slope ($H = 1.80$–1.86 vs. 1.73), a greater asymptotic value ($E_{max} = 74.9$–84.4 vs. 66.9), and a larger concentration with half of the asymptotic value ($EC_{50} = 30.7$–34.3 vs. 22.4) for CG and GG than for CC. We further calculate the additive and dominant effect trajectories over dosages at codn27 (Figure 2.4b); both effects change with dose in a concave shape, with a degree of change being larger for the additive effect than for the dominant effect.

2.4.2 Detection of Causal QTLs for Drug Response

We find that codon27 is significant in terms of its association with dobutamine response. However, this association may be due to the LD of codon27 (with two alleles G and C) with a latent casual QTL (with two hypothesized alleles Q and q). We implement LD-based functional mapping to detect this QTL. Table 2.7 lists the MLEs of four marker-QTL haplotypes, marker-allele frequencies, QTL-allele frequencies, and LD (D) when codon27 is used to map the dobutamine response QTL. The log-LR test of LD under hypotheses of equation (2.23) shows that codon27 is significant with the casual QTL ($P < 0.01$).

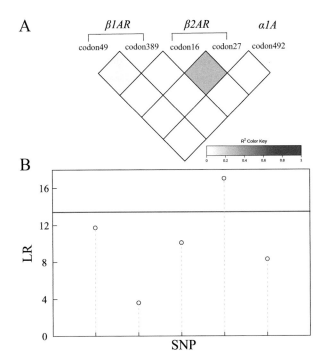

FIGURE 2.3
Population and quantitative genetic analyses of five SNPs from three candidate genes. (a) LD plot showing the pairwise distribution of nonrandom associations described by marker correlations (R^2). (b) The Manhattan plot of log-likelihood ratio (LR) tests for five SNPs. The horizontal line is the critical threshold determined from 1,000 permutation tests.

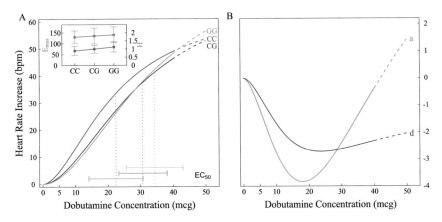

FIGURE 2.4
Functional mapping of drug response. (a) Genotypic curves of heart rate response to dobutamine for GG, CG, and CC, at the significant SNP codon27 from the β_2AR gene. The MLEs of three Hill parameters, E_{max}, H, and EC_{50}, and their standard errors for each genotype are given within the plot. (b) The dose-response curves of the additive and dominant effects at codon27.

TABLE 2.7

MLEs of Marker-QTL Haplotype Frequencies Composed of Allele Frequencies
and Marker-QTL Linkage Disequilibrium

	QTL		
Marker	**Q**	**Q**	
G	0.1748±0.0129	0.2048±0.0139	0.3796±0.0022
C	0.4108±0.0195	0.2059±0.0138	0.6167±0.0037
	0.5856±0.0241	0.4107±0.0197	

However, marked differences in allele frequencies between the marker and
QTL (0.380 vs. 0.411 and 0.617 vs. 0.586) imply that codon27 may not actually
be the causal QTL, but the marker is significantly associated with the QTL
with $D = 0.041 \pm 0.0088$ ($P < 0.05$). A further molecular study is needed to map
the genomic location of this QTL.

We calculate the conditional probabilities of each of three QTL genotypes, unconditional on a marker genotype, and assign a QTL genotype
to this marker genotype if the conditional probability of this QTL genotype is the highest. QTL homozygous genotypes QQ and qq are assigned
to marker genotypes CC and GG at 97% and 98%, respectively, but the QTL
heterozygote Qq is assigned to the marker heterozygote CG only at 65%
(Figure 2.5a), suggesting that it is more difficult to determine a real QTL
genotype from the marker heterozygote than the marker homozygotes.
The genotypic dose-response curves of the QTL detected are different
from those of the marker codon27 (Figure 2.5a vs. Figure 2.4a), although

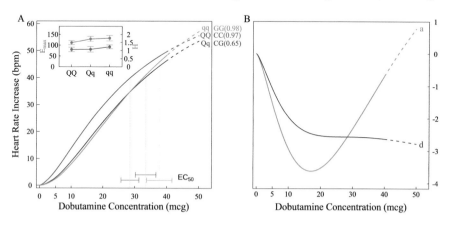

FIGURE 2.5
Causal QTL mediating drug response. (a) Genotypic curves of dobutamine response for three
genotypes at the QTL associated with codon27 from the β_2AR gene. The MLEs of three Hill
parameters, E_{max}, H, and EC_{50}, and their standard errors for each QTL genotype are given
within the plot. Numbers in parentheses are the conditional probability of a given QTL genotype given the marker genotype of codon27. (b) The dose-response curves of the additive and
dominant effects at the causal QTL.

curves of QTL genotypes and marker genotypes have a similar trend. Correspondingly, QTL genotypes have a lower slope of response curve, a smaller asymptotic value, and a smaller concentration at half of the asymptotic value than marker genotypes. We further calculate the additive and dominant effect curves of the QTL (Figure 2.5b), which have a different size from those from the marker, despite a similar dose-varying change trend between the QTL marker.

In summary, the current GWAS analysis uses a direct association strategy, i.e., assuming that the SNP under consideration is a causal QTL. However, by comparing the result from this strategy to that of a mixture-based mapping strategy (detecting the causal QTL by assuming that it is associated with the marker), the first strategy may not completely replace the second strategy. In other words, the direct association strategy can identify the occurrence of a casual QTL and estimate the trend of its genetic effects, but it may not precisely characterize the actual genetic effects of the causal QTL even if the marker-QTL association is statistically significant. To more accurately detect a causal QTL, the mixture-based model is needed.

2.4.3 Epistatic QTLs for Drug Response

Epistatic interactions have been thought to play an important role in pharmacological response to therapeutic interventions (Weigelt and Reis-Filho 2014). Functional mapping has been expanded to map epistatic QTLs for dynamic traits (Wu et al. 2004a). Consider two markers **A** and **B**, which form nine two-locus genotypes. We extend the likelihood of equation (2.12) to include these nine genotypes, each with a genotypic curve modeled by a mathematical equation. By testing differences in genotypic curves, we can claim whether the two markers are jointly associated with phenotypic variation. We use decomposition equations in Table 2.1 to estimate the additive and dominant genetic effects at each locus and additive×additive, additive×dominant, dominant×additive, and dominant×dominant epistatic effects between the two loci. Each of these effects can be tested through simulation studies.

We pair five SNPs to test whether any pairwise genetic interactions are significant for the trajectories of heart rate in response to dobutamine. By statistical testing, we find that codon27 (with two alleles C and G) from $\beta_2 AR$ significantly interacts with codon492 (with two alleles C and T) from $\alpha_1 A$ to govern dose-response curves. This suggests that epistasis between these two candidate genes plays an important role in affecting heart rate change. We find that homozygotes GG and CC at codon27 in combination with homozygote TT at codon492 have different dose-response curves than the other combination genotypes (Figure 2.6a).

A further test is performed to investigate how different components of epistasis affect drug response. We find that the four types of epistasis act in different ways, although all of them tend to change their effects periodically (Figure 2.6b). It appears that additive × additive epistasis and dominant ×

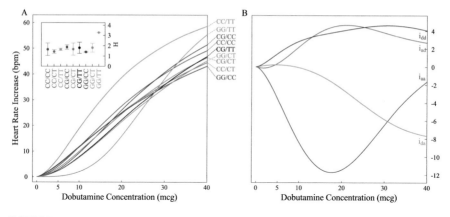

FIGURE 2.6

Epistatic detection of drug response. (a) Two-locus genotypic curves of response to dobutamine for nine genotypes at codon27 from the $\beta_2 AR$ gene and codon492 from the $\alpha_1 A$ gene. The MLEs of curve slope H and their standard errors for each genotype are given within the plot. (b) The dose-response curves of the additive × additive (i_{aa}), additive × dominant (i_{ad}), dominant × additive (i_{da}), and dominant × dominant (i_{dd}) epistatic effects at codon27 and codon492.

additive epistasis change their heart rate more dramatically than additive × dominant and dominant × dominant epistases. Through such genotypic comparisons, the genetic mechanisms underlying this dose-dependent change can be characterized.

2.5 Functional Mapping with High-Dimensional Predictors

Functional mapping was originally proposed on simple univariate linear regression, which associates dynamic phenotypes with genotypes at individual SNPs. However, this method ignores the effects of other SNPs and, thus, fails to capture the correlation information among SNPs while assessing one particular SNP and is subjected to a severe adjustment issue for multiple comparisons, reducing the precision and power of association detection for drug response. A way to overcome these issues is to analyze all SNPs simultaneously. Yet, in GWAS, a major challenge is often confronted in analyzing thousands of thousands of SNPs (p) on much fewer samples (n). In the current statistical literature, several models of variable selection have been available to handle such high-dimension data characterized by big p and small n, of which the least absolute shrinkage and selection operator (LASSO) has proved to be powerful and computationally feasible (Tibshirani 1996).

Li et al. (2015) integrated functional mapping and the Bayesian group LASSO to analyze multiple SNPs simultaneously, which can better unreal the developmental genetic mechanisms of trait formation. Their approach presents a two-stage procedure for multi-SNP modeling and analysis, by first producing a "preconditioned" response variable using supervised principal component analysis and then formulating a Bayesian Lasso to select a subset of significant sites. The Bayesian Lasso is implemented with a hierarchical model, in which scale mixtures of normal are used as prior distributions for the genetic effects, and exponential priors are considered for their variances and then solved by using the Markov chain Monte Carlo algorithm. This approach obviates the choice of the lasso parameter by imposing a diffuse hyperprior on it and estimating it along with other parameters and is particularly powerful for selecting the most relevant SNPs where the number of predictors exceeds the number of observations.

Li et al. (2014a) further proposed a variable selection framework for functional mapping of pairwise interactions in GWAS. This approach includes two stages. In the first stage, a two-stage sure independence screening procedure is implemented to generate a pool of candidate SNPs and interactions, which serve as predictors. The size of the reduced model is determined by a rate-adjusted thresholding estimation approach. In the second stage, a final set of significant predictors are identified by regularization regression methods, such as LASSO or smoothly clipped absolute deviation (SCAD). The biological relevance of Li et al.'s (2014a, 2015) approaches was validated by applying them to analyze body mass index from a well-known Framingham Heart GWAS data set, leading to the identification of significant loci that reside in known candidate genes coding alpha-ketoglutarate–dependent dioxygenase and other fat mass and obesity-associated proteins.

2.6 Concluding Remarks

Like complex diseases, variation in drug response is complex in terms of its multifactorial and interactive nature (Weinshilboum 2003; Weinshilboum and Wang 2006; Daly 2010; Wang et al. 2011; Zhang et al. 2020; Lozovsky et al. 2021). The identification of the genetic contribution to drug response has become one of the most active and promising subjects in modern genomics. Different from complex diseases, studying drug response needs to consider an additional layer of its complexity that reflects how drugs interact with the body through a cascade of biochemical and physiological pathways. Genetic mapping or association studies that integrate the mechanistic characterization of how the drug works to the body (PK) and how the body works to the drug (PD) can better enhance their capacity to chart the comprehensive picture of the genetic architecture of drug response.

Such integration has been made possible through functional mapping or functional GWAS (*f*GWAS) as a dynamic approach for dissecting developmental mechanisms into genetic mapping settings (Ma et al. 2002; Wu and Lin 2006, 2008; Lin et al. 2005a, b, 2007; Ahn et al. 2010; Das et al. 2012). The main theme of functional mapping is to integrate the mathematical equations that specify PK and PD reactions of drug response into a statistical mapping framework. Viewing drug response as a dynamic process, it can estimate and test the effects of genetic variants on changes in the concentration of a drug with time and drug efficacy with dose. More importantly, it can characterize how genetic variants modulate key pharmacological parameters that define the shape and pattern of dose-time-response curves (Wang et al. 2015a), providing an important avenue for translating genomic information into clinical practice. Functional mapping can not only dramatically enhance the biological, biomedical, and clinical relevance of genetic mapping but also augment the statistical precision and power of gene detection.

Functional mapping is very flexible to accommodate many issues typically occurring in pharmacogenetic research. For example, a drug may produce a side effect or toxicity in some tissue, while it is supposed to play a role in improving the function of the targeted tissues. To develop the most desirable drug, i.e., those of high efficacy but low toxicity, we need to understand the pleiotropic control of these two types of drug response (Xia 2017). Lin and Wu (2005) leveraged functional mapping to a bivariate space in which the commonality and difference of genes affecting drug efficacy and drug toxicity can be tested and identified. In the past, drug toxicity was regarded as being the most difficult to define, quantify, and predict (Sosnin et al. 2019). Yet, this has changed with the advent of sequencing technologies that can measure and define drug efficacy and drug toxicity from a transcriptomic perspective.

A desirable drug can effectively control disease, but when the disease becomes tolerant to the drug, a phenomenon, called drug resistance, results. It may exist either before drug treatment (intrinsic) or generate after therapy (acquired), both affected by genetic factors (Wang et al. 2019c). Functional mapping can be expanded to not only map genes for drug sensitivity but also characterize the genetic control mechanisms of drug resistance. Drug response is the consequence of interactions between genes and the environment. Functional mapping can be modified to map how genes interact with different types of environments to mediate drug efficacy and toxicity. It is also straightforward to include other genetic variants, including epigenetic marks, copy number variants, and rare-allele variants, to chart a more complete atlas of the pharmacogenetic architecture of drug response.

Existing approaches are mostly based on the marginal analysis of markers and drug response phenotypes, but this reductionism thinking cannot dissect the true effect of individual markers because the marginal effects are confounded by the effect of other markers. Joint analysis of all markers can overcome this issue, providing a more precise picture of how each gene acts and interacts with other genes to determine final phenotypes. The integration of functional mapping and variable selection produces a unique power to characterize a more complete landscape of genetic actions and interactions throughout the genome. Variable selection approaches have been available to tackle high-dimensional SNPs on much fewer samples. This enables functional mapping to shed light on the genetic architecture of inter-patient variation in complex drug responses (Li et al. 2014a, 2015; Jiang et al. 2015).

3

A Multiscale Model of Pharmacokinetic – Pharmacodynamic Mapping

3.1 Introduction

Human body's reaction to drugs varies dramatically from individual to individual. As such, pharmacogenetics and pharmacogenomics that document and catalogue genomic regions in relation to inter-individual variation have been a long-standing focus of studies in pharmacology and medicine (Weinshilboum 2003; Weinshilboum and Wang 2006; Daly 2010; Bailey and Cheng 2010; Wang et al. 2011; Gonzalez-Covarrubias et al. 2007). To better reveal the genetic architecture of how drugs affect the body, functional mapping integrates the mathematical aspects of pharmacokinetic-pharmacodynamic (PK-PD) reactions into pharmacogenetic characterization (Lin et al. 2005a, b, 2007, 2010; Wu and Lin 2008; Ahn et al. 2010; Mustavich et al. 2010; Wu et al. 2011a; Wang et al. 2013a, 2015a), which can greatly enhance both biologic and clinical relevance of pharmacogenetic dissection. Because of its implementation with advanced statistical methodologies, this approach can also increase the statistical power of pharmacogene detection, especially from a modest sample size, which is more commonly used in pharmacogenetic studies than disease genetic studies (Daly 2010; Motsinger-Reif et al. 2013).

Chapter 2 outlines a general framework for functional mapping as an approach to mapping pharmacogenes that affect the body's overall response to mediations. A single parameter is not adequately sufficient to comprehend drug response; rather drug response can be better characterized by its multifaceted features. For example, almost all drugs produce both favorable and unfavorable impacts on the body. Thus, the most desirable drug is of high efficacy and low toxicity at a given dose, but balancing drug efficacy and drug toxicity is challenged by their unknown pleiotropic genetic control (Giacomini et al. 2017). Lin and Wu (2005) extended functional mapping into a bivariate dimension at which both efficacy and toxicity can be jointly mapped. Although drug efficacy can be readily assessed, drug toxicity is quite difficult to define, quantify, and predict (Sosnin et al. 2019). Xia (2020) describes a transcriptomic definition for drug efficacy and drug toxicity, which can facilitate the integration of Lin and Wu's functional mapping to detect the pleiotropic control of these two processes in a transcriptomic context.

Drug efficacy can be measured by the endpoint measure of drug response, but it is important to measure a concentration-dependent effect that reveals changes in response to dosage. It is possible that a drug produces the same efficacy (E_{max}) for different patients, but the paths to produce such efficacy (described by drug potency EC_{50}) are patient-dependent. Thus, it is meaningful to map the pleiotropic control of drug efficacy vs. drug potency for designing an optimal dosage based on patients' genetic makeup. Pharmacologists' challenges with drug design and delivery are to determine how diseased cells from different patients respond to a drug or regime and when drug-resistant diseased cells start to emerge (Alaoui-Jamali et al. 2004). A profound understanding of drug susceptibility and drug resistance is crucial for resolving these challenges.

In this chapter, we expand functional mapping to its multivariate dimension at which the detailed mechanisms underlying the complexity of drug response can be understood. These multivariate approaches can particularly map and identify genes that mediate multifaceted response features of drug interventions and various pathways that cause end-point drug response. To demonstrate the utility of multivariate functional mapping, we apply it to analyze real examples for chronotherapy and hypertension mapping. The approach can be readily used in other fields with appropriate modifications.

3.2 Heterochronopharmacodynamics and Chronotherapy

The 2017 Nobel Prize in Physiology or Medicine was awarded to Jeffrey C. Hall, Michael Rosbash, and Michael W. Young for research that established key mechanistic principles on how circadian rhythms are regulated. Circadian rhythm, or biological clock, running over a period of around 24 hours in the human body, is tightly related to biological processes. Disruptions in biological rhythms can be associated with the sort of aberrant cell cycling, ultimately leading to disease, such as tumorigenesis (Sulli et al. 2019). An increasing number of pharmacological studies have associated circadian rhythm with PD reactions through revealing immune function and metabolism (Panda 2016; Kuhlman et al. 2017).

The study of how the efficacy of drugs changes according to the body's circadian rhythm, i.e., chronopharmacodynamics, has emerged as a vital and promising area of personalized medicine or individualized medicine (Lemmer 2007; Smolensky et al. 2015; Dallmann et al. 2016; Kaur et al. 2016; Ballesta et al. 2017; Kiessling and Cermakian 2017). PD variation can be viewed as an evolutionary process, in which key aspects of pharmacogenes implicated in pharmacological response and metabolism can be interpreted.

It has been increasingly recognized that the integration of some evolutionary concepts into pharmacological research can leverage pharmacogenetic research (Fuselli 2019).

Heterochrony is an important concept used to characterize the developmental mechanisms of evolution (Keyte and Smith 2014). In developmental evolutionary biology, it is defined as a dynamic change in the timing or rate of events from individual to individual. Variation in heterochrony can lead to changes and evolution in the form and process of development (Smith 2003; McNamara 2012). By integrating developmental, neontological, and palaeontological data based on a geometric morphometric approach, Bhullar et al. (2012) found that the heterochronic variation of paedomorphosis, a phenomenon by which descendants resemble the juveniles of their ancestors, is a forcing driver of several major evolutionary transitions in the origin of birds. A series of quantitative models based on functional mapping have been formulated to characterize the contributions of heterochrony to developmental variation (Sun et al. 2014, 2017; Jiang et al. 2015).

The effect of heterochrony on pharmacological response can date back to Levy's (1964) work in the 1960s where he found a mathematical link between the rate of decline of the pharmacological effect of drugs and their elimination rate. Levy's discovery has also led to the development of PD modeling that quantitatively integrates pharmacokinetics, pharmacological systems, and (patho-) physiological processes to better understand the strength and time-course of drug effects on the body (Felmlee et al. 2012).

Wei et al. (2018b) synthesized heterochrony and chronopharmacodynamics into a PK-PD paradigm to create a new terminology called heterochronopharmacodynamics (HCPD). HCPD enables the identification and quantification of key heterochronic parameters in the PK-PD process, which critically determine the pharmacogenetic variation of drug response. By the mathematical transformation of PK-PD equations, several key HCPD parameters can be estimated, including the timings or drug concentrations of maximum efficacy change rate, maximum efficacy change acceleration, and maximum efficacy change deceleration, from which to calculate the durations or concentration widows of three distinct PK-PD phases, lag, exponential, and stationary. The association analysis of these HCPD parameters with genome-wide genotypic data could provide new insight into how genes govern drug response by mediating key steps or events.

3.3 Heterochronopharmacodynamic Mapping

3.3.1 PD Model – The Hill Equation

A number of PD models have been constructed and evaluated to predict pharmacological/toxicological effects from drug exposure. These models have been instrumental for generating new insights and competing hypotheses of biochemical mechanisms that mediate drug responses and providing guidance for subsequent drug discovery, development, and pharmacotherapy. The Hill equation is the simple direct effect model, assuming that drug effects (E) change directly in proportion to plasma drug concentrations (C) (Giraldo 2003; Gesztelyi et al. 2012; Felmlee et al. 2012), expressed as

$$E(C) = E_0 + \frac{E_{max} C^H}{EC_{50}^H + C^H} \tag{3.1}$$

where E_0 is a baseline effect, E_{max} is the maximum possible effect, EC_{50} is the drug concentration producing half maximal effect, and H is the Hill coefficient describing the steepness of the concentration-effect relationship curve.

The pattern of how drug effects change with concentration can be visualized by estimating the model parameters (E_0, E_{max}, EC_{50}, H). Inter-individual variability in drug response can be broadly classified into four types as follows (Figure 3.1):

- High-low variation where one subject has a higher baseline and greater drug effects consistently across a full spectrum of drug concentration than the other
- Fast-slow variation where one subject has a greater slope of response than the other, although they start from the same baseline
- Long-short variation in which one subject can adapt to a long spectrum of dose than the other
- Reverse variation where drug response curves cross-over between two subjects

The Hill equation (3.1), also called the sigmoid Emax model, spans three distinct phases of curves, lag, exponential, and stationary or asymptotic (Figure 3.2). During the lag phase, drugs after administration are gradually absorbed and distributed within the body but do not metabolize heavily to function, although the synthesis of RNA, enzymes, and other molecules occurs under drug reaction. The exponential phase is a period characterized by the augment of drug metabolism during which drug effects are exponentially proportional to the present drug concentration. The rate of change of drug effects during the exponential phase and the concentration spectrum of this phase directly affect the outcome of drug efficacy or toxicity. At the stationary phase, drug effects approach their maximum value, tending to change little due to the depletion of drugs and the removal of substances from the body.

Each of these types may be controlled by a specific set of pharmacogenes. Functional mapping can be powerful to identify and discern these genes,

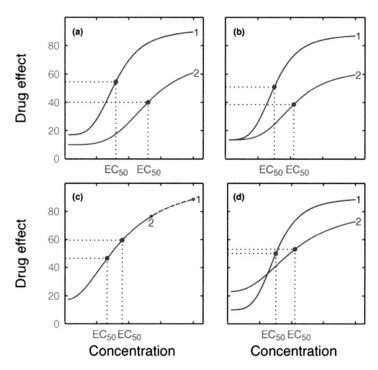

FIGURE 3.1
Types of variation in drug response modulated by HPD parameters. (a) High-low variation where one individual (#1) has a greater drug effect than the other (#2) during the full spectrum of concentration. (b) Fast-slow variation where one individual (#1) responds to drug concentration at a greater rate than the other (#2) although they start from the same baseline. (c) Long-short variation where one individual (#1) displays an extended spectrum (broken line) of drug concentration compared to the other (#2). (d) Reverse variation where one individual (#1) with a low baseline surpasses its high-baseline counterpart (#2) during changing concentrations.

called high-low genes, fast-slow genes, long-short genes, and reverse genes. Because of their different roles, a specific therapeutic strategy that implements each type of genes should be developed to maximize drug efficacy and minimize drug toxicity. For example, the high-response genotype at a fat-low gene needs a smaller dose to reach the same level of drug efficacy as the low-response genotype can reach; a smaller dose makes the former avoid the side-effect of the drug. In translational medicine, the identification of gene types becomes an important task to optimize drug dosing and scheduling.

3.3.2 Integrating Heterochrony into PD Modeling

Because of their different impacts on final pharmacological response, the distinction of lag, exponential, and stationary phases is essential for the design

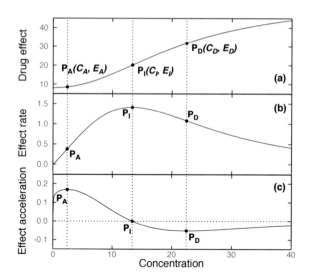

FIGURE 3.2
Curves of drug response (a), drug response rate (b), and drug response acceleration (c). Three (x, y)-coordinates on the curves, (C_A, E_A), (C_I, E_I), and (C_D, E_D), are shown, presenting the inflection point, the maximum acceleration and maximum deceleration of drug response curve, respectively.

of an optimal drug dose and an optimal time of drug administration. For example, if the exponential phase occurs within a short concentration spectrum, a small dose of drugs may be adequate to achieve their maximum pharmacological effects. If the concentration spectrum of the exponential phase is under genetic control, personalized drug delivery strategies can be made according to patients' genetic makeups.

The concept of heterochrony can be instrumental for better describing drug response and dissecting it into its lag, exponential, and stationary phases. By deriving the first, second, and third derivatives of the Hill equation with respect to concentration, it is expressed as

$$\frac{dE}{dC} = \frac{C^{H-1}E_{max}H \cdot EC_{50}^{H}}{(C^{H} + EC_{50}^{H})^{2}} \tag{3.2a}$$

$$\frac{d^{2}E}{dC^{2}} = \frac{C^{H-2}E_{max}H \cdot EC_{50}^{H}\left[C^{H}(1+H) - (H-1)EC_{50}^{H}\right]}{(C^{H} + EC_{50}^{H})^{3}} \tag{3.2b}$$

$$\frac{d^{3}E}{dC^{3}} = \frac{C^{H-3}E_{max}H \cdot EC_{50}^{H}\left[C^{2H}(2+3H+H^{2}) - 4C^{H}(H^{2}-1)EC_{50}^{H} + (2-3H+H^{2})EC_{50}^{2H}\right]}{(C^{H} + EC_{50}^{H})^{4}} \tag{3.2c}$$

Letting the second derivative of equation (3.2b) equal to zero, we solve the concentration as

$$C_I = \left[\frac{(H-1)EC_{50}^H}{H+1} \right]^{\frac{1}{H}} \tag{3.3}$$

which is the inflection point of the Hill curve, representing the concentration of drugs at which the rate of drug effect change reaches a maximum value. Letting the third derivative of equation (3.2c) equal to zero, we obtain two solutions of the concentration as

$$C_A = \left[\frac{EC_{50}^H \left(2(H^2-1) - H\sqrt{3(H^2-1)} \right)}{2+3H+H^2} \right]^{\frac{1}{H}} \tag{3.4a}$$

$$C_D = \left[\frac{EC_{50}^H \left(2(H^2-1) + H\sqrt{3(H^2-1)} \right)}{2+3H+H^2} \right]^{\frac{1}{H}} \tag{3.4b}$$

representing two points at which drug effect changes achieve the maximum acceleration, and maximum deceleration, respectively. The difference between these two concentrations,

$$W = C_D - C_A \tag{3.5}$$

describes a window of drug concentration during which drug effects change exponentially. In other words, W is the concentration window of drug response's exponential phase.

We are interested in drug effects at the points where drug response transmits from one phase to the next. Drug effects at C_I (at which drug effect reaches its maximum value), C_A (at which the exponential phase starts), and C_D (at which the exponential phase ends) can be derived as

$$E_I = E_0 + \frac{E_{max}(H-1)}{2H} \tag{3.6a}$$

$$E_A = E_0 - \frac{E_{max}\left(2 - 2H^2 + H^2\sqrt{3(H^2-1)}\right)}{\left(3 + 3H^2 - H\sqrt{3(H^2-1)}\right)} \qquad (3.6b)$$

$$E_A = E_0 - \frac{E_{max}\left(2 - 2H^2 - H^2\sqrt{3(H^2-1)}\right)}{\left(3 + 3H^2 + H\sqrt{3(H^2-1)}\right)} \qquad (3.6c)$$

In summary, these so-called heteropharmacodynamic (HPD) parameters that can describe the pattern of pharmacological response include (1) the (x, y)-coordinates of the inflection point of the Hill curve (C_I, E_I), (2) the (x, y)-coordinates of drug response acceleration curve (C_A, E_A), (3) the (x, y)-coordinates of drug response deceleration curve (C_D, E_D), (4) the concentration spectrum of the exponential phase of drug response (C_D–C_A), (5) the concentration associated with ½ E_{max} (EC_{50}), (6) the maximum drug effect at high concentrations (E_{max}), and (7) the slope of drug response (H). By fitting the Hill equation (3.1) to concentration-dependent drug effect data and substituting the estimated curve parameters into equations (3.3)–(3.6), these HPD parameters can be estimated.

3.3.3 Top-Down and Bottom-Up Mapping Approaches of HPD Genes

Given that the pharmacological response of drugs has a genetic component, the characterization of whether quantitative trait loci (QTLs) determine HPD parameters can provide mechanistic insight into the pharmacogenetic architecture of drug response. There are two approaches for mapping HPD parameters. The first approach establishes the genetic dependencies of drug response as a dynamic process in a top-down manner, whereas the second is a bottom-up approach that reconstructs drug response trajectories from QTL-based HPD parameters. The top-down approach walks from drug response to QTL, with a better capacity to chart the global pattern of pharmacogenetic control. The bottom-up approach, directed from QTL to drug response, is more powerful for characterizing the key HPD features of drug efficacy and toxicity. These two approaches represent different strategies of information processing and knowledge ordering.

Specifically, the top-down mapping approach treats drug response as a curve and map such curves by integrating PK-PD models into the maximum likelihood-based mapping setting. This approach, described in detail in Chapter 2, first detects significant QTLs and then tests the effect of these QTLs on HPD parameters. This approach has been used to map the so-called heterochrony QTLs (hQTLs) for plant development (Sun et al. 2014). A number of hQTLs have been identified for leaf growth in the common bean

(Jiang et al. 2015), stemwood growth in poplar (Xu et al. 2006), and shoot growth in woody ornamental plants (Sun et al. 2017). The bottom-up mapping approach is to estimate HPD parameters for individual subjects based on the procedure of Section 3.3.2, followed by mapping QTLs for these mathematical parameters by viewing them as a phenotypic trait. This approach has been used to map rate and event QTLs in plants (Baker et al. 2015; Zhang et al. 2017; Sun et al. 2018; Wei et al. 2018a).

Both mapping approaches can generate and test a number of competing hypotheses regarding pharmacogenetic mechanisms. Specifically, the following questions can be addressed:

1. How do genes control the timing at which drugs trigger a maximum efficacy?
2. How do genes mediate the time duration or concentration spectrum of maximum pharmacological effect?
3. Whether are there any genes that turn on or turn off the body's response to drugs? If there are such genes, where are they and how do they act and interact?
4. How do HPD-related genes alter their expression in response to life style, demographic factor, or developmental cue?
5. How do genes control differently three phases of PK-PD processes, lag, exponential, and stationary?

3.3.4 Identification of HPD QTLs

We analyze the real data from a pharmacogenetic association study of medical response to dobutamine, a drug developed to control congestive heart failure by increasing heart rate and cardiac contractility. This study, first reported in Lin et al. (2005a,b), reanalyzed by Wei et al. (2018b), and re-described in Chapter 2, included a group of 163 subjects (including males and females) in ages from 32 to 86 years. The patients had a wide range of baseline (untreated) heart rates. The subjects received increasing doses of dobutamine, from 0 (baseline) to 5, 10, 20, 30, and 40 mcg, at each of which their heart rates were recorded. The maximum doses vary among subjects because of different physiological limits. β-adrenergic receptors (βAR) may play a role in mediating the effect of dobutamine on cardiovascular function. This study genotyped five single-nucleotide polymorphisms (SNPs), located at codons 49 (Ser49Gly) and 389 (Arg389Gly) within the $\beta_1 AR$ gene, codons 16 (Arg16Gly) and 27 (Gln27Glu) within the $\beta_2 AR$ gene, and codon 492 (Arg492Cys) within the $\alpha_1 A$ gene. Here, we use the bottom-up mapping approach to test whether these SNPs are associated with HPD parameters or whether they are QTLs that control HPD variation.

We first corrected dose-dependent heart rate data by removing the effects due to age, sex, race, and body mass index (BMI). The Hill equation was then used to fit the corrected heart rate data for each subject. A bivariate ANOVA approach was used to test the association between each SNP and (x, y)-coordinates of (C_I, E_I), (C_A, E_A), and (C_D, E_D). Owing to inadequate data to fit the Hill equation, some subjects cannot obtain positive solutions for the coordinates of the inflection points of drug effect change acceleration curves, which thus were excluded from genetic association analysis. SNP codon27 within the $\beta_2 AR$ gene was found to be significantly associated with (x, y)-coordinates of (C_I, E_I) ($P=0.023$) and (C_D, E_D) ($P=0.028$). Thus, this SNP is regarded as a QTL that determines the dose-effect curve of dobutamine by mediating these HPD points. Using the estimated values of four Hill equation parameters, we draw the curves of heart rate change over different doses of dobutamine for three genotypes at this QTL (Figure 3.3a). From these curves, we can visually investigate how a QTL governs drug response through its mediation on HPD parameters.

A univariate ANONA was used to analyze and test the association between SNPs and single HPD parameters, E_{max}, EC_{50}, H, or W. We found that SNP at codon27 exerts a significant impact on the slope of drug response curve ($P=0.047$). As shown in Figure 3.3a, the slope of heart rate response curve varies remarkably among three genotypes at this QTL.

Lin et al. (2005a) developed a mixture model-based approach to detect the association of drug response with haplotype, a linear arrangement of DNA nucleotides on the same chromosome. By selecting the most likely haplotype that is most distinguishable from the rest, this approach can test how different nucleotides govern drug effects through their varying sequences on chromosomes. We implement Lin et al.'s haplotyping approach to identify haplotype variants associated with HDP parameters. Based on a pairwise haplotype analysis of five SNPs, we detect a significant haplotype effect composed of two SNPs within the $\beta_2 AR$ gene. Of four possible haplotypes constituted by these two SNPs, haplotype GG is detected to be a genetic determinant of heart rate response to dobutamine. For example, it affects (x, y)-coordinates of (C_I, E_I) and (C_D, E_D), and also maximum response value E_{max}. Using the Hill coefficients estimated, response curves of heart rates were drawn for three composite diplotypes constructed from different combinations of haplotype GG and the rest three haplotypes as a whole (Figure 3.3b), from which we can visualize how haplotype variants contribute to overall response-dose curves through the mediation of HPD variation.

3.3.5 Heterochronopharmacodynamic Dissection

The HPD concept is relevant for the determination of an optimal dose to achieve maximum efficacy and minimum toxicity. Since PD processes are rhythmically moderated by the circadian timing system over 24-hour day and night cycles (Kuhlman et al. 2017; Zhang et al. 2018), an optimal delivery

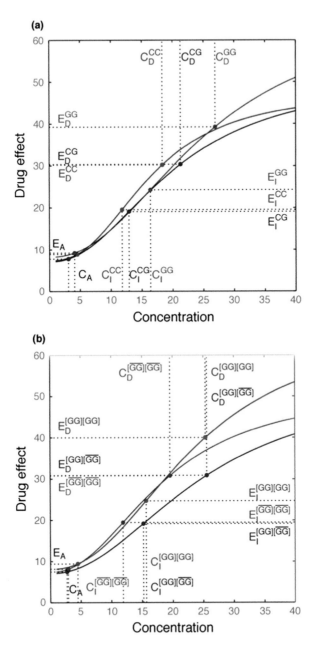

FIGURE 3.3
Genotypic differences in the curve of heart rate response to dobutamine at a QTL. (a) The QTL detected is a single SNP at codon 27 within the β2AR gene. (b) The QTL detected represents haplotype variants composed of two SNPs at codon 16 and 27 within the β2AR gene. Haplotype GG is a key determinant, whose combinations with the rest three haplotypes (collectively expressed by bars) form three composite diplotypes (Lin et al. 2005a). Genotypic differences in several key heteropharmacodynamic parameters are shown.

schedule may exist for the best therapy. Circadian timing, constituted of a network of genetic cellular circadian clocks, determines how a drug is absorbed, distributed, metabolized, and eliminated in the body and how this process causes pharmacological effects. One way for tailoring circadian drug delivery to individual circadian timing systems for optimizing treatment effects is the synthesis of HPD and its molecular clock control. This forms a new concept, heterochronopharmacodynamics (HcPD).

A chronopharmacodynamic equation can be manifested by a Hill equation, modulated in amplitude by a circadian chronosensitivity factor (Clairambault 2007). It is mathematically expressed as

$$E(c, t) = E_{max} \left\{ 1 + \cos\left(2\pi \left(\frac{t - \varphi}{T} \right) \right) \right\} \frac{c^H}{EC_{50}^H + c^H} \qquad (3.7)$$

where t is the time of drug reaction after administration, C, E_{max}, EC_{50}, and H are defined as above, $T=24\,h$ is the period of circadian drug sensitivity oscillations, and φ is the phase of the maximum activity of $E(C, t)$, in hours with reference to a fundamental 24-hour rhythm.

Consider a patient who is administered by the same drug at two different times, midnight (time 1) and 6 am (time 2). At both dosing times, drug effect changes over time in a 24-hour periodicity under a given concentration, although the pattern of this change depends on doing time. The dosing time at 6 am produces a higher drug effect under a low concentration than does the dosing time at midnight, whereas the drug effect of the dosing time at midnight is more responsible for drug concentration than that at 6 am (Figure 3.4a). At a given time after administration, drug response follows an S-shaped curve, with the pattern varying between dosing times. Because of different periods of rhythmic change, dosing time at midnight generates a great drug response than that dosing time at 6 am at one time after administration (e.g., $t=12$), whereas the inverse pattern was observed at the other time (e.g., $t=18$) (Figure 3.4b). Taken together, this hypothesized example suggests that different dosing times produce different drug effects through circadian timing systems, which is determined by HcPD.

HcPD can be described by several key parameters, including HPD parameters at different times after administration and amplitudes and phases of rhythmic drug response curves at different concentration levels. A great interpersonal variability in circadian timing system implicates the existence of QTLs for HcPD. By viewing each HcPD parameter as a phenotype, statistical models can be implemented to map HcPD QTLs throughout the genome.

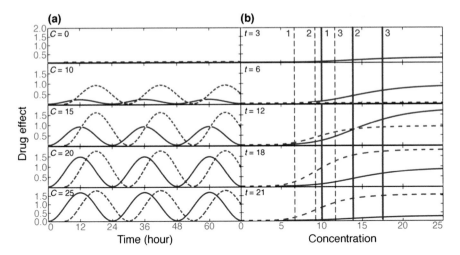

FIGURE 3.4

The diagrammatic representation of heterochronopharmacodynamics for the same patient administered by a drug at two dosing times, midnight (solid curve) and 6 am (dotted curve). (a) Drug effect changes as a function of time after administration at different concentrations. (b) Drug effect changes as a function of concentration at different times. Vertical slash lines present the timing of drug response acceleration (1), the timing of drug response inflection point (2), and the timing of drug response deceleration (3). Solid vertical lines and dotted vertical lines correspond to dosing times at midnight and 6 am, respectively.

3.4 Mapping Multifaceted Drug Reactions

3.4.1 Multifaceted Features of Drug Response: A Blood Pressure Example

As a complex physiological process involving various PD interactions, drug response is characterized by multifaceted features and, thereby, better described by multiple phenotypes. Similarly, a disease may not merely be related to a single physiological parameter, but more likely, is influenced by multiple aspects of comorbidities. For example, A growing body of evidence shows that the association of hypertension with the risk of cardiovascular disease is determined not only by either systolic blood pressure (SBP) or diastolic blood pressure (DBP), but also by the pulsatile component (described by pulse pressure, PP) and the steady component (described by mean arterial pressure, MAP) (Sesso et al. 2000; Safar 1989; Darne et al. 1989; Domanski et al. 1999; Palaniappan et al. 2002; Larstorp et al. 2012; Dart 2017; Melo et al. 2018). Several studies have been conducted to characterize hemodynamic determinants of these two components and the physiological mechanisms of how they impact heart function and disease (Vennin et al. 2017). The pulsatile component is determined by ventricular ejection fraction, large-artery stiffness, early pulse-wave reduction, and heart rate (Franklin et al. 1997), whereas the steady component is affected by left ventricular contractility, heart rate, and vascular resistance and elasticity averaged over time (Safar 1989). Current diagnostic protocols have used SBP and/or DBP, in conjunction with MAP and PP, to more comprehensively assess hypertension-related health risk (Palaniappan et al. 2002). For pharmacy sectors, a highly essential task is to develop and deliver specific medications for the simultaneous intervention for abnormal SBP and DBP as well as for PP and MAP according to patients' genetic makeups.

Previous studies of genetic mapping and association mapping have identified important QTLs that affect MAP and PP in animal and human populations (Wain et al. 2011; Hong et al. 2012; Koh-Tan et al. 2017; Padmanabhan and Joe 2017). In a meta-analysis of 150,134 individuals from 54 genome-wide association studies of European ancestry with 1000 Genomes Project-based imputation, Wain et al. (2017) identified a total of 48 genes that are involved in differences of SBP, DBP, and PP among humans. Chauvet et al. (2013) found that QTLs affect the MAP of the inbred rat through modularity and epistasis. However, results of these studies were obtained from a simple statistical method, whose implication may not be maximized in pharmacological practice. First, without integrating the MAP- and/or PP-related drug response, we lack a complete picture of BP genetics, making it difficult to comprehensively improve BP through drugs. Second, the MAP and PP responses to drugs are a dynamic process that follows PD and PK principles of drug effects and absorption in the body (Giraldo 2003; Wang et al. 2013a, 2015a). The incorporation of PD and PK processes can enhance our understanding of the mechanistic basis of drug response.

In Chapter 2, we described a univariate functional mapping framework for single dynamic traits. This model is conceptualized as a theory for computational pharmacogenetics and pharmacogenomics (Wu and Lin 2008; Ahn et al. 2010), which has been effectively used in practice (Lin et al. 2005a, b, 2007, 2010). This model enables Mustavich et al. (2010) to detect loci that control susceptibility to alcohol dependence, and Wang et al. (2015a) to identify important pharmacological genes for glucocorticoid intervention in asthma. Functional mapping has been upgraded to multivariate dimensions at which two or more than two dynamic traits can be mapped simultaneously to identify their underlying pleiotropic genetic control (Zhao et al. 2005b). Lin et al. (2006) used a bivariate functional mapping model to reveal how SBP and DBP respond differently to drugs.

Functional mapping has further been extended to map a composite trait that is derived from at least two individual traits (Sang et al. 2019b). Wang et al. (2019a) used this so-called composite functional mapping to characterize the genetic control of MAP and PP as two derivatives of SBP and DBP in response to change in drug dosage. In this section, we review a statistical procedure for mapping and identifying specific QTLs that govern MAP and PP curves and outline a number of clinically meaningful hypothesis tests used to address how a QTL determines the key events of PD and PK processes. We show how this composite model can be used to map pharmacological loci by analyzing a set of real data from dobutamine pharmacological studies.

3.4.2 Composite Functional Mapping

Clinical pharmacogenetic trial: A particular GWAS includes n patients who differ in age, race, sex, BMI, and other demographic factors, recruited from a human population. Consider a drug that is designed to improve BP, PP, and MAP. The drug is administered to each patient by a series of physiologically tolerable doses $(C_1, ..., C_T)$. Following each dosing, both SBP and DBP are monitored. Let $\mathbf{x}_{1i}=[x_{1i}(C_1), ..., x_{1i}(C_T)]$ and $\mathbf{x}_{2i}=[x_{2i}(C_1), ..., x_{2i}(C_T)]$ denote the vectors of measured SBP and DBP values for subject i, respectively. MAP $(\mathbf{y}_i)$ is approximated by one-third of SBP plus two-thirds of DBP at normal resting heart rates, whereas PP $(\mathbf{z}_i)$ of this subject is defined as the difference of DBP from SBP (Domanski et al. 1999). Then, we have

$$y_i = \left[x_{1i}(C_1) + 2x_{2i}(C_1), ..., x_{1i}(C_T) + 2x_{2i}(C_T) \right]/3 \qquad (3.8a)$$

$$\mathbf{z}_i = \left[x_{1i}(C_1) - x_{2i}(C_1), ..., x_{1i}(C_T) - x_{2i}(C_T) \right] \qquad (3.8b)$$

These two derived variables are used to map BP-QTLs. All the patients who participated in this study are genome-wide genotyped for thousands of thousands of SNPs, at each of which there are three different genotypes AA, Aa, and aa. Let n_2, n_1, and n_0 denote the observations of the three genotypes, respectively.

The drug-induced biochemical and distribution effects in the human body obey some basic kinetic rules that can be described by PD and PK equations. The Hill equation is one of the most commonly used PD models to illustrate and quantify drug dose-effect relationships (Giraldo 2003; Gesztelyi et al. 2012; Felmlee et al. 2012), shown in equation (3.1), where four parameters $(E_0, E_{max}, EC_{50}, \text{ and } H)$ describe the pattern of drug effect in response to dose change. In practice, we can remove the baseline effect to increase the precision of curve fitting by normalizing the longitudinal data.

Likelihood and estimation: To map BP-QTLs, we formulate the likelihood of derived variables (3.8a and b) at a given QTL as

$$L(\mathbf{y}, \mathbf{z}) = \prod_{i=1}^{n_2} f_2(\mathbf{y}_i, \mathbf{z}_i) \prod_{i=1}^{n_1} f_1(\mathbf{y}_i, \mathbf{z}_i) \prod_{i=1}^{n_0} f_0(\mathbf{y}_i, \mathbf{z}_i) \qquad (3.9)$$

where $f_j(\mathbf{y}_i, \mathbf{z}_i)$ is a bivariate longitudinal normal distribution for genotype j $(j=2$ for AA, 1 for Aa and 0 for $aa)$. This distribution has a form of

$$f_j(\mathbf{y}_i, \mathbf{z}_i) = \frac{1}{(2\pi)^T |\Sigma|^{\frac{1}{2}}} \exp\left[-\frac{1}{2}\left(\mathbf{y}_i - \boldsymbol{\mu}_{\hat{j}|i}^y\right)\Sigma^{-1}\left(\mathbf{z}_i - \boldsymbol{\mu}_{\hat{j}|i}^z\right)'\right] \quad (3.10)$$

which is specified by the vectors of genotypic means of MAP and PP for subject i who carries genotype j and covariance matrix. As derived variables of SBP and DBP, the mean vectors of MAP and PP can be modeled in terms of SBP and DBP that follow the Hill equations, i.e.,

$$\mu_{\hat{j}|i}^y(C_\tau) = \left\{ \frac{E_{maxj}^S C_\tau^{Hsj}}{3\left(EC_{50Sj}^{Hsj} + C_\tau^{Hsj}\right)} + \sum_{r=1}^{R}\alpha_r^S u_{ir}^S + \sum_{h=1}^{H}\sum_{l=1}^{L_h}\xi_{ihl}v_{hl}^S \right.$$

$$\left. + \frac{2E_{maxj}^D C_\tau^{HDj}}{3\left(EC_{50Dj}^{HDj} + C_\tau^{HDj}\right)} + \sum_{r=1}^{R}\alpha_r^D u_{ir}^D + \sum_{h=1}^{H}\sum_{l=1}^{L_h}\xi_{ihl}v_{hl}^D \right\}_{\tau=1} \quad (3.11a)$$

$$\mu_{\hat{j}|i}^z(C_\tau) = \left\{ \frac{E_{maxj}^S C_\tau^{Hsj}}{EC_{50Sj}^{Hsj} + C_\tau^{Hsj}} + \sum_{r=1}^{R}\alpha_r^S u_{ir}^S + \sum_{h=1}^{H}\sum_{l=1}^{L_h}\xi_{ihl}v_{hl}^S \right.$$

$$\left. - \frac{E_{maxj}^D C_\tau^{HDj}}{EC_{50Dj}^{HDj} + C_\tau^{HDj}} - \sum_{r=1}^{R}\alpha_r^D u_{ir}^D - \sum_{h=1}^{H}\sum_{l=1}^{L_h}\xi_{ihl}v_{hl}^D \right\}_{\tau=1} \quad (3.11b)$$

Equations (3.11a and b) include two parts: the first is the genotypic value specified by the Emax model and the second is the effect due to variate covariates. The Emax model is defined by the parameters $(E_{maxj}^S, E_{50Sj}, H_{Sj})$ for the SBP curve and $(E_{maxj}^D, E_{50Dj}, H_{Dj})$ for the DBP curve at genotype j. The covariate model specifies the effect of continuous and discrete covariates on SBP and DBP, respectively, including u_{ir} ($r=1, \ldots, R$), the value of the rth continuous covariate, such as age and BMI, for subject i; α_r, the effect of the rth continuous covariate; v_{sl} ($l=1, \ldots, L_s$, $s=1, \ldots, S$), the effect of the lth level for the sth discrete covariate, such as race, gender, and treatment, with $\sum_{i=1}^{L_s} v_{sl} = 0$, where L_s is the number of levels for the sth discrete covariate; and x_{isl} is an indicator variable of subject i who receives the lth level of the sth discrete covariate.

The longitudinal covariance matrix Σ_i of probability function (3.10) contains covariance matrices within and between two BP parameters. A variety of statistical approaches have been proposed to model the covariance structure. These approaches can be parametric, such as autoregressive, antedependent, autoregressive moving average, Brownian motion, and Ornstein-Uhlenbeck process, and also nonparametric, such as B-spline and Legendre orthogonal polynomials. A model-selection procedure is implemented to determine an optimal order of each approach and then the most parsimonious approach for covariance modeling (Zhao et al. 2005a; Yap et al. 2009; Li et al. 2010).

To obtain the MLEs of the unknown parameters in likelihood (3.9), a hybrid of the Nelder-Mead simplex and least squares methods can be implemented. The MLEs of the covariate effects are obtained by a least-square method, whereas the Emax parameters of three genotypes and covariance-structuring parameters are estimated by the simplex method.

Hypothesis tests: We provide a platform to test a number of hypotheses regarding the genetic control of how BP parameters respond to drug intervention. To test whether a significant QTL for BP exists, the following hypotheses are formulated:

$$H_0 : \left(E_{\text{max}j}^S, E_{50Sj}, H_{Sj} \right) = \left(E_{\text{max}}^S, E_{50S}, H_S \right) \text{ and } \left(E_{\text{max}j}^D, E_{50Dj}, H_{Dj} \right)$$

$$= \left(E_{\text{max}}^D, E_{50D}, H_D \right) \tag{3.12}$$

H_1: At leastoneof the equalities above does not hold

for any $j=2, 1, 0$. By calculating the log-likelihood ratio of the H_0 and H_1, we can claim whether or not a significant QTL has been detected. This can be done by comparing this ratio against the critical threshold determined by permutation tests.

Next, it is important to test how the QTL affects MAP and PP. This can be done by formulating the following null hypotheses:

$$H_0 : \frac{E_{\text{max}j}^S C_\tau^{Hsj}}{3\left(EC_{50Sj}^{Hsj} + C_\tau^{Hsj} \right)} + \frac{2E_{\text{max}j}^D C_\tau^{HDj}}{3\left(EC_{50Dj}^{HDj} + C_\tau^{HDj} \right)} \equiv \frac{E_{\text{max}}^S C_\tau^{Hs}}{3\left(EC_{50S}^{Hs} + C_\tau^{Hs} \right)} + \frac{2E_{\text{max}}^D C_\tau^{HD}}{3\left(EC_{50D}^{HD} + C_\tau^{HD} \right)} \tag{3.13}$$

$$H_0 : \frac{E_{\text{max}j}^S C_\tau^{Hsj}}{EC_{50Sj}^{Hsj} + C_\tau^{Hsj}} - \frac{E_{\text{max}j}^D C_\tau^{HDj}}{EC_{50Dj}^{HDj} + C_\tau^{HDj}} \equiv \frac{E_{\text{max}}^S C_\tau^{Hs}}{EC_{50S}^{Hs} + C_\tau^{Hs}} - \frac{E_{\text{max}}^D C_\tau^{HD}}{EC_{50D}^{HD} + C_\tau^{HD}} \tag{3.14}$$

If both null hypotheses (3.13) and (3.14) are rejected, this means that this QTL pleiotropically determine MAP and PP. Otherwise, this QTL may be specific for one of the two traits.

We can also test how the QTL governs DBP and SBP. These tests can be based on the comparison of Hill coefficients among genotypes. Specifically, we have

$$H_0 : \left(E_{\text{max}j}^S, E_{50Sj}, H_{Sj} \right) = \left(E_{\text{max}}^S, E_{50S}, H_S \right) \tag{3.15}$$

$$\left(E_{\text{max}j}^D, E_{50Dj}, H_{Dj} \right) = \left(E_{\text{max}}^D, E_{50D}, H_D \right) \tag{3.16}$$

If both null hypotheses (3.15) and (3.16) are rejected, this implies that the QTL is pleiotropic, triggering an effect on both DBP and SBP. Otherwise, it only affects one of the two BP parameters.

We can systematically characterize the genetic control of drug response as a dynamic process through BP parameters and their physiologically meaningful derived variables MAP and PP. The additional advantages of this model lie in its capacity to detect the genetic basis of key events that play a central role in the outcome of drug efficacy. Based on the Emax model (3.1), this model can test how the QTL determines maximum drug effect (E_{max}), the dose at which the drug effect achieves half of its maximal value (EC_{50}), the slope of drug response curve (H), and the dose at which drug-response change-rate is maximal (C_I), expressed as

$$C_I = \left[\frac{(H-1)EC_{50}^H}{H+1} \right]^{\frac{1}{H}}$$

We may be interested in testing genetic differences at any dose estimate, EC_p, which is the dose generating p-percentile of E_{max}, as an estimate of the maximal effective dose. For example, EC_{90} is of interest in dose–response analysis. EC_p is calculated as

$$EC_p = EC_{50} \left(\frac{p}{1-p} \right)^{\frac{1}{H}}$$

All these tests can be established on both DBP and SBP parameters.

3.4.3 Identification of Pleiotropic Pharmacogenes

We demonstrate the use of composite functional mapping by analyzing real data from Lin et al. (2005a,b) pharmacogenetic association study. By plotting all subjects' SBP and DBP values against different doses of dobutamine, we find different patterns of change between these two BP measures. In general, SBP increased with dose (Figure 3.5a), whereas DBP decreased with dose (Figure 3.5b). The average curves of both SBP and DBP can be fitted by the Hill equation (Adjusted $R^2 > 0.098$). By incorporating the Hill equation into equation (3.11a and b), we estimate the average curves of MAP (Figure 3.5c) and PP (Figure 3.5d). Both MAP and PP increase with dose, while the PP dose-related increase is expected given the dose-dependent SBP augmentation and DBP reduction. PP has a much greater rate of change than MAP. By comparing SBP, DBP, MAP, and PP, we find that the patterns by which these four types of BP measures respond to dobutamine are different. Also, dramatic differences

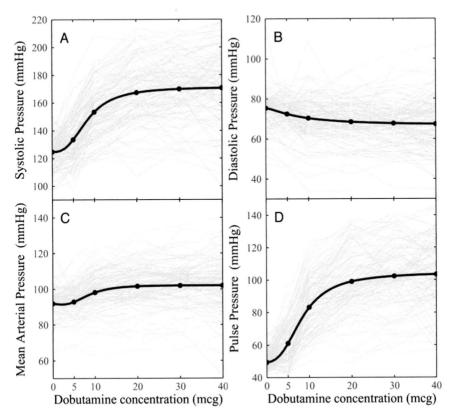

FIGURE 3.5
Response curves for systolic (SBP) (a) and DBP (b) to dobutamine in a pharmacogenomic study composed of 107 patients. From SBP and DBP, we obtained the curves of MAP (c) and PP (d). Thin green lines are response curves of individual subjects, and thick black lines are the mean curves fitted by the Hill equation. Dots are the doses of dobutamine at which SBP and SBP were measured.

noted among subjects in each type of BP parameters may imply the existence of genetic variants that affect specific inter-individual drug response.

Previous mapping studies with these data suggest that haplotype variants are a better determinant of pharmacological response to dobutamine than individual SNPs (Davidson 2000). As such, we incorporate the haplotype model into the likelihood (3.9). Consider a pair of SNPs with alleles A versus a, and B versus b, respectively, which form four possible haplotypes AB, Ab, aB, and ab. The haplotype model states that difference among these haplotypes is one important cause of the phenotypic variation of a complex trait (Liu et al. 2004). We use a risk haplotype to define a haplotype that is different from the remaining haplotypes. If AB is a risk haplotype and $\overline{AB}$ is the collective set of all remaining haplotypes, we can expect that diplotypes $AB|AB$, $AB|\overline{AB}$, and $\overline{AB}|\overline{AB}$ perform differently. It is possible to distinguish $AB|AB$, $\overline{AB}|\overline{AB}$, and $AB|\overline{AB}$ directly from all genotypes, except for the double heterozygote $AaBb$. If an individual carries $AaBb$, it is difficult to determine whether he/she is diplotype $AB|ab$ or diplotype $Ab|aB$. Lin et al. (2005a,b) implemented the EM algorithm to distinguish these two diplotypes so that their effect on drug response can be estimated. By assuming each haplotype as a risk haplotype, we estimated the likelihood value from (3.9). The optimal risk haplotype can be inferred from Akaike *information criterion* (AIC).

By testing each pair of SNPs from the same gene, the haplotype model identified a significant risk haplotype AC within the $\beta_1 AR$ gene for BP parameters in response to dobutamine (Figure 3.6). This haplotype affects MAP and PP in two fashions. First, diplotypes $(AC|AC, AC|\overline{AC})$ that contain at least one copy of the risk haplotype are dramatically different from the haplotypes $(\overline{AC}|\overline{AC})$, which do not contain the risk haplotype ($P<0.01$; Figure 3.6a and b). Second, and yet more interestingly, diplotype $(AC|AC)$

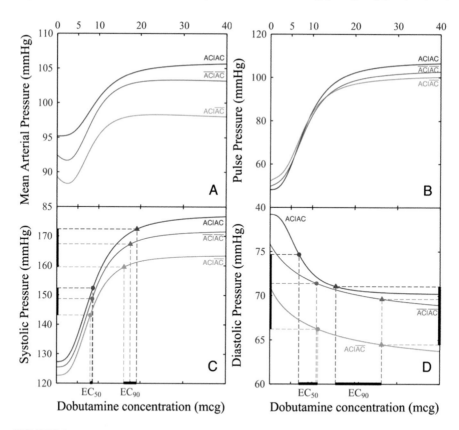

FIGURE 3.6
Genetic curves of MAP (a) and BP (b) in terms of three diplotypes $AC|AC$, $AC|\overline{AC}$, and $\overline{AC}|\overline{AC}$ between two SNPs within the $\beta_1 AR$ gene, estimated from the likelihood (2). The estimated Hill coefficients were used to draw SBP (a) and DBP curves (b) for each diplotype. The doses at which drug response reaches half of the maximum effect (EC_{50}, solid circles) and 90% of maximum effect (EC_{90}, solid triangles) are indicated.

with two copies of the risk haplotype differs at an even higher significance level ($P<0.001$) from diplotype ($AC|\overline{AC}$) with one copy of the risk haplotype. These results indicate that risk haplotype AC mediates MAP and PP not only through its existence but also through its frequency and interaction with non-risk haplotypes. Over the whole dobutamine-dose levels considered, diplotype $AC|AC$ correlates consistently with a larger MAP value than the other two diplotypes, whereas the diplotype $\overline{AC}|\overline{AC}$ correlates consistently with a larger MAP than $AC|\overline{AC}$. This suggests that the risk haplotype AC, by its interaction effect with the other haplotypes, can reduce MAP more effectively than the dobutamine dose can increase it (Figure 3.6a).

Compared with MAP, PP is found to be more sensitive to dobutamine (Figure 3.6b). Starting at a lower BP increment level (about 50 mmHg), among three diplotypes, $AC|AC$ reaches the largest PP (>100 mmHg) increment at a medium to high dose of dobutamine due to its highest slope of PP response to dobutamine. Among three diplotypes, diplotype $AC|\overline{AC}$ has the lowest slope, suggesting that the interaction between risk haplotype AC and any of the other haplotypes can inhibit the response of PP to dobutamine. Using the diplotype-dependent estimates of Hill coefficients under the likelihood function (3.9), we draw the curves of SBP and DBP (Figure 3.6c and d) from which we find that, among three diplotypes, diplotype $AC|AC$ exhibits the highest SBP and DBP over the entire range of dobutamine doses. Diplotype $AC|\overline{AC}$ has the lowest SBP and DBP, again suggesting the interaction between the risk haplotype AC and the other haplotypes as a critical determinant of BP parameters.

We further dissect the pattern of how the risk haplotype mediates BP. Three diplotypes start from slightly different baselines of SBP and display small differences in the dose reaching a half of maximum drug effect (EC_{50}), but they diverge dramatically in the persistence to response to dobutamine (Figure 3.6c). In spite of a smaller slope ($H=2.77$), $AC|AC$ reaches 90% of maximum drug effect at a much larger dose (EC_{90}), compared to diplotypes $\overline{AC}|\overline{AC}$ ($H=3.02$) and $AC|\overline{AC}$ ($H=3.17$). Unlike SBP, DBP exhibits remarkable differences among three diplotypes over an entire range of dobutamine doses (Figure 3.6d). Starting from a larger DBP baseline, diplotype $AC|AC$ is more responsive to dobutamine, at a greater steepness ($H=2.69$), than diplotypes $\overline{AC}|\overline{AC}$ ($H=0.98$) and $AC|\overline{AC}$ ($H=0.89$). The three diplotypes strikingly differ in the dose reaching a half of the maximum drug effect, whereas the difference in the dose at 90% of maximum drug effect is even more pronounced.

3.5 Concluding Remarks

How drugs exert their effects presents a multiscale strategy of drug-body interactions over time, space, and signals. As such, genetic mapping of drug response can be better conducted by multiscale modeling that links PK and PD information with evolutionary, physiological, and biochemic features to better establish and asses dose-concentration-response relationships. In this chapter, we focus on two dimensions of multiscale modeling–timing and multifaceted embodiments of pharmacological reactions, and their impacts on pharmacogenetic research.

Timing is everything in drug response because gene expression in its metabolic pathways needs to be well-timed to be effective. For example, drug efficacy and drug toxicity and their balance critically depend on the circadian rhythm of the body (Dallmann et al. 2016; Zhang et al. 2014, 2017), controlled by an inherent molecular clock network (Panda 2016; Kuhlman et al. 2017). Chronotherapy is a therapeutic strategy that capitalizes on the rhythmic change of the body to choose an optimal time for drug administration so that drug efficacy can be maximized and drug toxicity minimized (da Silva et al. 2016). As a potential clinical strategy, the application of chronotherapy critically relies on a profound genetic understanding of how circadian rhythms covary with drug response. The mechanistic basis of chronotherapy is established by chronopharmacokinetics and chronopharmacodynamics (Zhang et al. 2014). The implication of chronotherapy can be strengthened by integrating it with heterochrony, an evolutionary concept that defines how the timing or rate of developmental events determines the overall shape of developmental trajectories.

HcPD has been specifically proposed to study the timing and drug concentration window that determine the outcome of drug response. Functional mapping is combined with HcPD to address fundamental questions regarding the genetic mechanisms of pharmacological processes guided by evolutionary theory. This quantitative combination can provide guidance on tailoring drug treatment for individual patients by answering when these patients are more responsive to drugs and which dose window critically affect their pharmacological outcome. HcPD-based functional mapping can help pharmacologists not only determine an optimal dose of drugs for different patients based on their genetic blueprints, but also administer phase-dependent doses (i.e., a higher level used for exponential phase but a lower level used for lag and stationary phases) for the same patient.

A single criterion to evaluate drug response is obviously not sufficient for many reasons. First, drug response is the consequence of pharmacologically induced interactions among multiple physiological and biochemical factors, each under different control. Thus, it is sorely needed to characterize how genes mediate the strength and structure of such interactions in pharmacogenetic studies. Second, a drug may simultaneously cause multiple responses of the body, and it is such simultaneous responses that affect the balance between drug efficacy and drug toxicity. Third, much of variation in drug response can be attributed to cellular heterogeneity, i.e., distinct cell types and proportions, which can be measured by multi-omics variables. This chapter introduces the extension of functional mapping of drug response by taking into account its multifaceted features and illustrates the application of the extended model to study the genetics of blood pressure in response to a drug, aimed to gain useful information for personalized hypertension treatment.

Comorbidity risk due to hypertension is not only determined by absolute SBP and DBP values, but also the difference of SBP from DBP (i.e., PP or BP, reflecting arterial stiffness) and two thirds of DBP plus one third of SBP (i.e., MAP, reflecting left ventricular contractility and heart rate) (Padmanabhan and Joe 2017; Vennin et al. 2017). The use of drug intervention simultaneously designed for these four parameters can best prevent and treat cardiovascular disease, thereby improving quality of life and prolonging life expectancy. Composite functional mapping described is powerful for identifying, visualizing, and quantifying the genetic architecture of PP- and MAP-related drug responses. This framework can map individual QTLs for the pharmacological response of PP and MAP and also test whether and how PP and MAP are governed jointly by the same set of QTLs. Results from this testing are important for stratifying patients and tailoring theory therapy based on how the patients respond to PP and MAP treatments. This framework can also ask and answer a number of clinically meaningful hypotheses regarding pharmacological reactions and metabolism. It can identify and quantify how some key events of drug response affect drug-effect outcome.

4

Pharmacogenetic Mapping of Missing Longitudinal Data

4.1 Introduction

In pharmacogenomic studies, phenotypic data of interest to clinical practice are often longitudinal, where subjects are measured for drug response repeatedly throughout a period of time and/or a series of doses (Hogan and Laird 1997; Fitzmaurice and Laird 2000; McInnes and Altman 2021). However, it may occur that some subjects withdraw or remove from an assigned treatment due to physiological or other unavoidable reasons. In certain research areas, the proportion of dropouts is extremely high, e.g., as large as 70% (Follmann and Wu 1995). Based on whether there are missing data and how data are missing, all the subjects studied can be sorted into three categories (Figure 4.1): (1) the subjects who complete measurements of outcome responses from the first to intended completion time point, (2) the subjects whose responses are missing at one time but are then measured at a subsequent time(s), leading to the sparse structure of data for these subjects, and (3) the subjects who drop out from the study before the planned completion time, thus having an incomplete response (Daniels and Hogan 2008).

Functional mapping was originally proposed to map and identify genes that control dose-response curves with the data composed of the first category of subjects (Ma et al. 2002; Wu et al. 2004c; Wu and Lin 2006). Functional mapping can be readily modified to consider the second category of subjects measured with unevenly spaced time intervals (Hou et al. 2005, 2006) because the probability of the dropouts of these subjects does not depend on the unobserved response (ignorable dropout). The reasons for the dropouts of the third category of subjects include lack of efficacy, adverse effect, or death and, thus, their dropouts may be related to observed and unobserved outcomes. Functional mapping should incorporate these so-called non-ignorable or informative dropouts into the analysis, in order to draw a precise picture of the genetic architecture of longitudinal responses (Li and Wu 2012; Wang et al. 2013c).

Subject	SNP				Drug-Effect Parameter									
	1	2	...	m	t_1	t_2	t_3	t_4	t_5	t_6	t_7	t_8	t_9	t_{10}
1	AA	BB	...	MM	x	x	x	-	-	-	-	-	-	-
2	AA	Bb	...	MM	x	x	x	x	x	x	x	-	-	-
3	AA	bb	...	mm	x	x	x	x	x	-	-	-	-	-
4	Aa	BB	...	mm	x	x	x	x	x	x	x	x	-	-
5	Aa	Bb	...	Mm	x	x	x	x	x	x	x	-	-	-
6	Aa	bb	...	mm	x	x	x	x	x	x	-	-	-	-
7	aa	BB	...	Mm	x	x	-	-	-	-	-	-	-	-
8	aa	Bb	...	MM	x	x	x	x	x	-	-	-	-	-
9	aa	bb	...	Mm	x	x	x	x	x	x	x	x	x	x
10	aa	Bb	...	mm	x	x	x	x	x	x	x	x	x	x
Projected					x	x	x	x	x	x	x	x	x	x

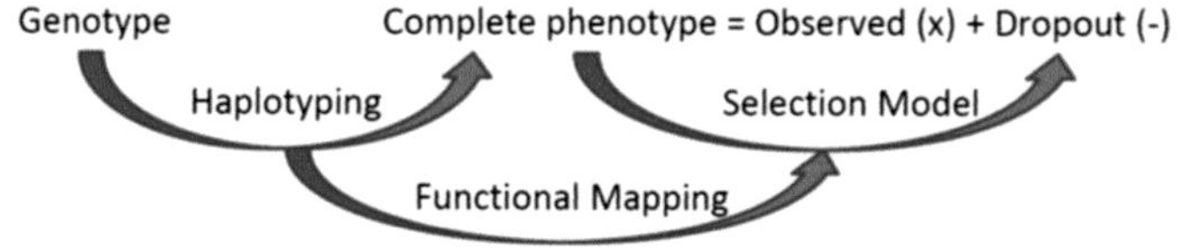

Genotype   Complete phenotype = Observed (x) + Dropout (-)

Haplotyping   Selection Model

Functional Mapping

FIGURE 4.1
Diagram of data structure in a pharmacogenetic association study, including marker data and longitudinal drug response data subject to dropout.

One strategy for handling non-ignorable dropouts is to model the joint distribution of the longitudinal process and the dropout process. Depending on how to factorize this joint distribution, modeling informative dropouts can be done in two ways (Hogan and Laird 1997; Little 1993, 1995; Wulfsohn and Tsiatis 1997). In the first way, we assume the occurrence of a pattern-dependent mechanism (pattern-mixture model), in which the distribution of longitudinal measures is a mixture of distributions for subjects within distinct sub-groups determined by the pattern of dropouts. In the second way, we assume that dropouts are outcome-dependent (selection model), in which the distribution of dropout indicators is conditioned on the values of longitudinal measures. Because of different assumptions use, both the pattern-mixture and the selection models should be implemented into functional mapping, allowing for choosing a better model fitted to a specific dataset so as to more effectively characterize the missing-data mechanisms of non-ignorable dropouts.

The purposes of this chapter are to review the fundamental statistical concepts and approaches for analyzing longitudinal data with non-ignorable dropouts and modify functional mapping based on pattern-mixture and selection models. We incorporate the principles of pattern-mixture and selection models to estimate and test the genetic effects of haplotypes on longitudinal responses subject to non-ignorable dropouts. For a detailed description of deriving functional mapping implemented with these two types of models, please refer to Li and Wu (2012) and Wang et al. (2013c), respectively.

4.2 Strategies for Modeling Non-Ignorable Dropout Data

4.2.1 The Factorization of Joint Distribution

From a statistical perspective, Little and Rubin (1987) defined data missing in a hierarchical manner: (1) missing completely at random (MCAR): the probability of non-response depends on neither observed nor unobserved longitudinal outcomes, (2) missing at random (MAR): non-response depends on the observed part but not on the unobserved part of the longitudinal responses, and (3) informative dropout (or non-ignorable non-response): the probability of dropout depends on the unobserved part of the longitudinal response. Under the MCAR, dropouts are randomly missing values, and, thereby, their analysis only needs to consider the observed data. As shown in Laird (2006), under the MAR, likelihood-based statistical inferences about the measurement process can ignore the dropout process. However, ignoring the informative dropout process will potentially result in biases in inferences about the measurement process. There has been a considerable body of literature available to model and analyze non-ignorable dropouts (Hogan and Laird 1997; Fitzmaurice and Laird 2000; Wu and Bailey 1989; Little 1993, 1995; Yu et al. 2004; Hsieh et al. 2006).

Let $\mathbf{y}_i$ denote the longitudinal measurements that have been taken in clinical pharmacogenetic studies, θ_0 denote the missing measurement, and D_i denote the failure time for subject i ($i=1, \ldots, N$), respectively. Then, under MCAR, missing at a random mechanism, and the informative dropout, the distribution of dropouts is expressed, respectively, as

$$f\left(D_i | \mathbf{y}_i, \mathbf{y}_i^m\right) = f\left(D_i\right) \tag{4.1a}$$

$$f\left(D_i | \mathbf{y}_i, \mathbf{y}_i^m\right) = f\left(D_i | \mathbf{y}_i\right) \tag{4.1b}$$

$$f\left(\mathbf{y}_i, D_i\right) = \int f\left(\mathbf{y}_i, \mathbf{y}_i^m\right) f\left(D_i | \mathbf{y}_i, \mathbf{y}_i^m\right) d\mathbf{y}_i^m \tag{4.1c}$$

It is straightforward to apply statistical methods for analyzing the first two types of dropouts. Yet, to handle the longitudinal data with non-ignorable dropouts, statistical inference by jointly modeling the longitudinal process and the dropout process is needed (Hogan and Laird 1997). Let ψ denote the parameter sets characterizing the joint distribution of $\mathbf{y}_i$ and D_i. By conditioning D_i on $\mathbf{y}_i$, the *selection model* specifies the joint density function as

$$f(\mathbf{y}_i, D_i; \Psi) = f(\mathbf{y}_i; \Psi_{\mathbf{y}}) f(D_i \mid \mathbf{y}_i; \Psi_{D\mid\mathbf{y}}) \tag{4.2}$$

whereas, by conditioning $\mathbf{y}_i$ upon D_i, the joint density function in a *mixture model* is expressed as

$$f(\mathbf{y}_i, D_i; \Psi) = f(D_i; \Psi_D) f(\mathbf{y}_i \mid D_i; \Psi_{\mathbf{y}\mid D}) \tag{4.3}$$

where $\psi_{\mathbf{y}}$ and ψ_D are the parameters that characterize the marginal distributions of $\mathbf{y}_i$ and D_i, respectively; and $\psi_{\mathbf{y}\mid D}$ and $\psi_{D\mid\mathbf{y}}$ are the parameters that characterize the conditional distribution of $\mathbf{y}_i$ given D_i and the conditional distribution of D_i given $\mathbf{y}_i$, respectively!

Generally speaking, the selection model can be appropriate for both survival and longitudinal settings, whereas the mixture model is mainly used in longitudinal studies. Both selection and mixture models are attractive because of their robustness in modeling the dropout process. Both models have such drawbacks as sensitivity to parametric assumptions and computational complexity. The selection model needs distribution assumptions for the dropout process, whereas the mixture model often needs simplifying assumptions to ensure the identifiability of parameters.

4.2.2 The Selection Model

From a view of longitudinal studies with informative dropouts, the primary appeal of the selection model is that it directly models the marginal distribution of $\mathbf{y}_i$, from which inference about longitudinal trends is made. The selection model approximates the dropout process as a function of $\mathbf{y}_i$, which may be used to characterize the missing data mechanism. The selection model is also useful in characterizing the relationship between a longitudinally measured surrogate marker and an event process. However, it does not seem well suited to estimating the unconditional distribution of the dropout process.

The selection model allows the failure time distribution to depend directly on elements of $\mathbf{y}_i$, which is the outcome-dependent selection model, or on $\mathbf{y}_i$ through individual random effects used to describe its distribution, which is the random effects–dependent selection model. In some cases, the dropout can also depend on some covariates that describe the longitudinal process. The outcome-dependent selection model is suited to situations with a fixed discrete set of measurement time $(t_{i1},\ldots,t_{iT_i})$ for $\mathbf{y}_i$ ($i=1$, ..., N) in which dropout depends on the most recent missing outcome or both observed and missing outcomes. In an outcome-dependent selection model proposed by Diggle and Kenward (1994), the probability of dropout at time t_r is a function of both longitudinal outcome history prior to t_r and the unobserved $y_i(t_r)$. Longitudinal outcomes follow a multivariate normal distribution $\mathbf{y}_i \sim N(W_i\beta, \mathbf{\Sigma})$ and dropout probability is modeled with a logistic regression, expressed as

$$\text{logit}\left[\text{pr}\left\{D = t_\tau \mid D \geq t_\tau, H_i(t_\tau), y_i(t_\tau), V_i\right\}\right] = \phi_0 + \phi_1' H_i(t_\tau) + \phi_2 y_i(t_\tau) + \phi_3' Z_i \quad (4.4)$$

where $\psi_y = (\beta, \mathbf{\Sigma})$ and $\psi_{D|y} = (\phi_0, \phi_1', \phi_2', \phi_3')$; $H_i(t_\tau) = (y_i(t_1) \ldots, y_i(t_{\tau-1}))$; Z_i and W_i contain other covariates which may be mutually exclusive, overlapping, or identical. In this formulation, if $\phi_2 \neq 0$, the dropout depends on $y_i(t_r)$ so that the missing is non-ignorable. If $\phi_2 = 0$, the dropout only depends on observed responses so the missing is MAR; if $\phi_1 = \phi_2 = 0$, the missing mechanism is MCAR since $\mathbf{y}_i$ and D_i are independent. But fitting this model is computationally intensive and there is no explicit algorithm for it. Note that this formulation only accommodates a monotone dropout and the measurement times are a fixed set for all subjects.

In some cases, dropouts may be more directly related to a longitudinal trend. For example, patients are typically removed from the study if the treatment has no effect or a severe adverse effect over a fixed period of time. These situations imply that the dropout process depends on an underlying disease progression related to $\mathbf{y}_i$, rather than on actual outcomes. Here, we should use the random effects dependent selection model that allows the event time distribution and longitudinal data to depend on a common set of latent random effects. In this case, $\mathbf{y}_i$ is viewed as a continuous process, which has values at any time.

The linear mixed effects model for longitudinal measurements is attractive in this situation since it does not require $\mathbf{y}_i$ to be observed at the same set of occasions or to have the same dimension. The model is formulated as

$$\mathbf{y}_i \mid \theta_i = \mathbf{X}_i \beta + \mathbf{Z}_i \theta_i + \mathbf{e}_i \quad (4.5)$$

and

$$f(D_i \mid \mathbf{y}_i, \theta_i; \Psi_{D|y}) = f(D_i \mid \theta_i; \Psi_{D|y}) \quad (4.6)$$

where $\mathbf{X}_i$ is the design matrix of fixed effects β; $\mathbf{Z}_i$ is the design matrix of random effects θ_i;

$$\mathbf{Z}_i = \begin{bmatrix} 1 & t_{i1} \\ \vdots & \vdots \\ 1 & t_{iT_i} \end{bmatrix}$$

$\mathbf{e}_i$ is the measurement error and independent of θ_i, $e_i(t) \sim N(0, \sigma^2)$ $(t = t_{i1}, \ldots, t_{iT_i})$ and $\theta_i \sim N(0, V)$. In a simple case where $\mathbf{y}_i$ follows a linear time trend, $\theta_i = (\theta_{0i}, \theta_{1i})'$ represents an individual's random intercept and slope.

In this model, we have

$$f\left(\theta_i \mid \mathbf{y}_i, \mathbf{y}_i^m\right) = \int_{\theta_i} f(D_i \mid \theta_i, \mathbf{y}_i, \mathbf{y}_i^m) f\left(\theta_i \mid \mathbf{y}_i, \mathbf{y}_i^m\right) d\theta_i$$

$$= \int_{\theta_i} f(D_i \mid \theta_i) f\left(\theta_i \mid \mathbf{y}_i, \mathbf{y}_i^m\right) d\theta_i$$

(4.7)

which depends on $\mathbf{y}_i^m$ since $f\left(\theta_i \mid \mathbf{y}_i, \mathbf{y}_i^m\right)$ depends on $\mathbf{y}_i^m$ in general. Based on the previous definition, this implies that the dropout process is non-ignorable.

Wu and Carroll (1988) first proposed a random effects model for longitudinal data in the presence of informative censoring, in which the individual random effects include intercepts and slopes and dropouts only occur at discrete time points where the probability of dropouts is modeled using a probit regression on random effects. Wulfsohn and Tsiatis (1997) proposed such a random effect–dependent selection model:

$$y_i(t_{i\tau}) = \theta_{0i} + \theta_{1i}\, t_{i\tau} + e_i(t_{i\tau})$$

(4.8)

where $\theta_{\tau i} = (\theta_{0i}, \theta_{1i})'$ is the random effects vector, distributed as $N(\theta, V)$ and $e_i(t_{i\tau}) \sim N(0, \sigma^2)$ is the measurement error. θ_i and $e_i(t_{i\tau})$ are independent. The Cox model was used to model the dropout process where the hazard of dropouts depends on the longitudinal data through its current unobserved true value:

$$\lambda(t \mid \theta_i, \mathbf{y}_i, t_{i\tau}) = \lambda(t \mid \theta_i) = \lambda_0(t)\exp\{\beta(\theta_{0i} + \theta_{1i}t_{i\tau})\}$$

(4.9)

The parameter β quantifies the relationship between failure time and longitudinal covariates. Henderson et al. (2000) extended Wulfsohn and Tsiatis' (1997) model by assuming that the measurement and event processes are conditionally independent if both are conditional on a latent bivariate Gaussian process. DeGruttola and Tu (1994) modeled the random effects and failure time as a multivariate normal distribution. Follman and Wu (1995) extended the linear mixed model for longitudinal data to generalized linear mixed effects model.

4.2.3 The Pattern-Mixture Model

In formulating the pattern-mixture model, the conditional distribution of longitudinal data given failure time and the marginal distribution of the failure time is modeled. The goal of such modeling is that we can adjust the inference about the joint density function for the effects of outcome-related dropouts. According to different situations, dropout time D_i may be considered a qualitative or quantitative covariate for the longitudinal measures.

Little (1995) proposes a pattern-mixture model where for each potential dropout outcome, there is a different pattern for $\mathbf{y}_i$. So, D_i here is a qualitative covariate. The author assumes that $\mathbf{y}_i$ follows a multivariate normal distribution conditional on dropout time D_i. If all potential dropout time is $\mathbf{t}_i=(t_{i1}, \ldots, t_{iT_i})$, dropout time follows a multinomial distribution and $\mathbf{y}_i|(D_i=t_{it}) \sim N(\mu_{it}, \Sigma_{it})$. This model needs some simplifying assumptions to ensure the identifiability of parameters. The random effects mixture model considers the dropout a random effect for the longitudinal process. In a random effects mixture model proposed by Pawitan and Self (1993), the failure time process is treated as a Weibull distribution. Guo et al. (2004) proposed a random pattern-mixture model by generalizing the definition of the pattern. Their pattern is defined according to a good surrogate for the dropout process. For example, the pattern can be defined according to a baseline or time-varying covariate, or time to dropout as the original. They treated the pattern-specific parameters as nuisance parameters and modeled them as random. A constraint is then imposed on the pattern by linking it to the time to dropout using a random-effects survival model (Clayton and Cuzick 1985).

4.3 Haplotyping Drug Response Using the Pattern-Mixture Model

4.3.1 Pharmacogenetic Dropout Example

To better describe our problem, we start with a pharmacogenetic study (Lin et al. 2015a, b, 2007). This study included 163 subjects, measured for heart rate repeatedly after the treatment of dobutamine (Figure 4.2). The patients received increasing doses of dobutamine until they achieved a target heart rate response or a predetermined maximum dose. Of these subjects studied, 112 (69%) completed the tests of heart rate at all the six dose levels; the others dropped out before the completion of the trial because heart rates at any higher dose level were beyond their physiological limits. A total of 31 (19%), 15 (9%), and 5 (3%) subjects dropped out after receiving four, three, and two injections, respectively. Because the dropouts of these subjects were likely related to the outcome, they are called non-ignorable dropouts. Under MCAR, functional mapping can be readily implemented to map the genetic architecture of dobutamine response with such sparse data. Here, we explore whether mapping power can increase if we treat missing data as informative dropouts. In this section, we analyze this data using functional mapping implemented pattern-mixture models.

Haplotype diversity has been thought to be associated with drug response (Saito et al. 2007; McInnes et al. 2020). To map haplotypes (linear combinations of alleles at different loci located in a similar genomic region) mediate

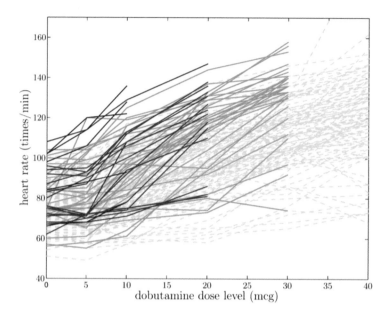

FIGURE 4.2
The dobutamine drug response experiment data. The curves in dashed lines are the complete responses covering all dose levels, whereas the curves in solid lines are the incomplete responses showing non-ignorable dropouts from different dosages.

dobutamine response, we consider two sets of SNP pairs, i.e., codon49 with two alleles Ser49 (A) and Gly49 (G) and codon389 with two alleles Arg389 (C) and Gly389 (G) within the $\beta_1 AR$ gene on chromosome 10, as well as codon16 with two alleles Arg16 (A) and Gly16 (G) and codon27 with two alleles Gln27 (C) and Glu27 (G) within the $\beta_2 AR$ gene on chromosome 5. Without loss of generality, we consider two SNPs, **A** (with alleles A and a) and **B** (with alleles B and b). The capital and small alleles are symbolized as 1 and 0, respectively. The two SNPs considered produce four haplotypes AB, Ab, aB, and ab, whose frequencies are expressed as p_{11}, p_{10}, p_{01}, and p_{00}, respectively. In the population, a total of ten diplotypes, $AB|AB$, $AB|Ab$, $AB|aB$, $AB|ab$, $Ab|Ab$, $Ab|aB$, $Ab|ab$, $aB|ab$, and $ab|ab$, are formed by randomly uniting maternally- and paternally derived haplotypes.

In most practical association studies, we can only observe genotypes (i.e., a combination between alleles at individual SNPs). For the double heterozygote $AaBb$, it has two possible diplotypes $AB|ab$ and $Ab|aB$ that are not directly observable. If a specific haplotype or diplotype impacts on drug response, we need to develop a mixture model for inferencing this effect based on observed genotype data. As can be seen, genotypes $AABB$, $AABb$, $AAbb$, $AaBB$, $Aabb$, $aaBB$, $aaBb$, and $aabb$ are consistent with their diplotypes, whereas genotype $AaBb$ is not. We formulate a multinomial distribution of nine possible genotypes in which the probabilities of diplotype-consistent genotypes are expressed as the product of the frequencies of the two underlying haplotypes for a Hardy-Weinberg equilibrium (HWE) population and the probability of the diplotype-inconsistent genotype is a mixture of two diplotype frequencies (Liu et al. 2004). The EM algorithm is implemented to obtain the maximum likelihood estimates (MLEs) of unknown haplotype frequencies $\hat{\Omega}_p = (\hat{p}_{11}, \hat{p}_{10}, \hat{p}_{01}, \hat{p}_{00})$, which are used to formulate the likelihood of drug response phenotypes in terms of haplotype effects (Liu et al. 2004).

4.3.2 Functional Mapping with Non-Ignorable Dropouts

Pattern-mixture models analyze non-ignorable dropout data by constructing a likelihood on the joint distribution of the complete response and dropout mechanism and factoring the joint likelihood as the marginal distribution of the mechanism multiplied by the conditional distribution of the response given the mechanism (Wu and Bailey 1989; Little 1993, 1995). Pattern-mixture models have now been used in many applications for which longitudinal non-ignorable missing data are common (Fitzmaurice and Laird 2000; Hogan and Laird 1997). We integrate pattern-mixture models within the framework of functional mapping through explicit modeling of the missing data distribution by first identifying different patterns of missing data and then including parameters in the outcomes model that capture these patterns.

Li and Wu (2012) derived a procedure for incorporating the pattern-mixture model into functional mapping. Let $\mathbf{y}_i = (C_{i1}, \ldots, C_{iT_i})$ denote the vector of heart rates for subject i measured at different subject-specific dose levels. Let D_i denote the pre-specified dose at which subject i drops out based on this subject's physiological limit. Given its uncertainty, the maximum dose (C_i) this subject can tolerate is right censored relative to his/her dropout dose (D_i). The indicator of censoring is denoted by $\Delta_i = I(D_i < C_i)$, which is zero if D_i is censored and one otherwise. The observed dropout dose is expressed as $\tilde{D}_i = \min(D_i, C_i)$, where $\tilde{D}_i$ has possible values from $S = \{s_1, \ldots, s_L\}$.

For two adjacent SNPs, four haplotypes AB, Ab, aB, and ab form nine observable genotypes, where the double heterozygote $AaBb$ has two diplotypes $AB|ab$ and $Ab|aB$. We want to characterize which haplotype, i.e., risk haplotype, exerts an effect on drug response. This risk haplotype combines with the other three (non-risk) haplotypes to form three composite diplotypes (Liu et al. 2004; Lin et al. 2005a, b). Let Q_i denote the composite diplotype of subject i ($Q_i = 2$ for the homozygote composite diplotype composed of two risk haplotypes, 1 for the heterozygote composite diplotype composed of a risk haplotype and a non-risk haplotype, and 0 for the homozygote composite diplotype composed of two non-risk haplotypes).

We construct a mixture-based likelihood for heart rate data and genotypic data because the double heterozygote genotype contains two indistinguishable diplotypes (whose frequencies are differently determined by $2\hat{p}_{11}\hat{p}_{00}$ and $2\hat{p}_{10}\hat{p}_{01}$, respectively). A general form of this likelihood (assuming that there is censoring in dropout time) is written as

$$L_c\left(\Omega_q\right) = \prod_{i=1}^{N}\prod_{l=1}^{L}\sum_{j=0}^{2} f\left(\mathbf{y}_i \mid D_i = s_l, Q_i = j\right) f\left(D_i = s_l \mid Q_i = j\right) f\left(Q_i = j\right) \quad (4.10)$$

where Ω_q is the quantitative genetic parameters that fit the multivariate normal distribution $f\left(\mathbf{y}_i \mid D_i = s_l, Q_i = j\right)$ of subject i with composite diplotype j dropping out at s_l, expressed as

$$f\left(\mathbf{y}_i \mid D_i = s_l, Q_i = j\right) = (2\pi)^{-\frac{T_i}{2}} |\Sigma_i|^{-\frac{1}{2}} \exp\left\{-\frac{1}{2}\left(\mathbf{y}_i - \boldsymbol{\mu}_{j|il}\right)\Sigma_i^{-1}\left(\mathbf{y}_i - \boldsymbol{\mu}_{j|il}\right)'\right\} \quad (4.11)$$

characterized by composite diplotype-specific mean vectors $\boldsymbol{\mu}_{j|il}$ and subject-specific covariance matrix Σ_i. We use the Hill equation to model genotypic dose-response curves of each composite diplotype. Thus, we have

$$\boldsymbol{\mu}_{j|il} = \left(E_{0jl} + \frac{E_{maxjl}C_{i1}^{H_{jl}}}{EC_{50jl}^{H_{jl}} + C_{i1}^{H_{jl}}}, \ldots, E_{0jl} + \frac{E_{maxjl}C_{iT_i}^{H_{jl}}}{EC_{50jl}^{H_{jl}} + C_{iT_i}^{H_{jl}}}\right)$$

where $\{E_{0jl}, E_{maxjl}, EC_{50jl}, H_{jl}\}$ are the Hill parameters specific to subject i carrying composite diplotype j that drops out at s_l. We use SAD(1) to model the covariance matrix Σ_i (Zhao et al. 2005a). In the likelihood of equation (4.10), $f\left(D_i = s_l \mid Q_i = j\right)$, denoted as π_{jl}, is assumed to be multinominal with possible outcomes from $S = \{s_1, \ldots, s_L\}$, and $f\left(Q_i = j\right)$ is the probability of subject i to carry composite diplotype j.

An integrative EM and Newton-Raphson algorithm is implemented to estimate the unknown parameters Ω_q. After the MLEs of Ω_q are obtained, $\text{var}(\hat{\Omega}_q)$ is calculated from the Fisher information matrix. A detailed procedure for parameter estimation was described in Li and Wu (2012).

4.3.3 Hypothesis Tests

As claimed by Lin et al. (2005a), an optimal risk haplotype can be selected from four haplotypes based on a model selection criterion. Thus, the significance of the genetic effect of the selected risk haplotype presents a multiple testing problem. Tradition approaches to correcting for multiple comparisons, such as the false discovery rate control, can be used for risk haplotype discovery. For drug response data with informative dropouts, we need to consider additional hypotheses as follows. Note that for all the tests, we have composite diplotype notation $j=2, 1, 0$ and dropout-dose notation $l=1, \ldots, L$.

Ignorability test of dropout: Whether the dropout can be ignored is the first question to address, in order to better utilize the data. This can be tested by formulating the hypotheses

$$H_0 : \left\{ E_{0jl}, E_{\text{max}jl}, EC_{50jl}, H_{jl} \right\} \equiv \left\{ E_0, E_{\text{max}}, EC_{50}, H \right\} \text{ and } \pi_{jl} \equiv \pi_l$$

$$H_1 : \left\{ E_{0jl}, E_{\text{max}jl}, EC_{50jl}, H_{jl} \right\} \equiv \left\{ E_{0l}, E_{\text{max}l}, EC_{50l}, H_l \right\} \text{ and } \pi_{jl} \equiv \pi_l$$

(4.12)

where the H_0 states that the dropout is ignorable in terms of longitudinal curves and dropout doses, whereas the H_1 states that the dropout is informative, i.e., different patterns of dropout lead subjects to have different longitudinal curves. These hypotheses are based on a mean pattern of all subjects studied by assuming no genetic effects on longitudinal curves and dropouts.

Genetic tests with ignorable dropout: If the dropout is ignorable, by accepting the H_0 of test (4.12), we test the existence of a significant haplotype effect first on the distribution of dropout doses, and then on the distribution of longitudinal curves. The genetic effect of haplotype on the distribution of dropout doses can be tested according to

$$H_0 : \left\{ E_{0jl}, E_{\text{max}jl}, EC_{50jl}, H_{jl} \right\} \equiv \left\{ E_0, E_{\text{max}}, EC_{50}, H \right\} \text{ and } \pi_{jl} \equiv \pi_l$$

$$H_1 : \left\{ E_{0jl}, E_{\text{max}jl}, EC_{50jl}, H_{jl} \right\} \equiv \left\{ E_0, E_{\text{max}}, EC_{50}, H \right\}$$

(4.13a)

If there is a haplotype effect on the distribution of dropout doses, then whether this haplotype effect impacts longitudinal curves can be tested according to

$$H_0 : \left\{ E_{0jl}, E_{\text{max}jl}, EC_{50jl}, H_{jl} \right\} \equiv \left\{ E_0, E_{\text{max}}, EC_{50}, H \right\}$$

$$H_1 : \left\{ E_{0jl}, E_{\text{max}jl}, EC_{50jl}, H_{jl} \right\} \equiv \left\{ E_{0j}, E_{\text{max}j}, EC_{50j}, H_j \right\}$$

(4.13b)

If the null hypothesis of test (4.13b) is rejected, this suggests that the haplotype has a pleiotropic effect on dropout times and longitudinal curves. If there is no haplotype effect on the distribution of dropout doses, then whether this haplotype effect impacts longitudinal curves can be tested according to

$$H_0 : \left\{ E_{0jl}, E_{\text{max}jl}, EC_{50jl}, H_{jl} \right\} \equiv \left\{ E_0, E_{\text{max}}, EC_{50}, H \right\} \text{ and } \pi_{jl} \equiv \pi_l$$

$$H_1 : \left\{ E_{0jl}, E_{\text{max}jl}, EC_{50jl}, H_{jl} \right\} \equiv \left\{ E_{0j}, E_{\text{max}j}, EC_{50j}, H_j \right\} \text{ and } \pi_{jl} \equiv \pi_l$$

(4.13c)

Genetic tests with non-ignorable dropout: If the dropout is non-ignorable, by rejecting the H_0 at equation (4.13c), we also need to test how haplotypes impact longitudinal curves and dropout doses. For the genetic effect of haplotype on the distribution of dropout doses, we test

$$H_0 : \left\{E_{0jl}, E_{\max jl}, EC_{50jl}, H_{jl}\right\} \equiv \left\{E_{0l}, E_{\max l}, EC_{50l}, H_l\right\} \text{ and } \pi_{jl} \equiv \pi_l$$

$$H_1 : \left\{E_{0jl}, E_{\max jl}, EC_{50jl}, H_{jl}\right\} \equiv \left\{E_{0l}, E_{\max l}, EC_{50l}, H_l\right\}$$

(4.14a)

If there is a haplotype effect on the distribution of dropout doses, then whether this haplotype effect impacts longitudinal curves can be tested according to

$$H_0 : \left\{E_{0jl}, E_{\max jl}, EC_{50jl}, H_{jl}\right\} \equiv \left\{E_{0l}, E_{\max l}, EC_{50l}, H_l\right\}$$

$$H_1 : \left\{E_{0jl}, E_{\max jl}, EC_{50jl}, H_{jl}\right\} \neq \left\{E_{0l}, E_{\max l}, EC_{50l}, H_l\right\}$$

(4.14b)

If there is no haplotype effect on the distribution of dropout doses, then whether this haplotype effect impacts longitudinal curves can be tested according to

$$H_0 : \left\{E_{0jl}, E_{\max jl}, EC_{50jl}, H_{jl}\right\} \equiv \left\{E_{0l}, E_{\max l}, EC_{50l}, H_l\right\} \text{ and } \pi_{jl} \equiv \pi_l$$

$$H_1 : \left\{E_{0jl}, E_{\max jl}, EC_{50jl}, H_{jl}\right\} \neq \left\{E_{0l}, E_{\max l}, EC_{50l}, H_l\right\} \text{ and } \pi_{jl} \equiv \pi_l$$

(4.14c)

For all tests above, test statistics are approximately χ^2 with degrees of freedom equal to the difference in parameter number between the H_1 and H_0.

4.3.4 The Identification of Significant Haplotypes

As shown in Figure 4.2, the dropout dose set is $S = \{s_1, s_2, s_3, s_4\} = \{10, 20, 30, 40\}$. Assume that there is no censoring on dropout doses, $\Delta_i = 1$ for $i = 1, \ldots, N$. We use three schemes to jointly model dropout and longitudinal curve data: Scheme I has four differently modeled dropout patterns; Scheme II has dropouts at dose levels 10, 20, and 30 modeled in the same way. We find significant haplotype effects due to codon16 and codon27 within the β_2AR gene on chromosome 5. Schemes I and II identify haplotype GG as an optimal risk haplotype. Figure 4.3 shows the composite diplotype-specific response curves of heart rate to dobutamine under Schemes I (Figure 4.3a) and II (Figure 4.3b). The comparison of AIC values calculated between the two shows that Scheme II with 29 parameters (5,980) is a better fit to the data than Scheme I with 50 parameters (6,100). It is observed that composite diplotype GG|GG has a similar trend of heart rate for both the completers and dropouts. For this reason, we pose an additional constraint by setting composite genotype GG|GG to be equal across different dropout patterns. This model, Scheme

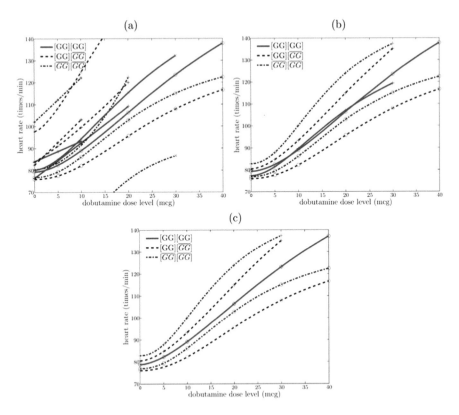

FIGURE 4.3
The response curves of heart rate to dobutamine for different composite diplotypes, [GG][GG] (solid), [GG][GG-] (dashed), and [GG-][GG-] (dash-dotted), derived from gene $\beta_2 AR$, under model Scheme I (A), II (B), and III (C), respectively.

III, is better than Scheme II in terms of AIC values. Also, since Scheme III is nested in Scheme II, we calculate the likelihood ratio of Scheme III over Scheme II, with a p-value of 0.912 confirming the choice of Scheme III.

All the subsequent analyses are based on Scheme III. With hypothesis test (3.1), we could test if the dropout was informative under Scheme III. The resulting likelihood ratio test statistic is $-2(-2{,}902.4+2{,}884.1)=36.6$, corresponding to the p-value of 2.2×10^{-7} for a $\chi^2_{df=4}$ distribution. This suggests that dropout is informative and it is crucial to integrate this information into the analysis. Given that the dropout is non-ignorable, we perform a hypothesis test based on test (4.14a) to find whether risk haplotype GG|GG exerts a significant effect on dropout doses. It was found that dropout doses do not depend on risk haplotype GG ($p=0.849$). A further test for longitudinal curves based on (4.14c) suggests that risk haplotype GG has a significant effect on the response curve of heart rate to dobutamine ($p=0.0329$).

Since the dropouts are non-ignorable, it is not surprising to see that the dropouts respond to dobutamine more rapidly than the completers. However, it is interesting to find that dramatic differences occur in the pattern of genetic control between the completers and dropouts (Figure 4.3c). In the completers, the composite diplotype with double risk haplotypes GG|GG is the most sensitive in drug response, followed by the composite diplotype with double non-risk haplotypes, and the composite diplotype with one risk haplotype and one non-risk haplotype; in the dropouts, the last two composite diplotypes show much greater sensitivity than the first one. Table 4.1 tabulates the MLEs of four drug response parameters (E_0, E_{max}, EC_{50}, H) for different dropout types and covariance-structuring parameters under Scheme III. As

TABLE 4.1

MLEs of Parameters that Define the Model with Non-ignorable Dropouts

Dropout Pattern	Composite Diplotype	Parameter	MLE	STD
Dropout	$Q=0$	E_0	78.74	1.2103
		E_{max}	120.33	32.0615
		EC_{50}	41.47	12.8841
		H	1.66	0.2168
	$Q=1$	E_0	80.49	0.9548
		E_{max}	131.57	57.7866
		EC_{50}	36.68	15.4237
		H	1.71	0.2545
	$Q=2$	E_0	82.80	1.0628
		E_{max}	72.58	11.3941
		EC_{50}	17.55	2.7767
		H	2.07	0.2272
Completer	$Q=0$	E_0	78.74	1.2103
		E_{max}	120.33	32.0615
		EC_{50}	41.47	12.8841
		H	1.66	0.2168
	$Q=1$	E_0	76.18	0.6552
		E_{max}	62.82	10.0181
		EC_{50}	29.53	5.0611
		H	2.00	0.2841
	$Q=2$	E_0	76.91	0.5506
		E_{max}	59.62	6.9851
		EC_{50}	22.73	2.7717
		H	2.06	0.2488
Covariance modeling		ϕ	0.96	0.0131
		σ_e^2	62.06	1.9352
		π_1	0.3147	0.0224

Standard deviations (STD) of the MLEs are estimated by Louis' approach shown by the estimates of their standard errors, many parameters can be reasonably well estimated, except for E_{max}.

4.3.5 Comparison with Traditional Functional Mapping

We compare results by functional mapping implemented with the pattern-mixture model and by traditional functional mapping. First, we perform functional mapping only using the subjects (98) who completed the study. This approach does not detect a significant haplotype effect for two SNPs from gene $\beta_1 AR$, but a significant haplotype effect on heart rate curves is found for two SNPs from gene $\beta_2 AR$ ($p=0.040$). Yes, this significance level is lower than that by pattern-mixture–based functional mapping ($p=0.033$). Haplotype GG within gene $\beta_2 AR$ is detected to be a risk haplotype based on the likelihoods calculated by assuming each of four possible haplotypes, AC, AG, GC, and GG, as a risk haplotype.

Second, we perform functional mapping using all subjects (143) who have heart rate data, assuming that the dropout is noninformative. Under this assumption, both incompleters and completers are treated equally. This approach does not detect any significant risk haplotype for both candidate genes ($p>0.085$), suggesting that this treatment reduces the power of gene identification. Taken together, when the association studies contain dropouts, it is important to test their non-ignorability because joint modeling of drug response curves and informative dropouts can improve the power of functional mapping than considering drug response curves alone. Moreover, non-ignorable dropout is a biological trait on its own merit and, thereby, it is of great significance to reveal its genetic architecture and its pleiotropic control shared with drug response.

4.4 Haplotyping Drug Response Using the Selection Model

4.4.1 Likelihood and Estimation

In this section, we implement functional mapping with the selection model to consider the effect of non-ignorable dropouts. A detailed description of this implementation was described by Wang et al. (2013c). Among all subjects participating in a longitudinal association study, some can complete the entire clinical trial, but others drop out from the study during the period of the trial due to some physiological limits. We use the same notation as described in Section 4.5. Drug response over different dosages can be fitted by the Hill equation. Yet, for the purpose of easy illustration, we assume a linear trend. The implementation of the more complex Hill equation is straightforward, although this will be computationally more expensive.

Given subject i, let $\mathbf{y}_i = (C_{i1}, \ldots, C_{iT_i})$ denote the vector of its heart rates measured at a series of dose levels. The phenotypic value of drug response for subject i at a particular dose is written as

$$y_i(C_{it}) = (a_2 + b_2 C_{it})I(Q_i = 2)$$
$$+ (a_1 + b_1 C_{it})I(Q_i = 1) + (\theta_{0i} + \theta_{1i}C_{it}) + e_i(C_{it}) \qquad (4.15)$$

where Q_i is the indicator for subject i to carry a particular composite diplotype, (a_2, b_2) and (a_1, b_1) are the curve parameters for the two composite diplotypes, i.e., one composed of two risk haplotypes and the other composed of one risk haplotype and one non-risk haplotype, respectively, which are treated as a fixed effect, $\theta_i = (\theta_{0i}, \theta_{1i})'$ are subject-specific random effects for the composite diplotype composed of two non-risk haplotypes, with θ_i being assumed to have a bivariate Gaussian distribution $N(e, V)$, or

$$\begin{pmatrix} \theta_{0i} \\ \theta_{1i} \end{pmatrix} \sim N\left(\begin{pmatrix} \theta_0 \\ \theta_1 \end{pmatrix}, \begin{pmatrix} \sigma_{00} & \sigma_{10} \\ \sigma_{01} & \sigma_{11} \end{pmatrix} \right)$$

and the error term $e_i(C_{it})$, distributed as $N(0, \sigma_e^2)$, is mutually independent among different dose levels. Note that in this formulation, $\mathbf{y}_i$ is characterized by a linear mixed effects model. When Q_i is not observed, there are missing covariates in this model. The distribution of Q_i is obtained using the same multinomial likelihood function in the preceding section.

For the event time distribution, we use the extended Cox proportional model to model the hazard of failure and, similar to that in Wulfsohn and Tsiatis (1997), the hazard depends on longitudinal covariate $\mathbf{y}_i$ through the underlying true value at that time, i.e.,

$$\lambda\left(C_{it} \mid \theta_i, y_i(C_{it}), Q_i \right)$$
$$= \lambda_0(C_{it}) \exp\left\{ \beta\left[(a_2 + b_2 C_{it})I(Q_i = 2) + (a_1 + b_1 C_{it})I(Q_i = 1) + \theta_{0i} + \theta_{1i}C_{it} \right] \right\} \qquad (4.16)$$

where the baseline hazard function $\lambda_0(C)$ is left unspecified. So, the longitudinal and event time distributions share the same latent random process θ_i and the same fixed effect a_2, b_2, a_1, b_1.

For the selection model, the joint distribution of longitudinal ($\mathbf{y}$) and event time data can characterize the informative dropout. Let L^o denote the joint likelihood function of observed data. We factorize this likelihood function as the product of the marginal distribution of $\mathbf{y}$ (which is easily obtained) and the conditional distribution of event times given $\mathbf{y}$, i.e.,

$$L^0 = L_y^0 \times L^0\left(\tilde{D}, \Delta \mid \mathbf{y}\right)$$

$$= \prod_{i=1}^{N} \sum_{Q_i=0}^{2} \left\{ \int_{-\infty}^{+\infty} \left[\prod_{\tau=1}^{T_i} f\left(y_{i\tau} \mid Q_i, a_1, b_1, a_2, b_2, \theta_i, \sigma_e^2\right) \right] f\left(\theta_i \mid \boldsymbol{\theta}, V\right) \quad (4.17)$$

$$\times f\left(\tilde{D}_i, \Delta_i \mid Q_i, \lambda_0, \beta, a_1, b_1, a_2, b_2, \theta_i\right) d\theta_i f\left(Q_i \mid G_i, \hat{\Omega}_p\right) \right\}$$

where

$$f\left(y_{i\tau} \mid Q_i, a_1, b_1, a_2, b_2, \theta_i, \sigma_e^2\right)$$

$$= \left(2\pi\sigma_e^2\right)^{-1/2} \exp\left\{ -\frac{1}{2\sigma_e^2}\left(y_{i\tau} - \sum_{z=1}^{2}\left(a_z + b_z C_{i\tau}\right)I\left(Q_i = z\right) - \theta_{0i} - \theta_{1i}C_{i\tau} \right)^2 \right\}$$

$$f\left(\theta_i \mid \boldsymbol{\theta}, V\right) = \left(2\pi|V|\right)^{-1/2} \exp\left\{ -\frac{1}{2}(\theta_i - \boldsymbol{\theta})' V^{-1}(\theta_i - \boldsymbol{\theta}) \right\}$$

$$f\left(\tilde{D}_i, \Delta_i \mid Q_i, \lambda_0, \beta, a_1, b_1, a_2, b_2, \theta_i\right)$$

$$= \left[\lambda_0\left(\tilde{D}_i\right) \exp\left\{ \beta\left(\sum_{z=1}^{2}\left(a_z + b_z\tilde{D}_i\right)I\left(Q_i = z\right) + \theta_{0i} + \theta_{1i}\tilde{D}_i \right) \right\} \right]^{\Delta_i}$$

$$\times \exp\left[-\int_0^{\tilde{D}_i} \lambda_0(u)\exp\left\{ \beta\left(\sum_{z=1}^{2}\left(a_z + b_z u\right)I\left(Q_i = z\right) + \theta_{0i} + \theta_{1i}u \right) \right\} du \right]$$

and $f\left(Q_i \mid G_i, \hat{\Omega}_p\right)$ is the probability of composite diplotype Q_i given marker genotypes G_i and estimated haplotype frequencies $\hat{\Omega}_p$.

The parameters $\left(a_2, b_2, a_1, b_1, \boldsymbol{\theta}, V, \sigma_e^2\right)$ and β can be estimated using a parametric maximum likelihood and $\lambda_0(u)$ estimated using a nonparametric maximum likelihood. The baseline hazard $\lambda_0(u)$ takes mass at each failure time, and the dimension of λ_0 is equal to the number of unique failure times. The EM algorithm is implemented to estimate the MLEs of the parameters.

4.4.2 Asymptotic Sampling Variances

After the point estimates of parameters are obtained, we need to derive the asymptotic variance-covariance matrix and evaluate the sampling errors of the estimates. This model is complex. A naive approach to this is proposed. It is to use numerical derivative (Numerical Recipe). The partial derivative of a given function with respect to some parameters x and y is given by:

$$\frac{\partial^2 f}{\partial x \, \partial y}$$

$$= \frac{\left[f\left(x+h_1, y+h_2\right) - f\left(x+h_1, y-h_2\right) \right] - \left[f\left(x-h_1, y+h_2\right) - f\left(x-h_1, y-h_2\right) \right]}{4h_1 h_2}$$

(4.18)

If x and y are the same parameters, the above formula simplifies to

$$\frac{\partial^2 f}{\partial x^2} = \frac{f(x+h) - 2f(x-h) + f(x)}{h^2}$$

where f is the log-likelihood function and x and y are any parameters of interest in the current model. Taking the inverse of the negative values of the partial derivative matrix, we can obtain the estimate of the asymptotic sample covariance matrix.

4.4.3 Computer Simulation

To examine whether functional mapping implemented with the selection model can improve mapping efficiency, we perform computer simulations. We simulate the phenotypic value of a longitudinal trait at seven evenly spaced doses $C = (0, 1, 2, 3, 4, 5, 6)$, allowing a certain proportion of subjects to be dropped out in a non-ignorable manner. The middle dose ($C=3$) at which there is an averaged variance is used to calculate the heritability of longitudinal curves. We assume that the population from which a set of samples are drawn for haplotype mapping is at HWE. We simulate 2-SNP haplotypes that encode the variation in longitudinal response. The allele frequencies at the two SNPs and their linkage disequilibrium (LD) in the population are assumed as in Table 3.1. By assuming one of the four haplotypes as a risk haplotype, we specify three different composite diplotypes, with corresponding frequencies determined by allele frequencies and LD, and diplotype-specific response curve parameters given in Table 3.2. The phenotypic value of longitudinal response is simulated from equation (4.15). Event times are generated by the hazard model of equation (4.16) with Weibull baseline hazard function $\lambda_0(C) = 0.001C$. The event time is censored at dose level $C=6$. Note that typically in a drug response study, we usually do not record the precise dropout dose and only know that after some dose level the drop-outed subjects have no observations. For example, if subject i only has observations at dosages 0, 1, 2, we would consider this subject that drops out at dosage 2; i.e., the dropout dosage is the last dose that the subject has an observation.

TABLE 4.2

MLEs of SNP Allele Frequencies ($p_1^{(1)}, p_1^{(2)}$) and Linkage Disequilibrium (D)

	$p_1^{(1)}$	$p_1^{(2)}$	D
Given	0.6	0.6	0.03
MLE	0.601	0.602	0.029
STD	0.0368	0.0378	0.217

Standard errors (STD) of the MLEs were calculated from 100 simulation replicates

The means of MLEs of all parameters Ω_p and Ω_q and standard errors of their MLEs over 100 simulation replicates are tabulated in Tables 4.1 and 4.2. The estimates include population genetic parameters (Ω_p), i.e., allele frequencies and LD, quantitative genetic parameters (Ω_q), i.e., composite diplotype-specific curve parameters and covariance matrix-structuring parameters. The MLEs of the population genetic parameters are quite unbiased and precise since they are estimated from a simple multinominal likelihood function. The estimates of the quantitative genetic parameters under a sample size of 100 and heritability of 0.4 are also reasonably precise, as indicated by the small standard errors of the estimates (Table 4.2). The selection model can successfully detect the risk haplotype. The same simulated data are analyzed by traditional functional mapping that assumes MCAR and MAR dropouts. As can be seen, the two approaches display similar precision for parameter estimation (Table 4.2). The most significant merit of the selection model lies in the characterization of missing mechanisms that gain more insight into the genetic architecture of drug response. The selection model has additional power to test the common genetic basis of dropout time events and response outcome, helping medical doctors determine an optimal window of dosing for individual patients based on their genetic makeup (Table 4.3).

4.5 Concluding Remarks

Functional mapping has proven to be powerful for mapping drug response in terms of its capacity to integrate the pharmacokinetic and pharmacodynamic processes of drug-body interactions into a mapping setting. The prerequisite of its application is to repeatedly measure pharmacological parameters of drug effects at a series of time points or dose levels. To well fit time-varying concentration changes or concentration-varying response changes by functional mapping, an adequate number of time points or dosages (say six or more) are required. However, in practical clinics, some subjects do not complete a full range of drug administration routes owing to physiological or other unavoidable reasons, leading to data missing. By assuming that the dropout occurs at random or completely at random, Hou et al. (2005, 2006)

TABLE 4.3

MLEs of the Parameters Describing the Longitudinal Curve and Dropout
Process from Selection Model-Incorporated Functional Mapping

	Given	Dropout Model		Traditional Model	
		MLE	STD	MLE	STD
θ_0	11.3	11.3012	0.2695	11.3016	0.2698
θ_1	0.8	0.7992	0.0342	0.7991	0.0344
σ_{00}	1	0.9824	0.1407	0.9827	0.1409
σ_{01}	0.02	0.0183	0.0134	0.0183	0.0135
σ_{11}	0.02	0.0189	0.0026	0.0189	0.0026
a_1	−1	−1.0124	0.3311	−1.0138	0.3325
b_1	−0.04	−0.0356	0.0404	−0.0353	0.0405
a_2	−2.3	−2.2637	0.3050	−2.2625	0.3042
b_2	−0.1	−0.0952	0.0410	−0.0956	0.0413
σ^2	0.0029	0.0029	0.0002	0.0029	0.0002
β^e	0.2	0.1745	0.1136	–	–

The standard errors (STD) of the MLEs were calculated from 100 simulation replicates

modified functional mapping by considering a more heterogeneous situation in which longitudinal traits for each subject are measured at an unequally spaced time/dose intervals, different subjects have different measurement patterns, and the residual correlation within subjects is nonstationary. This modification is very powerful to map highly sparse data, where individual subjects only have a few observations but at alternative time points or dose levels. The observations of all subjects together project on a dense spectrum of measurements, allowing for the application of functional mapping.

However, if data missing does not occur at random rather depends on the unobserved part of the longitudinal response, a phenomenon, called informative dropout or non-ignorable dropout, arises. For those dropouts, Hou et al.'s modifications do not work to map drug response. In this chapter, we describe the modifications of functional mapping by integrating the missing mechanisms of non-ignorable dropouts. The modifications are based on two alternative models, the pattern-mixture model that specifies the conditional distribution of the unobserved measurements given the observed ones in a given pattern, and the selection model that specifies the distribution of dropout indicators conditioned on the values of repeated measures. The pattern-mixture model can not only map genetic variants for longitudinal responses but also identify genes that mediate informative dropouts. Through computer simulation, Li and Wu (2012) found that pattern-mixture–based functional mapping performs better than Hou et al.'s sparsity data–implemented functional mapping, both of which are more advantageous than functional mapping that only considers completers. The application of the pattern-mixture model to a pharmacogenetic association study confirms this simulation results.

The strength of the selection model lies in the modeling of the event time. By conditioning on the longitudinal data, we can better capture the event distribution. In many clinical trials or survival studies, this method is used to find a biomarker for disease development. Given the different assumptions used, the selection model is an alternative to the pattern-mixture model in mapping longitudinal drug response with informative dropouts. In general, the selection model can study both longitudinal response and dropout as an event, whereas the pattern-mixture model is used in longitudinal studies. In practice, which one should be used can be determined by considering the design of clinical trials and the feature of data collected.

In human genetic studies, there are many other variables (besides the time and genetic information) that may influence the experiment, such as age, sex, and lifestyle. These variables should be included in the model as covariates, thus allowing one to characterize various variations more precisely. Also, as a demonstration, we describe the model on the basis of two SNPs. There is no technical difficulty in extending the model to include more than two SNPs, allowing a genome-wide search for the distribution and effect of multi-SNP haplotypes and their genetic interactions.

By including the dropout time as a covariate for the longitudinal development, we can now study the genetic control of the longitudinal curve more precisely with selection or pattern-mixture models. They can be used to shed light on the genetic architecture of inter-patient variation in complex longitudinal responses with incomplete data and provide scientific guidance about the design of efficient and effective clinical trials for biomedical and health studies. All these will greatly help to translate genetic information into clinical trials, promoting the practical use of "clinical genomics."

5

Systems Mapping of Drug Response

5.1 Introduction

Genetic mapping or association studies aim to dissect complex traits into their underlying genetic components. The majority of approaches used focus on the dissection of genetic architecture into various genetic and epigenetic elements and the identification of key elements that interrogate genetic architecture. There are also several other approaches developed from a different perspective, which dissect complex traits into their developmental events through mathematical and statistical models and map genetic variants responsible for developmental trajectories. These approaches, called functional mapping, have proven to be more statistically powerful for the detection of trait genes and more biologically meaningful for genetic discoveries (Ma et al. 2002; Wu and Lin 2006; Wu at et al. 2004a, b, c; Li and Sillanpää 2015). Originated in plant genetic mapping, functional mapping has shown its applications to pharmacogenetic and pharmacogenomic studies by integrating mathematically derived pharmacokinetic (PK) and pharmacodynamic (PD) mechanisms (Lin et al. 2005a, b, 2007; Wu and Lin 2008; Ahn et al. 2010; Wu et al. 2011b; Wang et al. 2015a, 2019a; Wei et al. 2018b).

Functional mapping has developed to a point, at which complex traits are mapped by dissolving them into their physiological, structural, or metabolic components according to the design principle of biological systems, followed by mapping individual components and their functional interconnections. Wu et al. (2011a) first named this approach systems mapping, whose central hypothesis is that phenotypic formation is the consequence of developmental interactions and coordination among various elements on a time-space scale. Given their robustness in manipulating the complexity of system dynamics, differential equations have been implemented into systems mapping to quantify and predict the genetic control of phenotypic formation (Sun and Wu 2015a, b). Compared to functional mapping, systems mapping is equipped with a capacity to tackle the complex aspects of developmental interactions, making results more interpretable in biology. Owing to the parsimonious modeling of dynamic systems, systems mapping displays tremendous statistical power and computational flexibility. Systems mapping has shown its implications for genetic mapping of viral dynamics (Luo et al. 2010), circadian rhythm (Liu et al. 2007; Fu et al. 2010, 2011; Sun and Wu 2015a, b), plant growth (Wu et al. 2011a; Fu et al. 2017; Cao et al. 2017), and drug resistance dynamics (Guo et al. 2011).

As a complex trait involving a series of biochemical interactions between drugs and body chemistry, drug response can be better described and studied by a dynamic system (Jusko et al. 1995). The past three decades have seen tremendous efforts to identify and map pharmacogenetic variants for drug response (Weinshilboum 2003; Daly 2009, 2010; Ge et al. 2009; Klein et al. 2009; Shuldiner et al. 2009; Manolio 2010; Roden et al. 2011; Wang et al. 2015a; Primorac et al. 2020). These studies characterize pharmacogenes by mapping a direct genotype-phenotype relationship, which fails to reveal a black box behind the biochemical processes from drug administration to the emergence of drug effect. Beyond this, systems mapping explores and models the genetic regulation involved in the mechanistic and kinetic details of drug absorption and drug metabolism. Ahn et al. (2010) argue that mechanistic exploration can increase our ability to predict which medical treatments will be safe and effective for a specific patient and which ones will not be. Systems mapping could provide critical information for personalized medicine or precision medicine, allowing physicians to select a therapy or treatment protocol in a quantitative and precise way based on a patient's genetic profile (Kraft and Hoffmann 2012; van der Wouden et al. 2020). The integration of systems mapping into precision medicine may not only minimize harmful side effects to ensure a more successful outcome, but can also help to reduce costs compared with a "trial-and-error" approach to disease treatment.

In this chapter, we describe the principle of systems mapping and show how it is used to map drug response from a mechanistic perspective. After a drug is administered, it is absorbed and transported to a specialized site of action where the drug interacts with targets, such as receptors and enzymes, through metabolic activation and is then excreted (Jusko et al. 1995; Weinshilboum 2003; Mager et al. 2003). Such processes of drug reactions and drug effects in the human body can be described by two independent but related mechanisms, PK, and PD (Figure 1.1; Jusko et al. 1995; Meibohm and Derendorf 1997; Macheras and Iliadis 2006; Wu and Lin 2008). A variety of mathematical equations, including ordinary differential equations (ODEs) and stochastic differential equations (SDEs), have been derived to specify PK-PD changes of drug response (Mager et al. 2003; Kristensen et al. 2005; Wang et al. 2008, 2015b; Donnet and Samson 2013). Systems mapping integrates the mathematical aspects of PK-PD processes into a genomic mapping framework, by which we can test the pattern of genetic control for biochemical pathways of drug response through the underlying mathematical curves.

5.2 ODE Modeling of PK/PD Machineries

Interactions between drug and body molecules can be viewed as a biological system in which the drug is absorbed, distributed, and metabolized by receptors and enzymes through PK/PD processes. Compartmental analysis provides a method for mathematical modeling of PK/PD links by assuming that drug response is divided into a series of homogeneous compartments where the compartments interact via exchanging material. This method capitalizes on a system of ODEs that describes continuous biological process, interconnects different compartments, and traces the distributional behavior of the drug between the plasma and other organs (Wang et al. 2008). More precisely, ODEs can describe changes in drug concentrations in each compartment at a rate which is usually proportional to the blood flow to that compartment (Macheras and Iliadis 2006).

Suppose that a system of first-order ODEs can describe the PK/PD machineries, expressed as

$$\frac{dy}{dt} = g(y, A, B; \varphi), \quad y(t_0) = y_0, t \geq t_0 \tag{5.1}$$

where y is an m-dimensional dependent variable vector, g is the structural model in which A and B are the functions of t, and φ is a q-dimensional vector of unknown model parameters. Below, we show how equation (5.1) can be used to describe PK and PD machineries.

Using exploratory data analysis and knowledge of drug physiology, Wang et al. (2008) built up a system of ODEs for drug response based on the first-order absorption and Michaelis-Menten elimination and a one-compartment indirect response, expressed as

$$\begin{cases} \dfrac{dQ}{dt} = -\dfrac{V_{max}}{k_m + Q}Q \\[2mm] \dfrac{dC}{dt} = \dfrac{V_{max}Q}{(k_m + Q)V} - \dfrac{V_{max}}{k_m + C}C \\[2mm] \dfrac{dR}{dt} = k_{in}\left(1 + \dfrac{E_{max}C^H}{EC_{50}^H + C^H}\right) - k_{out}R \end{cases} \tag{5.2}$$

where t is the time, an independent variable varying between 0 and 300 minutes, Q is the amount of drug in the gastrointestinal (GI) tract (mg), C is the plasma drug concentration (mg/L), and R is drug response that can be viewed as blood pressure, body temperature, or other pharmacologic response. A Michaelis-Menten equation describes the initial rate of reaction as a function of the substrate concentration, with the reaction reaching a certain maximum

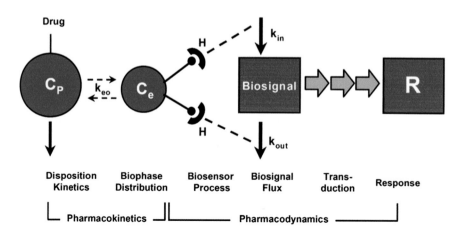

FIGURE 5.1

Key components of drug interactions specified by PK and PD models. When a drug is administrated to the human body, it reacts in a biological fluid (e.g., plasma), undergoing a kinetic change of drug concentration (C_p) proportional by a factor k_{eo} to biophase concentration (C_e), and then produces the pharmacological response (R) through a series of processes, such as biosensor (Hill function or H), biosignal flux (production, k_{in}, or removal, k_{out}), and transduction. Adapted from Jusko et al. (1995) and Mager et al. (2003).

rate as the substrate concentration increases, where k_m is the Michaelis-Menten constant, V_{max} is the maximum rate of the reaction, and V is the volume of distribution. A large volume of distribution is usually associated with the extensive distribution of the drug into body tissues and fluids. In contrast, a small volume of distribution often implies limited drug distribution (Brunton et al. 2006). The PK parameters include k_m and V_{max} and the PD parameters include k_{in} and k_{out}, the zero- and first-order rate constant for production and loss of an effect, respectively (Figure 5.1; Jusko et al. 1995; Mager et al. 2003), and H, E_{max} and EC_{50}, a slope of the effect-concentration curve (or Hill coefficient), the maximum effect of the drug and the drug concentrations producing 50% of the maximum stimulation, respectively. The Q-C-R system, the overall behavior of which is described by ODE parameters arrayed in (k_m, V_{max}, V, k_{in}, k_{out}, H, E_{max}, EC_{50}), can reflect the process of drug response.

5.3 Systems Mapping: Model and Algorithm

5.3.1 Clinical Design

Assume that a random sample of n subjects is drawn from a natural population at Hardy-Weinberg equilibrium. All these samples are genotyped for DNA markers throughout the genome. After a drug is administrated, these subjects are measured for the amount of drug in the GI tract (Q) (mg), the plasma concentration of drug (C) (mg/L), and the pharmacologic response of drug (R), such as blood pressure or heart rate, at a series of time points. Considering the reality of pharmacological trials, we allow the phenotypic measures of the subjects to be taken at irregular, unequally spaced intervals, with subject-dependent measurement schedules. Our purpose here is to describe the model framework of systems mapping and, thereby, consider the drug response data that have been corrected for the effects due to covariates such as race, sex, life style among others by data standardization.

5.3.2 Likelihood and Estimation

Let $\mathbf{y}_i = (\mathbf{y}_{Qi}; \mathbf{y}_{Ci}; \mathbf{y}_{Ri}) \equiv (y_{Qi}(t_{i1}), \ldots, y_{Qi}(t_{iT_i}); y_{Ci}(t_{i1}), \ldots, y_{Ci}(t_{iT_i}); y_{Ri}(t_{i1}), \ldots, y_{Ri}(t_{iT_i}))$ are the phenotypic values measured for subject i ($i=1, \ldots, n$) at time points $(t_{i1}, \ldots, t_{iT_i})$, including amounts of drug in the GI tract (Q), the plasma concentrations of drug (C), and drug effect (R). Consider an SNP with three genotypes AA, Aa, and aa, the observations of which are denoted as n_2, n_1, and n_0 ($n_2+n_1+n_0=n$), respectively. The likelihood of $\mathbf{y}_i$ at this SNP is formulized as

$$L(\mathbf{y}) = \sum_{i=1}^{n_2} f_2\left(\mathbf{y}_i; \mu_{2|i}, \Sigma_i\right) \sum_{i=1}^{n_1} f_1\left(\mathbf{y}_i; \mu_{1|i}, \Sigma_i\right) \sum_{i=1}^{n_0} f_0\left(\mathbf{y}_i; \mu_{0|i}, \Sigma_i\right) \qquad (5.3)$$

where $f_j\left(\mathbf{y}_i; \mu_{j|i}, \Sigma_i\right)$ is a tri-variate longitudinal (multivariate) normal probability density function with expected mean vector $\mu_{j|i}$ for subject i that belongs to QTL genotype j ($j=2$ for AA, 1 for Aa, 0 for aa), expressed as

$$\mu_{j|i} = \left(\mu_{Qj|i}; \mu_{Cj|i}; \mu_{Rj|i}\right)$$

$$\equiv \left(\mu_{Qj|i}(t_{i1}), \ldots, \mu_{Qj|i}(t_{iT_i}); \mu_{Cj|i}(t_{i1}), \ldots, \mu_{Cj|i}(t_{iT_i}); \mu_{Rj|i}(t_{i1}), \ldots, \mu_{Rj|i}(t_{iT_i})\right)$$
$$(5.4)$$

and subject-dependent symmetrical tri-variate covariance matrix Σ_i, expressed as

$$\Sigma_i = \begin{pmatrix} \Sigma_{Qi} & \Sigma_{QCi} & \Sigma_{QRi} \\ \Sigma_{CQi} & \Sigma_{Ci} & \Sigma_{CRi} \\ \Sigma_{RQi} & \Sigma_{RCi} & \Sigma_{Ri} \end{pmatrix} \qquad (5.5)$$

with elements on diagonal being ($T_i \times T_i$) covariance matrices of time-dependent Q, C, and R variables and those off diagonal being a ($T_i \times T_i$) covariance matrix between a pair of variables.

In systems mapping of drug response, where Q, C, and R variables are assumed to obey the dynamic system (5.2), the derivatives of the genotypic means of these variables can be expressed by this system. Thus, we fit geno-typic means (5.4) with genotype-specific ODE parameters (k_{mj}, V_{maxj}, k_{inj}, k_{outj}, H_j, E_{maxj}, EC_{50j}) that specify this system for each genotype. Let $\mu_{kj|i}(t, u_{kj|i})$ denote the time-varying genotypic derivative of variable k ($k=Q$, C or R) for subject i belonging to QTL genotype j, i.e.,

$$\mu_{kj|i}\left(t, u_{kj|i}\right) = \frac{du_{kj|i}}{dt}$$

where $u_{kj|i}$ is the genotypic mean of variable k for subject i (with genotype j) at an arbitrary point in a time course. Based on the Runge-Kutta scheme, the value of $u_{kj|i}$ in iteration $l+1$ is determined by the present value plus the weighted aver-age of 4 deltas (where each delta is the product of the size of the interval and an estimated slope), expressed as

$$u_{kj|i}^{\{l+1\}} = u_{kj|i}^{\{l\}} + \frac{1}{6}\left(R_{1kj|i} + 2R_{2kj|i} + 2R_{3kj|i} + R_{4kj|i}\right)$$

where $R_{1kj|i} = h\mu_{kj|i}\left(t^{\{l\}}, u_{kj|i}^{\{l\}}\right)$ is the delta based on the slope at the begin-ning of the interval, using $u_{kj|i}^{\{l\}}$; $R_{2kj|i} = h\mu_{kj|i}\left(t^{\{l\}} + \frac{1}{2}h, u_{kj|i}^{\{l\}} + \frac{1}{2}h\,R_{1kj|i}\right)$ is the delta based on the slope at the midpoint of the interval, using $u_{kj|i}^{\{l\}} + \frac{1}{2}hR_{1kj|i}$; $R_{3kj|i} = h\mu_{kj|i}\left(t^{\{l\}} + \frac{1}{2}h, u_{kj|i}^{\{l\}} + \frac{1}{2}hR_{2kj|i}\right)$ is another delta based on the slope at the midpoint, but now using $u_{kj|i}^{\{l\}} + \frac{1}{2}h\,R_{2kj|i}$, and $R_{4kj|i} = h\mu_{kj|i}\left(t^{\{l\}} + h, u_{kj|i}^{\{l\}} + h\,R_{3kj|i}\right)$ is the delta based on the slope at the end of the interval. The Runge-Kutta fourth-order algorithm with step size $h=0.1$ is used to approximate the solution in high accuracy given a trial set of parameter values and initial conditions.

We fit the covariance structure by using a parsimonious and flexible approach, such as an autoregressive, antedependence, autoregressive mov-ing average, or nonparametric and semiparametric approaches (Yap et al. 2009; Li et al. 2010). Because of its favorable properties, a tri-variate SAD(1) model can be used in systems mapping (see Wu and Hou 2005, 2006; Zhao et al. 2005a, b; Jiang et al. 2018b). Below, we provide the closed forms of the inverse and determinant of the SAD(1)-structured covariance matrix.

We use simple notation to simplify the description. Given two variables x and y, we denote their residual errors at time t ($t=1, \ldots, T$) by $e_1(t)$ and $e_2(t)$ (the variances of which are $\sigma_x^2(t)$ and $\sigma_y^2(t)$) and innovation errors $\varepsilon_1(t)$ and $\varepsilon_2(t)$ (the variances of which are $\delta_x^2(t)$ and $\delta_y^2(t)$ and the correlation of which is $\phi(t)$). Let ρ_x (ρ_y) denote the coefficient of the first-order antedependence for x (y) variable and ψ_x (ψ_y) denote the coefficient of the first antedependence of x (y)

on y (x). For a bivariate SAD(1)-structured covariance matrix Σ, it is positive definite if and only if a unique low triangle matrix $\mathbf{L}$ and a diagonal matrix Σ_ε exist such that $\mathbf{L\Sigma L}^T = \Sigma_\varepsilon$, where we have

$$
\mathbf{L} = \begin{pmatrix} \mathbf{I} & 0 & \cdots & 0 & 0 \\ -\mathbf{V} & \mathbf{I} & \cdots & 0 & 0 \\ 0 & -\mathbf{V} & \cdots & 0 & 0 \\ \vdots & \vdots & \ddots & \vdots & \vdots \\ 0 & 0 & \cdots & -\mathbf{V} & \mathbf{I} \end{pmatrix}, \Sigma_\varepsilon = \begin{pmatrix} \Sigma_\varepsilon(1) & 0 & \cdots & 0 \\ 0 & \Sigma_\varepsilon(2) & \cdots & 0 \\ \vdots & \vdots & \ddots & \vdots \\ 0 & 0 & \cdots & \Sigma_\varepsilon(T) \end{pmatrix},
$$

with

$$
\mathbf{V} = \begin{pmatrix} \rho_x & \psi_x \\ \psi_y & \rho_y \end{pmatrix} \text{ and } \mathbf{I} = \begin{pmatrix} 1 & 0 \\ 0 & 1 \end{pmatrix}
$$

Given that matrix $\mathbf{L}$ is nonsingular and matrix Σ_ε is positive semidefinite, it can be shown that

$$
|\Sigma|^{-1/2} = |\Sigma_\varepsilon|^{-1/2} = \prod_{t=1}^{T}\left[\sqrt{1 - \varphi^2(t)}\delta_x(t)\delta_y(t) \right]^{-1} \text{ and}
$$

$$
\Sigma^{-1} = \mathbf{L}^T\Sigma_\varepsilon^{-1}\mathbf{L}
$$

$$
= \begin{pmatrix} \Sigma_\varepsilon^{-1}(1) + \mathbf{V}^T\Sigma_\varepsilon^{-1}(2)\mathbf{V} & -\mathbf{V}^T\Sigma_\varepsilon^{-1}(1) & \cdots & 0 & 0 \\ -\Sigma_\varepsilon^{-1}(2)\mathbf{V} & \Sigma_\varepsilon^{-1}(2) + \mathbf{V}^T\Sigma_\varepsilon^{-1}(3)\mathbf{V} & \cdots & 0 & 0 \\ 0 & -\Sigma_\varepsilon^{-1}(3)\mathbf{V} & \cdots & 0 & 0 \\ \vdots & \vdots & \ddots & \vdots & \vdots \\ 0 & 0 & \cdots & -\Sigma_\varepsilon^{-1}(T-1)\mathbf{V} & \Sigma_\varepsilon^{-1}(T) \end{pmatrix}
$$

$$
= \Lambda_1 + \Lambda_2 + \Lambda_3 + \Lambda_3^T
$$

where

$$
\Lambda_1 = \begin{pmatrix} \Sigma_\varepsilon^{-1}(1) & 0 & \cdots & 0 \\ 0 & \Sigma_\varepsilon^{-1}(2) & \cdots & 0 \\ \vdots & \vdots & \ddots & \vdots \\ 0 & 0 & \cdots & \Sigma_\varepsilon^{-1}(T) \end{pmatrix}
$$

$$\Lambda_2 = \begin{pmatrix} \mathbf{V}^T\mathbf{\Sigma}_\varepsilon^{-1}(2)\mathbf{V} & 0 & \cdots & 0 & 0 \\ 0 & \mathbf{V}^T\mathbf{\Sigma}_\varepsilon^{-1}(3)\mathbf{V} & \cdots & 0 & 0 \\ \vdots & \vdots & \ddots & \vdots & \vdots \\ 0 & 0 & \cdots & \mathbf{V}^T\mathbf{\Sigma}_\varepsilon^{-1}(T)\mathbf{V} & 0 \\ 0 & 0 & \cdots & 0 & 0 \end{pmatrix}$$

$$\Lambda_3 = \begin{pmatrix} 0 & 0 & \cdots & 0 & 0 \\ -\mathbf{\Sigma}_\varepsilon^{-1}(2)\mathbf{V} & 0 & \cdots & 0 & 0 \\ 0 & -\mathbf{\Sigma}_\varepsilon^{-1}(3)\mathbf{V} & \cdots & 0 & 0 \\ \vdots & \vdots & \ddots & \vdots & \vdots \\ 0 & 0 & \cdots & -\mathbf{\Sigma}_\varepsilon^{-1}(T)\mathbf{V} & 0 \end{pmatrix}$$

Combining two variables $\mathbf{x}_i = (x_i(1), ..., x_i(T))$ and $\mathbf{y}_i = (y_i(1), ..., y_i(T))$ into one vector, $\mathbf{z}_i = (\mathbf{z}_i(1); ...; \mathbf{z}_i(T)) \equiv (x_i(1), y_i(1); ..., x_i(T), y_i(T))$, we divide the quadratic form $\mathbf{z}_i \mathbf{\Sigma}^{-1} \mathbf{z}_i^T$ into the following three parts:

$$\mathbf{z}_i \mathbf{\Sigma}^{-1} \mathbf{z}_i^T = \mathbf{z}_i \Lambda_1 \mathbf{z}_i^T + \mathbf{z}_i \Lambda_2 \mathbf{z}_i^T + 2\mathbf{z}_i \Lambda_3 \mathbf{z}_i^T$$

where

$$\mathbf{z}_i \Lambda_1 \mathbf{z}_i^T = \sum_{t=1}^{T} \mathbf{z}_i(t) \mathbf{\Sigma}_\varepsilon^{-1}(t) \mathbf{z}_i^T(t)$$

$$\mathbf{z}_i \Lambda_2 \mathbf{z}_i^T = \sum_{t=1}^{T-1} \mathbf{z}_i(t) \mathbf{V} \mathbf{\Sigma}_\varepsilon^{-1}(t+1) \mathbf{V}^T \mathbf{z}_i^T(t)$$

$$\mathbf{z}_i \Lambda_3 \mathbf{z}_i^T = \sum_{t=1}^{T-1} \mathbf{z}_i(t+1) \mathbf{\Sigma}_\varepsilon^{-1}(t+1) \mathbf{V}^T \mathbf{z}_i^T(t)$$

The above procedure can be readily extended to derive the closed forms of the determinant and inverse of covariance matrix among three variables.

Fitted by a system of ODEs and SAD(1), the likelihood given in equation (5.3) is solved by implementing a hybrid of the fourth-order Runge-Kutta algorithm and the Simplex algorithm. Ultimately, we obtain the MLEs of genotype-dependent ODE parameters and SAD(1)-structuring parameters.

5.3.3 Hypothesis Tests

Next, we need to test whether a given SNP functions as a QTL, which is significantly associated with the PK-PD process. This can be conducted by formulating the null and alternative hypotheses as follows:

$H_0 : (k_{mj}, V_{maxj}, V_j, k_{inj}, k_{outj}, H_j, E_{maxj}, EC_{50j})^0 (k_m, V_{max}, V, k_{in}, k_{out}, H, E_{max}, EC_{50})$

H_1: At least one equality in the H_0 does not hold

(5.6)

for $j=2, 1, 0$. Under each hypothesis, we estimate the MLEs of model parameters and plug in these MLEs into the likelihood. Let L_0 denote the likelihood under the null hypothesis, i.e., there is no QTL, and L_1 denote the likelihood under the alternative hypothesis, i.e., there is a QTL. The likelihood ratio (LR) is calculated as

$$LR = -2(\ln L_0 - \ln L_1)$$ (5.7)

which is compared with the critical threshold determined empirically from permutation tests. We claim that an SNP is a significant QTL if its LR is larger than the threshold.

In the PK/PD models, different parameters have different mechanistic interpretations. Systems mapping allows the genetic control of each parameter or parameter combination to be tested. In practice, it is interesting to test how a QTL differently control PK and PD processes. This can be tested by the two hypotheses as follows:

$$H_0 : (k_{mj}, V_{maxj}, V_j)^0 (k_m, V_{max}, V) \text{ vs. } H_1 : (k_{mj}, V_{maxj}, V_j)^1 (k_m, V_{max}, V)$$ (5.8)

$$H_0 : (k_{inj}, k_{outj}, H_j, E_{maxj}, EC_{50j})^0 (k_{in}, k_{out}, H, E_{max}, EC_{50}) \text{ vs.}$$
$$H_1 : (k_{inj}, k_{outj}, H_j, E_{maxj}, EC_{50j})^1 (k_{in}, k_{out}, H, E_{max}, EC_{50})$$ (5.9)

If the null hypotheses of both equations (5.8) and (5.9) are rejected, this means that this is a pleiotropic QTL that simultaneously controls PK and PD processes. If the null hypothesis of equation (5.8) is rejected but the null hypothesis of equation (5.9) is accepted, this means that this QTL is PK-specific. Likewise, whether this QTL is PD-specific can be tested.

5.3.4 Computer Simulation

We perform Monte Carlo simulation to examine the statistical properties of systems mapping for drug response. Consider a panel of n subjects randomly drawn from an equilibrium human population. The panel is genotyped for genome-wide SNPs. The sampled subjects are administered by a drug to treat a disease. To simulate PK-PD phenotypic data, we assume that the time-dependent genotypic means at an SNP are determined by equation (5.2), plus

TABLE 5.1

ODE Parameters and Covariance-Structuring SAD(1) Parameters Used to Simulate the Measurement Data of the Q-C-R Drug Response System

	ODE Parameters							
	K_m	V_{max}	V	K_{in}	k_{out}	E_{max}	H	EC_{50}
AA	0.70	0.70	5.0	0.30	0.20	10	0.80	1.0
Aa	0.60	0.60	4.0	0.40	0.30	6	0.60	0.7
Aa	0.65	0.65	4.5	0.25	0.15	8	1.30	0.8
	SAD(1) Parameters							
	ρ_Q	ρ_C	ρ_Q	ψ_Q	ψ_C	ψ_R	ϕ_{QC}	ϕ_{CR}	ϕ_{CR}
$H^2=0.1$	1.3	1.3	1.3	0.6	0.002	0.02	0.5	0.6	0.7
$H^2=0.4$	1.2	1.2	1.2	0.5	0.001	0.03	0.5	06	0.7

the residual errors that follow a multivariate normal distribution with mean vector **0** and subject-specific covariance Σ_i with the SAD(1) structure. The size of variance is determined by a given heritability (H^2). The phenotypic data are the amount of the drug in the GI tract (Q) (mg), the plasma concentration of the drug (C) (mg/l), and drug response (R) at T time points after drug administration. To make the simulated Q-C-R system approach the reality, we choose and determine clinically meaningful PK and PD parameters (k_m, V_{max}, V, k_{in}, k_{out}, H, E_{max}, EC_{50}) for three different genotypes from real pharmacological studies (Kristensen et al. 2005; Wang et al. 2008), which are given in Table 5.1. Our simulation includes multiple scenarios by changing (n, T, H^2) on their spaces.

We use the procedure as described above to estimate the model parameters that define the likelihood of equation (5.3). All parameters related to PK and PD processes can be reasonably well estimated for the heritability of $H^2=0.1$ and a given sample size of $n=200$ (Table 5.2). As expected, the precision of parameter estimation increases when heritability increases to 0.4. These results confirm our previous estimates for different biological systems, such as circadian rhythm, by systems mapping (Fu et al. 2010). Figure 5.2 shows how well ODEs of equation (5.1) fit the simulated data. To further show how the dynamic behavior of PK and PD processes can be characterized by systems mapping, we use the estimated ODE parameters to draw genotype-dependent time-varying change curves for each process, in a comparison with those by true parameters (Figure 5.3). We find that systems mapping can generally well capture PK and PD behaviors even when there is a modest heritability (0.1) (Figure 5.3a). The accuracy and precision of curve estimates can increase dramatically with heritability (Figure 5.3b). In general, a sample size of 200 is needed to obtain the reasonable estimation precision of PK-PD systems for each genotype at an SNP.

TABLE 5.2

MLEs of Genotype-Dependent PK-PD ODE Parameters and Covariance-Structuring SAD(1) Parameters and the Standard Deviations (in Parentheses) from Simulated Data under Different Heritabilities and a Sample Size of $n=200$

	AA		Aa		aa	
Parameters	True	MLE (SE)	True	MLE (SE)	True	MLE (SE)
$H^2=0.1$						
k_m	0.700	0.078 (0.052)	0.600	0.562 (0.044)	0.650	0.626 (0.059)
V_{max}	0.700	0.703 (0.002)	0.600	0.601 (0.002)	0.650	0.649 (0.002)
V	5.000	5.437 (0.284)	4.000	3.823 (0.210)	4.500	4.385 (0.292)
k_{in}	0.300	0.291 (0.013)	0.400	0.336 (0.019)	0.250	0.275 (0.022)
k_{out}	0.200	0.194 (0.008)	0.300	0.252 (0.014)	0.150	0.165 (0.013)
E_{max}	10.000	9.345 (0.379)	6.000	5.659 (0.330)	8.000	8.275 (0.614)
H	0.800	0.771 (0.030)	0.600	0.613 (0.078)	1.300	1.248 (0.152)
EC_{50}	1.000	0.962 (0.085)	0.700	0.615 (0.141)	0.800	1.065 (0.236)
d_Q	1.300	1.292 (0.008)	1.300	1.292 (0.008)	1.300	1.292 (0.008)
d_C	1.300	1.292 (0.009)	1.300	1.292 (0.009)	1.300	1.292 (0.009)
d_R	1.300	1.292 (0.008)	1.300	1.292 (0.008)	1.300	1.292 (0.008)
$\hbar_Q$	0.600	0.613 (0.033)	0.600	0.613 (0.033)	0.600	0.613 (0.033)
$\hbar_C$	0.002	0.002 (0.000)	0.002	0.002 (0.000)	0.002	0.002 (0.000)
$\hbar_R$	0.500	0.020 (0.001)	0.500	0.020 (0.001)	0.500	0.020 (0.001)
ϕ_{QC}	0.500	0.499 (0.049)	0.500	0.499 (0.049)	0.500	0.499 (0.049)
ϕ_{QR}	0.600	0.600 (0.045)	0.600	0.600 (0.045)	0.600	0.600 (0.045)
ϕ_{CR}	0.700	0.703 (0.031)	0.700	0.703 (0.031)	0.700	0.703 (0.031)
$H^2=0.4$						
k_m	0.700	0.670 (0.037)	0.600	0.570 (0.019)	0.650	0.628 (0.046)
V_{max}	0.700	0.699 (0.002)	0.600	0.600 (0.001)	0.650	0.650 (0.001)
V	5.000	4.832 (0.205)	4.000	3.858 (0.088)	4.500	4.384 (0.235)
k_{in}	0.300	0.315 (0.015)	0.400	0.376 (0.026)	0.250	0.256 (0.033)
k_{out}	0.200	0.210 (0.001)	0.300	0.282 (0.020)	0.150	0.154 (0.019)
E_{max}	10.000	9.484 (0.378)	6.000	6.263 (0.019)	8.000	8.084 (0.424)
H	0.800	0.786 (0.032)	0.600	0.619 (0.424)	1.300	1.252 (0.136)
EC_{50}	1.000	0.986 (0.088)	0.700	0.689 (0.136)	0.800	0.912 (0.177)
ρ_Q	1.200	1.213 (0.014)	1.200	1.213 (0.014)	1.200	1.213 (0.014)
ρ_C	1.200	1.213 (0.014)	1.200	1.213 (0.014)	1.200	1.213 (0.014)
ρ_R	1.200	1.213 (0.014)	1.200	1.213 (0.014)	1.200	1.213 (0.014)
ψ_Q	0.500	0.508 (0.014)	0.500	0.508 (0.014)	0.500	0.508 (0.014)
ψ_C	0.001	0.001 (0.000)	0.001	0.001 (0.000)	0.001	0.001 (0.000)
ψ_R	0.300	0.030 (0.001)	0.300	0.030 (0.001)	0.300	0.030 (0.001)
ϕ_{QC}	0.500	0.492 (0.042)	0.500	0.492 (0.042)	0.500	0.492 (0.042)
ϕ_{QR}	0.600	0.596 (0.042)	0.600	0.596 (0.042)	0.600	0.596 (0.042)
ϕ_{CR}	0.700	0.699 (0.027)	0.700	0.699 (0.027)	0.700	0.699 (0.027)

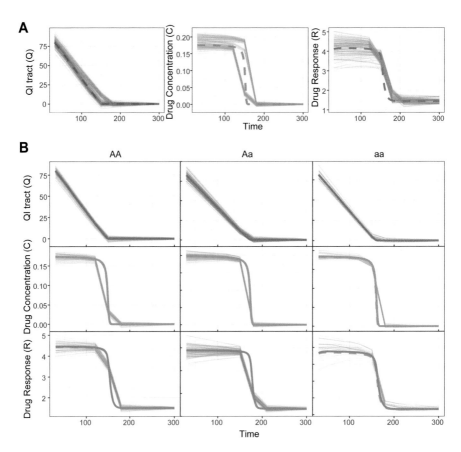

FIGURE 5.2
The goodness-of-fitness of a coupled PK-PD ODE model to simulated data. (a) curve fitness under the null hypothesis (there is no QTL). (b) curve fitness under the alternative hypothesis (this is a QTL with three genotypes *AA, Aa,* and *aa*). The data are simulated under $H^2 = 0.4$ and a sample size of $n = 200$.

5.4 Stochastic Systems Mapping

5.4.1 Why Stochastic Modeling in Drug Response

Substantial interindividual variability occurs in drug efficacy and toxicity for most patient populations. For example, while many patients are beneficial for a drug, there often exist a proportion of patients who does not respond, responds only partially, or encounters adverse drug reactions to drugs (Eichelbaum et al. 2006). In some circumstance, drug concentrations in plasma can differ by more than 600-fold between two patients of the same

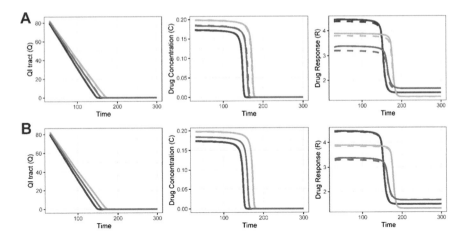

FIGURE 5.3
Estimated PK-PD curves (dash line) for three different QTL genotypes *AA, Aa,* and *aa,* in a comparison with the true curves (solid line), under $H^2=0.1$ (a) and 0.4 (b) and a sample size of $n=200$.

weight treated with the same drug dosage. This variation can be attributed to a drug's physicochemical (e.g., passive diffusion) and biochemical properties (e.g., interactions with metabolizing enzymes and transporters) (Iyengar et al. 2012; Yamashita and Hashida 2013), jointly determined by genes and the environment (Evans and McLeod 2013; Weinshilboum 2003; Ben-David et al. 2018).

Genetic and environmental factors affect the response of individuals to a drug by altering its absorption, distribution, metabolism, and interactions with molecular targets within the PK and PD machinery (Iyengar et al. 2012). As a theory that can reveal the mechanisms and processes of drug reactions in the body, PK/PD principles have been applied to the safe and effective therapeutic management of drugs for an individual patient (Yamashita and Hashida 2013). By treating drug-body interactions as a dynamic system, a number of ODEs have been developed to characterize the dynamic behavior of PK/PD processes (Mager et al. 2003; Macheras and Iliadis 2006; Wang et al. 2008). These ODEs have been instrumental for the prediction of drug response from the physiology and biochemistry of drug action (Lu et al. 2021; Truong et al. 2022). As illustrated in the preceding section, the integration of PK/PD-based ODEs into systems mapping provides a powerful tool to unravel the genetic architecture of drug response.

Since ODEs are derived under the assumption that observed kinetics and dynamics are driven through internal deterministic mechanisms, their applications may be limited in real pharmacological processes in which random fluctuations affect the relationship between drug effect and drug concentration (Kristensen et al. 2005). Tremendous efforts have been made to extend the deterministic models to SDEs, where one or more of the terms are modeled as a stochastic process (Ditlevsen and Gaetano 2005; Donnet and Samson 2013; Ben-David et al. 2018). D'Argenio and Park (1997) and Ramanathan (1999a, b) are among the first who incorporated random fluctuations into the PK/PD models. More sophisticated stochastic models that include multiple compartments, nonlinear or time-inhomogeneous absorption or elimination have been available through collective work of many mathematical biologists (Ferrante et al. 2005; Tornøe et al. 2004; Ditlevsen and Gaetano 2005; Picchini et al. 2006). The approaches for estimating the curve parameters that specify a group of SDEs using observed data at discrete time points have been proposed (Sørensen 2004). Donnet et al. (2010) developed a Bayesian method to estimate SDE-based mixed model parameters using PK/PD data, typical of high sparsity and subject-dependent measure schedule. A review of the estimation of SDEs in PK/PD models is given by Donnet and Samson (2013).

In this section, we introduce an SDE-based systems mapping model for characterizing the pharmacogenetic architecture of drug response. The main part of the model was described in Wang et al. (2013d). The application of the model to a real data analysis was reported in Gan (2021). The advantages of SDE-based system mapping include its capacity to more precisely elucidate the genetic control mechanisms of drug response by integrating random fluctuations. We implement an EM algorithm to estimate genotype-specific SDE parameters that characterize the process of drug reactions. The model allows the interplay between pharmacogenes and PK/PD processes to be tested in a quantitative way. Results from computer simulation suggest that this model has reasonably good statistical properties and can be used in practice. This model could potentially help pharmaceutic researchers choose optimal drugs and drug dosage by matching the genetic makeup of individual patients and their living environment.

5.4.2 Stochastic Modeling of Dynamic Systems

Consider a dynamic system that can be described by m traits or variables with time-varying continuous changes. The global interrelationship among these traits and its impact on system behavior can be quantified by a set of nonlinear ODEs, expressed as

$$\frac{d\mathbf{x}_t}{dt} = \mathbf{f}(\mathbf{x}_t, t, \theta), \quad \mathbf{x}(t_0) = \mathbf{x}_0(\theta) \tag{5.10}$$

where $\mathbf{x}_t = (x_{t1}, \ldots, x_{tm})$ denote the values of m traits at time t, θ is the parameter vector, and $\mathbf{f}$ is a function that specifies the underlying dynamic features of the system. The values of traits at time $t=0$, $\mathbf{x}(t_0)$, are the initial values that can be described by the parameter vector θ.

The ODE model in equation (5.10) is powerful for describing a deterministic system, but it fails to disentangle the complexity of a stochastic system in which some parts, e.g., traits and/or their relationships, are perturbed by random errors (Leander et al. 2014). To capture these random perturbations, we need to add to this model a stochastic part, referred to as the system noise or diffusion. In so doing, we extend ODEs to SDEs. The system noise can capture all the unknown phenomena that are unobservable to the deterministic model. A general SDE model is written as

$$d\mathbf{x}_t = \mathbf{f}(\mathbf{x}_t, t, \theta)dt + \Sigma(\mathbf{x}_t, t, \theta)d\mathbf{w}_t, \ \ \mathbf{x}(t_0) = \mathbf{x}_0(\theta) \tag{5.11}$$

where the second term is the system noise composed of scale terms $\Sigma(\mathbf{x}_t, t, \theta)$ and $\mathbf{w}_t$, a standard q-dimensional Wiener process (also known as Brownian motion). Note that $\Sigma = 0$ corresponds to the ODE model (5.10).

The dynamic system can be measured by sampling it at discrete time points ($t_1, \ldots, t_{k-1}, t_k, t_{k+1}, \ldots, t_T$). Measurement errors follow Gaussian white noise process. Let $\mathbf{y}_k = \left(y_1(t_k), \ldots, y_m(t_k)\right)$ denote the vector of variable values measured at time t_k. The measured system can be described by

$$d\mathbf{x}_k = \mathbf{f}\left(\mathbf{x}_{t_k}, t_k, \theta\right)dt + \Sigma(\mathbf{x}_t, t, \theta)d\mathbf{w}_{t_k}, \ \ k = 1, \ldots, T \tag{5.12a}$$

$$\mathbf{y}_k = \mathbf{h}\left(\mathbf{x}_{t_k}, t_k, \theta\right) + \mathbf{e}_k \tag{5.12b}$$

where $\mathbf{h}$ is a function describing the measurement structure and $\mathbf{e}_k$ is an l-dimensional white noise process with $\mathbf{e}_k \sim N\left(0, \mathbf{S}(t_k, \theta)\right)$.

5.4.3 Parameter Estimation of SDEs

We introduce a probabilistic approach for estimating the parameters in θ that define the SDE model of equation (5.11) from a set of measurements. This approach aims to find the parameters that maximize the likelihood function of a given set of measurements. We describe this approach mostly following Leander et al. (2014). Let $\boldsymbol{y}_T = (\mathbf{y}_T, \ldots, \mathbf{y}_k, \ldots, \mathbf{y}_1)$ denote the whole set of measurements. Let

$$\boldsymbol{y}_k \triangleq \left\{y_k, \ldots, y_1\right\} \tag{5.13}$$

denote the set of measurements up to time point t_k. The likelihood function of the whole measurements is written as

$$L\left(\theta; \boldsymbol{y}_T\right) \triangleq p(\boldsymbol{y}_T \mid \theta) \tag{5.14}$$

which is a conditional probability of $\boldsymbol{y}_T$ given the parameter vector θ. By repeatedly using the Bayes law, the likelihood function can be rewritten as

$$L(\theta;\boldsymbol{y}_T) = \left(\prod_{k=2}^{T} p(\mathbf{y}_k \mid \boldsymbol{y}_{k-1}, \theta) \right) p(\boldsymbol{y}_1 \mid \theta) \tag{5.15}$$

Although it is computationally infeasible to evaluate this likelihood function, it may be reasonable to assume that the conditional densities can be approximated by Gaussian densities since the increments of Wiener processes that drive the differential equations are Gaussian (Kristensen and Madsen 2010). These densities of the output variables are characterized by their means and covariances, expressed as

$$\hat{\boldsymbol{y}}_{k|k-1} \triangleq \mathrm{E}\left\{ \mathbf{y}_k \mid \boldsymbol{y}_{k-1}, \theta \right\} \tag{5.16}$$

$$\mathbf{R}_{k|k-1} \triangleq \mathrm{Var}\left\{ \mathbf{y}_k \mid \boldsymbol{y}_{k-1}, \theta \right\} \tag{5.17}$$

With these means and covariances, we express the likelihood function of equation (5.15) as

$$L(\theta;\boldsymbol{y}_T) = \prod_{k=2}^{T} \left(\frac{\exp\left(-\frac{1}{2} \epsilon_k^T \mathbf{R}_{k|k-1}^{-1} \epsilon_k \right)}{\sqrt{\det\left(\mathbf{R}_{k|k-1} \right)} \left(\sqrt{2\pi} \right)^l} \right) p(\boldsymbol{y}_1 \mid \theta) \tag{5.18}$$

where $\epsilon_k = \mathbf{y}_k - \hat{\boldsymbol{y}}_{k|k-1}$. By taking the negative logarithm, we have the negative log-likelihood as

$$\mathcal{L}(\theta) = \mathcal{L}(\theta;\boldsymbol{y}_T) = -\ln\left(L(\theta;\boldsymbol{y}_T) \right)$$

$$= \frac{1}{2} \sum_{k=1}^{T} \left(\ln(\det\left(\mathbf{R}_{k|k-1} \right)) + \epsilon_k^T \mathbf{R}_{k|k-1}^{-1} \epsilon_k + l\ln\left(2\pi \right) \right) \tag{5.19}$$

which is to be minimized with respect to the parameter vector θ. Note that $\mathbf{R}_{1|0}$ corresponds to the initial covariances. Several local minima may exist for the function (5.19) because it depends on the parameters θ in a nonlinear way. Optimization techniques need to be carefully implemented to obtain a global minimum.

5.4.4 Extended Kalman Filter (EKF)

In order to estimate the residuals ϵ_k and output covariances $\mathbf{R}_{k|k-1}$, we need to estimate the state $(\hat{\mathbf{x}}_{k|k})$ and covariance of the system $(\mathbf{P}_{k|k})$ given measurements and the underlying structure of the system. Since the states change randomly due to the stochastic fluctuations in the Wiener process, we implement the EKF, which is a state estimator in nonlinear continuous-discrete state space models with the form given in equations (5.12a) and (5.12b) (Jazwinski 1970). For a linear dynamic system, the Kalman filter can provide an optimal estimate of the state for a given parameter vector θ (Kalman 1960). When the system is nonlinear, the EKF uses a first-order linear approximation of the model under the assumption that there is no state-dependent expression of the system noise Σ.

The EKF estimates the conditional expectation of the state $\hat{\mathbf{x}}_{k|k} = E\{\mathbf{x}_{t_k} | \mathbf{y}_k, \theta\}$ and its covariance $\mathbf{P}_{k|k} = \text{Var}\{\mathbf{x}_{t_k} | \mathbf{y}_k, \theta\}$. This process is described as follows. Given initial conditions $\hat{\mathbf{x}}_{1|0} = \mathbf{x}_0$ and $\mathbf{P}_{1|0} = \mathbf{P}_0$ and linearization:

$$\mathbf{A}_t = \frac{\partial \mathbf{f}}{\partial \mathbf{x}_t}\Big|_{\mathbf{x}_t = \hat{\mathbf{x}}_{t|k}} \tag{5.20}$$

$$\mathbf{C}_t = \frac{\partial \mathbf{h}}{\partial \mathbf{x}_t}\Big|_{\mathbf{x}_t = \hat{\mathbf{x}}_{t|k-1}} \tag{5.21}$$

the states and state covariances between two consecutive measurement time points can be predicted according to

$$\frac{d\hat{\mathbf{x}}_{t|k}}{dt} = \mathbf{f}\left(\hat{\mathbf{x}}_{t|k}, t, \theta\right), \quad t \in [t_k, t_{k+1}] \tag{5.22}$$

$$\frac{d\mathbf{P}_{t|k}}{dt} = \mathbf{A}_t \mathbf{P}_{t|k} + \mathbf{P}_{t|k} \mathbf{A}_k^T + \Sigma\Sigma^T, \quad t \in [t_k, t_{k+1}] \tag{5.23}$$

In a general case, $\mathbf{A}_t = \mathbf{A}_t\left(\hat{\mathbf{x}}_{t|k}, \theta\right)$, which implies that

$$\frac{d\mathbf{A}_t}{d\theta_u} = \frac{\partial \mathbf{A}_t}{\partial \hat{\mathbf{x}}_{t|k}} \frac{d\hat{\mathbf{x}}_{t|k}}{d\theta_u} + \frac{\partial \mathbf{A}_t}{\partial \theta_u}$$

From the predicted states and state covariances, the output prediction equations can be formulated as

$$\hat{\mathbf{y}}_{k|k-1} = \mathbf{h}\left(\hat{\mathbf{x}}_{k|k-1}, t_k, \theta\right) \tag{5.24}$$

$$\mathbf{R}_{k|k-1} = \mathbf{C}_k \mathbf{P}_{k|k-1} \mathbf{C}_k^T + \mathbf{S} \tag{5.25}$$

Also, in a general case $\mathbf{C}_k = \mathbf{C}_k\left(\hat{\mathbf{x}}_{t|k}, \theta\right)$, from which we have

$$\frac{d\mathbf{C}_k}{d\theta_u} = \frac{\partial \mathbf{C}_k}{\partial \hat{\mathbf{x}}_{t|k}} \frac{d\hat{\mathbf{x}}_{t|k}}{d\theta_u} + \frac{\partial \mathbf{C}_k}{\partial \theta_u}$$

From the state covariances $\mathbf{P}_{k|k-1}$ and measurement covariances $\mathbf{R}_{k|k-1}$, the Kalman gain is given by

$$\mathbf{K}_k = \mathbf{P}_{k|k-1}\mathbf{C}_k^T\mathbf{R}_{k|k-1}^{-1} \tag{5.26}$$

Finally, the states and its covariances are updated according to

$$\hat{\mathbf{x}}_{k|k} = \hat{\mathbf{x}}_{k|k-1} + \mathbf{K}_k\epsilon_k \tag{5.27}$$

$$\mathbf{P}_{k|k} = \mathbf{P}_{k|k-1} - \mathbf{K}_k\mathbf{R}_{k|k-1}\mathbf{K}_k^T \tag{5.28}$$

The Kalman gain $\mathbf{K}_k$ combines the state covariance and output covariance. If there is no system noise, we have $\Sigma = 0$ so that we trust the model completely. If there is no measurement variance, we have $\mathbf{S}=0$ so that we trust the measurements completely. Because the measurements are longitudinal, the covariance matrix of measurement errors S contains a certain structure which can be fitted by a parsimonious approach, such as autoregressive models, antedependence models, autoregressive moving average models, and nonparametric and semiparametric approaches (Yap et al. 2009; Li et al. 2010).

5.4.5 Differentiation of EKF Equations

The parameter vector θ that explains the underlying structure of the stochastic system can be estimated by minimizing the nonlinear objective function $\mathcal{L}(\theta)$ of equation (5.19). The objective function $\mathcal{L}(\theta)$ is differentiated with respect to the uth component of the parameter vector θ. We have

$$\frac{\mathcal{L}(\theta)}{d\theta_u} = \frac{1}{2}\sum_{k=1}^{T}\left(\frac{d\epsilon_k^T}{d\theta_u}\mathbf{R}_{k|k-1}^{-1}\epsilon_k + \epsilon_k^T\frac{d\mathbf{R}_{k|k-1}^{-1}}{d\theta_u}\epsilon_k + \epsilon_k^T\mathbf{R}_{k|k-1}^{-1}\frac{d\epsilon_k}{d\theta_u} + \frac{d\ln(\det(\mathbf{R}_{k|k-1}))}{d\theta_u} \right) \tag{5.29}$$

Since

$$\frac{d\mathbf{R}^{-1}}{d\theta_u} = -\mathbf{R}^{-1}\frac{d\mathbf{R}}{d\theta_u}\mathbf{R}^{-1}$$

and

$$\frac{d\ln(\det(\mathbf{R}_{k|k-1}))}{d\theta_u} = Tr\left(\mathbf{R}_{k|k-1}^{-1}\frac{d\mathbf{R}_{k|k-1}}{d\theta_u} \right)$$

the uth component $\dfrac{\mathcal{L}(\theta)}{d\theta_u}$ of the gradient has the final expression:

$$\frac{\mathcal{L}(\theta)}{d\theta_u} = \frac{1}{2}\sum_{k=1}^{T}\left(\frac{d\epsilon_k^T}{d\theta_u}\mathbf{R}_{k|k-1}^{-1}\epsilon_k - \epsilon_k^T\mathbf{R}_{k|k-1}^{-1}\frac{d\mathbf{R}_{k|k-1}^{-1}}{d\theta_u}\epsilon_k\right.$$

$$+\ \epsilon_k^T\mathbf{R}_{k|k-1}^{-1}\frac{d\epsilon_k}{d\theta_u} \tag{5.30}$$

$$+\ d\ln\left(\det\mathbf{R}_{k|k-1}\right)d\theta_u$$

To calculate this gradient, we need to calculate the partial derivatives $\dfrac{d\epsilon_k}{d\theta_u}$

and $\dfrac{d\mathbf{R}_{k|k-1}}{d\theta_u}$, which are obtained from the sensitive analysis of the EKF equation. The sensitive equations can be yielded from the differentiation of the state predictions in equations (5.22) and (5.23), expressed as

$$\frac{d}{dt}\frac{d\hat{\mathbf{x}}_{t|k}}{d\theta_u} = \frac{\partial\mathbf{f}}{\partial\hat{\mathbf{x}}_{t|k}}\frac{d\hat{\mathbf{x}}_{t|k}}{d\theta_u} + \frac{\partial\mathbf{f}}{\partial\theta_u},\quad t\in[t_k,t_{k+1}] \tag{5.31}$$

$$\frac{d}{dt}\frac{d\mathbf{P}_{t|k}}{d\theta_u} = \frac{d\mathbf{A}_t}{d\hat{\mathbf{x}}_{t|k}}\mathbf{P}_{t|k} + \mathbf{A}_t\frac{d\mathbf{P}_{t|k}}{d\theta_u} + \frac{d\mathbf{P}_{t|k}}{d\theta_u}\mathbf{A}_t^T + \mathbf{P}_{t|k}\frac{d\mathbf{A}_t^T}{d\theta_u} + \frac{d\Sigma\Sigma^T}{d\theta_u},\quad t\in[t_k,t_{k+1}] \tag{5.32}$$

Likewise, we obtain the derivatives of the output prediction in equation (5.24) and (5.25) as

$$\frac{d\hat{\mathbf{y}}_{k|k-1}}{d\theta_u} = \frac{\partial\mathbf{h}}{\partial\hat{\mathbf{x}}_{k|k-1}}\frac{d\hat{\mathbf{x}}_{k|k-1}}{d\theta_u} + \frac{\partial\mathbf{h}}{\partial\theta_u} \tag{5.33}$$

$$\frac{d\mathbf{R}_{k|k-1}}{d\theta_u} = \frac{d\mathbf{C}_k}{d\theta_u}\mathbf{P}_{k|k-1}\mathbf{C}_k^T + \mathbf{C}_k\frac{d\mathbf{P}_{k|k-1}}{d\theta_u}\mathbf{C}_k^T + \mathbf{C}_k\mathbf{P}_{k|k-1}\frac{d\mathbf{C}_k^T}{d\theta_u} + \frac{\partial\mathbf{S}}{\partial\theta_u} \tag{5.34}$$

We differentiate the Kalman gain in equation (5.26) and the residual $\epsilon_k = \mathbf{y}_k - \hat{\mathbf{y}}_{k|k-1}$ as

$$\frac{d\mathbf{K}_k}{d\theta_u} = \frac{d\mathbf{P}_{k|k-1}}{d\theta_u}\mathbf{C}_k^T\mathbf{R}_{k|k-1}^{-1} + \mathbf{P}_{k|k-1}\frac{d\mathbf{C}_k^T}{d\theta_u}\mathbf{R}_{k|k-1}^{-1} + \mathbf{P}_{k|k-1}\mathbf{C}_k^T\frac{d\mathbf{R}_{k|k-1}^{-1}}{d\theta_u} \tag{5.35}$$

$$\frac{d\epsilon_k}{d\theta_u} = -\frac{d\hat{\mathbf{y}}_{k|k-1}}{d\theta_u} \tag{5.36}$$

Lastly, we differentiate the updating state and state covariance in equations (5.27) and (5.28) as

$$\frac{d\hat{\mathbf{x}}_{k|k}}{d\theta_u} = \frac{d\hat{\mathbf{x}}_{k|k-1}}{d\theta_u} + \frac{d\mathbf{K}_k}{d\theta_u}\epsilon_k + \mathbf{K}_k\frac{d\epsilon_k}{d\theta_u} \tag{5.37}$$

$$\frac{d\mathbf{P}_{k|k}}{d\theta_u} = \frac{d\mathbf{P}_{k|k-1}}{d\theta_u} - \frac{d\mathbf{K}_k}{d\theta_u}\mathbf{R}_{k|k-1}\mathbf{K}_k^{\mathrm{T}} - \mathbf{K}_k\frac{d\mathbf{R}_{k|k-1}}{d\theta_u}\mathbf{K}_k^{\mathrm{T}} - \mathbf{K}_k\mathbf{R}_{k|k-1}\frac{d\mathbf{K}_k^{\mathrm{T}}}{d\theta_u} \quad (5.38)$$

Equations (5.31)–(538) give the differentiated filters. By applying these filters, we can estimate the gradient for the likelihood function of equation (5.19), together with the ordinary filter equations. Since the approximation of the gradient is not based on finite differences, this estimation procedure can lead to a more robust optimization procedure

5.4.6 Likelihood Function of Stochastic Systems Mapping

Systems mapping aims to identify specific QTLs that mediate the PK-PD system subject to stochastic perturbations. Suppose there is a mapping population of n subjects genotyped for a panel of SNPs. The subjects are repeatedly measured for a set of m pharmacological traits at a series of time points. These traits constitute a complex PK-PD system subject to stochastic perturbations. Consider an SNP with three genotypes, AA, Aa, and aa, the observations of which are n_2, n_1, and n_0, respectively. Let $y_{Ti}=(\mathbf{y}_{Ti}, \ldots, \mathbf{y}_{ki}, \ldots, \mathbf{y}_{1i})=\mathbf{y}_i$ denote the whole set of pharmacological measurements for subject i ($i=1, \ldots, n$). The likelihood function of phenotypic values for m traits at this SNP is formulated as

$$L\left(\mathbf{y}_1, \ldots, \mathbf{y}_n\right) = \prod_{i=1}^{n_2} p_2(\boldsymbol{y}_{Ti} \mid \theta_2) \prod_{i=1}^{n_1} p_1(\boldsymbol{y}_{Ti} \mid \theta_1) \prod_{i=1}^{n_0} p_0(\boldsymbol{y}_{Ti} \mid \theta_0) \quad (5.39)$$

where $p_j(\boldsymbol{y}_{Ti} \mid \theta_j)$ is the conditional probability of $\boldsymbol{y}_{Ti}$ given the parameter vector θ_j for genotype j ($j=2$ for AA, 1 for Aa, 0 for aa). We implement the EKF approach as described in Section 5.4.4 to estimate the output states and state covariances for each genotype. Thus, genotype-dependent parameter vector θ_j is estimated, which specifies the stochastic PK-PD system for each genotype.

Whether there exist significant QTLs affecting stochastic drug response can be tested by formulating the null and alternative hypotheses as follows:

$$H_0 : \theta_2 = \theta_1 = \theta_0$$

H_1: At least one of the equalities above does not hold

Under each hypothesis, we calculate the likelihood values and use these values to calculate the log-LR as a test statistic. The critical threshold can be determined through permutation tests. The parameter vector θ contains a set of parameters each describing a different feature of the stochastic system. We can also test whether a QTL determines a particular parameter, say θ_u, through the following hypotheses:

$$H_0 : \theta_{u2} = \theta_{u1} = \theta_{u0}$$

H_1: At least one of the equalities above does not hold

The log-LR under these two hypotheses is calculated and compared to the critical threshold determined from simulation studies.

The two hypothesis tests above provide a general procedure of testing the genetic control of the global behavior of the PK-PD system as well as the genetic control of specific features of the system. As a complex biological process, drug response is the consequence of a cascade of biochemical, physiological, and biophysical interactions, in each of which stochastic noises may pervasively occur (McKinstry-Wu et al. 2019; Hayford et al. 2021). As such, stochastic systems mapping, implemented with various hypothesis tests, is a critical tool for precisely dissecting the pharmacogenetic architecture of drug response.

5.4.7 Computer Simulation

Wang et al. (2013d) performed simulation studies to investigate the statistical properties of stochastic systems mapping used to identify QTLs for PK/PD responses. Tornøe et al. (2007) derived a stochastic first-order elimination one-compartment PK model and an indirect response PD model, which is coupled in the form,

$$\begin{cases} dC_t = -k_e C_t dt + \gamma_C dw_{Ct} \\[2mm] dR_t = \left[k_{in} - k_{out} \left(1 + \frac{C_t}{EC_{50}} + C_t \right) R_t \right] dt + \gamma_R dw_{Rt} \end{cases} \tag{5.40}$$

where C_t is the state variable for the plasma concentration of a drug at time t; R_t is the state variable for the PD response at time t; k_e is the elimination constant, EC_{50} is the drug concentration causing 50% of maximal stimulation; γ_C and γ_R are two diffusion coefficients for the PK and PD, respectively; and w_{Ct} and w_{Rt} are two independent standard Wiener processes. The PD parameters include k_{in} and k_{out}, the zero- and first-order rate constant for production and loss of an effect, respectively (Mager et al. 2003). Parameters in the SDE models (5.40) are $(k_e, k_{in}, k_{out}, EC_{50}, \gamma_C, \gamma_R) = (\theta, \gamma)$, where $\theta = (k_e, k_{in}, k_{out}, EC_{50})$ are the parameters corresponding to the drift terms and $\gamma = (\gamma_C, \gamma_R)$ are the parameters corresponding to the diffusion terms.

As an example, Wang et al. (2013d) simulated a PK-PD system, only controlled by a causal QTL that is associated with a molecular marker. Assume a random sample of 200 and 500 subjects from an equilibrium human population, in which frequencies of marker alleles and QTL alleles are $p=0.6$ for M vs. $1 - p = 0.4$ for m and $q=0.7$ for A vs. $1 - q = 0.3$ for a. The marker-QTL linkage disequilibrium is $D=0.05$. All subjects are assumed to receive the administration of a drug to treat a disease. The PK-PD phenotypic data, the plasma concentration of drug (C) (mg/l), and drug effect (R) at six time points after a drug is administered were simulated by summing time-dependent genotypic means for QTL genotypes, AA, Aa, and aa, determined by equation (5.40) and the residual errors. The residual variances are determined under two heritability levels: 0.1 and 0.4.

Different from the likelihood of equation (5.39), we formulate a mixture-based likelihood for phenotypic data under the marker-QTL disequilibrium and then implement the EM algorithm and Kalman filter procedure to estimate the model parameters. Wang et al. (2013d) found that stochastic systems mapping provides reasonably good estimates of all parameters (including SDE parameters, residual variances, marker and QTL allele frequencies, and marker-QTL linkage disequilibrium) with a sample size of $n=500$ (Table 5.3).

TABLE 5.3

MLEs of SDE Parameters, Residual Variances, Marker and QTL Allele Frequencies, and Marker-QTL Linkage Disequilibrium and Their Standard Errors (in Parentheses) from a Simulated Natural Population of 500 Subjects under Heritabilities of $H^2=0.1$ and 0.4

			MLE (SE)							
			$H^2=0.4$				$H^2=0.1$			
Parameter	Geno type	True	SDE		ODE		SDE		ODE	
k_e	AA	1.00	1.019	(0.013)	1.012	(0.018)	1.006	(0.035)	1.028	(0.037)
	Aa	0.80	0.772	(0.015)	0.780	(0.023)	0.807	(0.028)	0.759	(0.035)
	aa	0.50	0.514	(0.009)	0.518	(0.017)	0.525	(0.024)	0.516	(0.029)
k_{in}	AA	1.00	0.962	(0.031)	1.029	(0.038)	1.036	(0.058)	0.968	(0.064)
	Aa	1.50	1.539	(0.035)	1.527	(0.052)	1.495	(0.081)	1.531	(0.079)
	aa	2.00	1.907	(0.047)	1.916	(0.064)	1.951	(0.098)	1.926	(0.107)
k_{out}	AA	0.10	0.103	(0.003)	0.092	(0.011)	0.099	(0.015)	0.093	(0.018)
	Aa	0.30	0.304	(0.005)	0.291	(0.013)	0.288	(0.022)	0.286	(0.025)
	aa	0.20	0.209	(0.005)	0.212	(0.009)	0.190	(0.017)	0.215	(0.031)
EC_{50}	AA	5.00	5.243	(0.316)	5.195	(0.427)	5.140	(0.528)	5.283	(0.564)
	Aa	3.00	3.043	(0.283)	3.052	(0.358)	3.077	(0.450)	3.142	(0.518)
	aa	1.00	1.047	(0.179)	0.949	(0.221)	0.980	(0.396)	1.053	(0.430)
γ_C		0.10	0.108	(0.008)	–		0.112	(0.025)	–	
γ_R		0.50	0.516	(0.017)	–		0.519	(0.041)	–	
σ_C		0.08	0.085	(0.004)	0.076	(0.005)	–		–	
		0.20	–		–		0.226	(0.027)	0.217	(0.026)
σ_R		0.72	0.717	(0.012)	0.724	(0.015)	–		–	
		1.76	–		–		1.699	(0.081)	1.825	(0.093)
P		0.60	0.592	(0.005)	0.595	(0.005)	0.605	(0.016)	0.593	(0.018)
Q		0.70	0.693	(0.013)	0.708	(0.014)	0.684	(0.037)	0.712	(0.039)
D		0.05	0.065	(0.008)	0.061	(0.009)	0.068	(0.019)	0.059	(0.017)

Parameter estimates by the ODE model are also given.

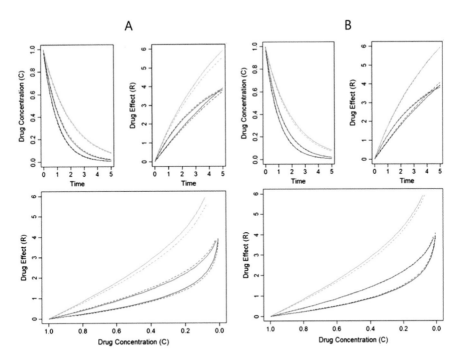

FIGURE 5.4
Genetic variation in PK and PD processes estimated from a couple of simulated dynamic phe-notypic variables with heritability of 0.1 (a) and 0.4 (b) by stochastic systems mapping. Broken lines are the estimated PK and PD curves for three genotypes at a hypothesized QTL, *AA* (black), *Aa* (red), and *aa* (green), which are broadly consistent with the true curves indicated by solid lines. The plots include PK process in which drug concentration decreases with time, PD process in which drug effect increases with time, and cycle limit of PK and PD response.

Increasing heritability can dramatically improve the accuracy and pre-cision of parameter estimation, suggesting that precise measurements of PK/PD phenotypes are crucial for better estimation of parameters. The estimated SDE parameters were used to draw dynamic curves of PK and PD responses over time as well as dynamic relationships between these two processes (Figure 5.4). We find that the estimates curves are broadly consistent with the true curves obtained from given SDE values, confirming the precision of systems mapping. PK/PD responses can be better estimated when the underlying heritability increases from 0.1 to 0.4. The model can also test whether the QTL pleiotropically control the PK and PD.

The simulated data are also analyzed by ODE-based systems mapping. It is not surprising that the estimation precision of allele frequencies, LD, and residual variances does not differ dramatically between ODE- and SDE-based mapping models (Table 5.3). However, genotype-dependent model parameters that describe PK-PD curves are estimated at higher precision by stochastic systems mapping than deterministic systems mapping. This suggests that analyzing stochastically perturbed data can be benefitted from the stochastic model.

5.4.8 Application of Stochastic Systems Mapping

As a proof of concept, we apply SDE-based systems mapping to analyze a real data in a forest tree (Gan 2021). The data was derived from a mapping population of Euphrates poplar containing 273 seedlings of a full-sib family, grown in a homogeneous environment (Zhang et al. 2017; Sang et al. 2019b). To adapt to a saline and drought desert, Euphrates poplar has evolved to grow a strong taproot that can reach deep water tables. Taproot growth is sensitive to random change in soil moisture and salination, which can be better mapped by stochastic systems mapping. The population was genotyped for 8,279 SNPs that are grouped to 19 *Populus* chromosomes. To analyze this data, we modify the SDE to accommodate to a growth trait, expressed as

$$dg_t = rg_t\left(1 - \frac{g_t}{K}\right)dt + \sigma_w dw_t \qquad (5.41)$$

where g_t is the trait value at time t, r is the relative growth rate, K is the asymptotic value of g_t when t tends to be infinite, σ_w is the scaling term, and w_t is independent standard Wiener process (Jazwinski 1970). Term $\sigma_w dw_t$ is the system noise. To make a comparison, we also analyze the same data by ODE-based systems mapping, expressed as

$$dg_t = rg_t\left(1 - \frac{g_t}{K}\right)dt \qquad (5.42)$$

The models in equations (5.41) and (5.42) are incorporated into systems mapping by which we can test whether different genotypes at a marker differ in growth trajectories. Note that we use SAD(1) to model the residual covariance matrix.

We illustrate growth trajectories of taproot growth for all full-sib seedlings (Figure 5.5). We use both ODE and SDE to fit the mean growth curve. According to Bayesian Information Criterion (BIC) values calculated, SDE performs better than ODE, suggesting that stochasticity occurs for taproot growth even in a well-controlled environment. Stochastic systems mapping identifies 19 taproot growth QTLs mostly distributed in chromosomes 6 and 9 (Figure 5.6a and b). Heritabilities explained by a QTL at different time points are calculated and illustrated as a function of time (Figure 5.6c). While some QTLs explain a consistently small heritability over time, others show a dramatic time-varying change in heritability, suggesting that

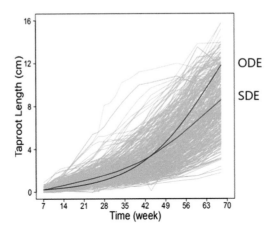

FIGURE 5.5
Taproot growth trajectories for 273 seedlings from a full-sib of Euphrates poplar. The mean trajectory is fitted by an SDE (red line) and ODE (blue line), respectively.

QTLs affect taproot growth in different manners. Gene enrichment analysis shows that all these QTLs detected reside within the genomic regions of known candidate genes, suggesting the biological relevance of the stochastic model. For example, QTL nn_np_5701 detected on chromosome 9 is located

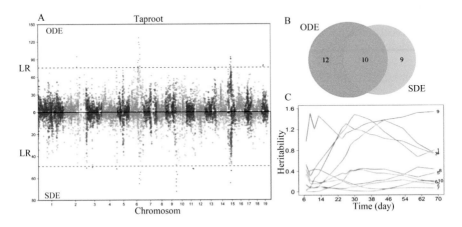

FIGURE 5.6
(a) Manhattan plots of significance tests for taproot growth using SNPs across 19 Euphrates poplar chromosomes by ODE- (upper) and SDE-based systems mapping (lower). Dotted horizontal lines are the critical thresholds at the 5% significance level determined from 100 permutation tests. (b) Venn diagram for QTLs detected by ODE and SDE models. (c) The trajectories of heritability explained by each of 10 randomly chosen QTLs.

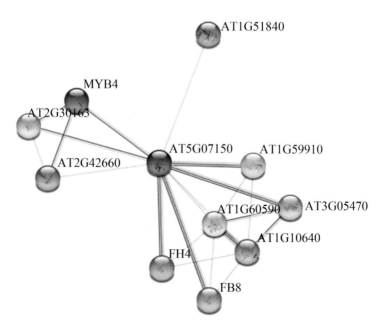

FIGURE 5.7
Genetic interaction network of *AT5G07150* (nn_np_5701) with other functional genes.

within gene *AT5G07150* encoding serine-threonine protein kinase 2 mRNA expressed in root tissues. *AT5G07150* forms an interaction network with many other genes to mediate root apical growth and the sprouting of root hairs (Figure 5.7).

The deterministic ODE model identifies 22 QTLs (Figure 5.6a), of which 10 are also detected by the SDE model (Figure 5.6b). Most of the QTLs (18) detected by the ODE model can also be explained by candidate genes. Given these findings, we suggest that ODE- and SDE-based systems mapping represent two alternative approaches for QTL mapping. If the effect of a QTL is sensitive to random noises, the SDE model should be used. However, to detect those developmentally stable QTLs, the ODE model should be a better choice, because the SDE model may overfit the data in this case. In practice, both ODE and SDE models should be simultaneously used, given that the QTLs detected by both models are biologically relevant. If a QTL is simultaneously detected by both ODE and SDE models, this may imply that this QTL is perturbed to an extent, above which the ODE model is not powerful enough to detect it but below which the SDE model is an overfit. Which model is better for such QTLs should be determined according to information criteria (e.g., AIC or BIC) and empirical rule.

5.5 Concluding Remarks

Systems mapping has proven to be a powerful tool for mapping genes that control complex phenotypes (Fu et al. 2010, 2011; Luo et al. 2010; Guo et al. 2011; Wu et al. 2011a; Sun and Wu 2015a; Cao et al. 2017). In this chapter, we show that systems mapping can be applied to map pharmacogenes for drug response by integrating differential equations for PK and PD modeling. A key feature of PK- and PD-based systems mapping is that it allows us to make systematic inference on all model components within a unified parametric model framework (Fu et al. 2013). Systems mapping is capable of testing the genetic control of the biochemical and metabolic mechanisms underlying drug response, thus displaying great potential to be implicated for personalized medicine.

Systems mapping in pharmacogenetic and pharmacogenomic studies was derived from a pressing need for comprehending the multifactorial inheritance of drug response, and it has been benefitted from a multidisciplinary interplay among genetics, pharmacology, chemistry, statistics, mathematics, and computer science. It first dissects the pharmacological response of a drug into its biochemical components according to the pathways of how the drug is absorbed and transported to target tissues in the human body, where it is metabolized and reacts with receptors and enzymes, and then models the interconnections and coordination of these components using robust mathematical equations. By linking these processes with molecular markers, systems mapping uses computing algorithms to identify specific genes involved in each and every step from drug absorption to drug metabolism to drug efficacy. Next, systems mapping should be integrated with synthetic biology to reconstruct and simulate a new drug reaction system that optimizes personalized drug delivery based on key biochemical pathways contributing to drug effects.

In practical clinical trials, PK/PD variables may not be measured under a completely controlled condition, inevitably leading to imprecision of pharmacological data. Also, PK/PD data are often highly sparse and unbalanced due to irregular measurement intervals. ODE modeling is less powerful to handle these heterogeneous data. This challenge can be addressed by a different type of models, SDEs, which embrace more complex variations in the dynamics (Jazwinsky 1970; Kristensen and Madsen 2010; McKinstry-Wu et al. 2019). Wang et al. (2013d) made a first attempt to implement SDEs into systems mapping for mapping PK/PD genes or QTLs.

All biological systems, including pharmacological processes, evolve under stochastic forces. The advantage of SDEs lies in its capacity to model random influences by taking into account the subsystems of the real world that cannot be sufficiently isolated from effects captured by ODEs (Jazwinsky 1970). Systems mapping implemented with SDEs can particularly model and investigate the influence of random noise in the PK/PD dynamics through genes. In pharmacological studies, both internal and external factors may lead to the erratic behavior of drug reactions. SDE-implemented systems mapping can model variations due to these factors, enhancing the model predictions and results interpretation. Wang et al. (2013d) performed computer simulation to assess this stochastic mapping model, showing its usefulness for the identification of pharmacological QTLs in practice. Maximum likelihood approaches are implemented as model-fitting algorithms of systems mapping, but other approaches, such as weighted least squares or Bayesian, can also be used in helping select the best-fit model to real data sets.

In this chapter, we only describe a general framework for systems mapping under deterministic and stochastic models. The implications of ODE- and SDE-based systems mapping for practical pharmacogenetic studies can be made possible by accommodating it to various situations. In statistics, systems mapping can be extended to accommodate possible model misspecification by implementing more flexible nonparametric functions in the ODEs and SDEs that quantify model uncertainty. As an increasingly used strategy for pharmacogenetic research (Ge et al. 2009; Shuldiner et al. 2009; Daly 2010; Wu et al. 2011b), GWAS encounter a critical issue of joint analysis and modeling of a large number of markers. Leveraging systems mapping by high-dimensional models can increase our capacity to comprehend the genetic architecture of complex traits (Li et al. 2011a, 2014a, 2015). Pharmacogenes affect final phenotypes of drug response by perturbing the abundances of transcripts, proteins, and metabolites that form a sequential order of biochemical pathways toward cell physiology and drug reactions (Wang et al. 2014). Thus, an integrative approach of systems biology and systems mapping will provide an unprecedented opportunity to find and construct cellular regulatory networks causing drug effects (Imoto et al. 2007; van der Wijst et al. 2018; Lee et al. 2020a). Taken all these together with the analysis and modeling of data from GWAS, systems mapping with appropriate extensions will help to drive the drug discovery processes, predict rare adverse events, and catalyze the practice of precision medicine.

Part 2

Network Pharmacogenetics

6

Network Mapping of Drug Response

6.1 Introduction

Candidate-gene and genome-wide association studies (GWAS) have been widely used and will continue to be used as a powerful tool for pharmacogenetic research (Daly 2010; Motsinger-Reif et al. 2013; McInnes et al. 2021), but these two approaches have not been very successful in identifying replicable and valid biomarkers of pharmacological treatment response. Although several genes that code drug-metabolizing enzymes (e.g., CYP2D6, CYP2C19) have been identified (Sistonen et al. 2009; Hicks et al. 2017), a complete genome-wide landscape of genetic control over the pharmacodynamics and pharmacokinetics of medications remains elusive, making the translation of pharmacogenetics/-genomics into clinical practice less successful across a wide range of disorders. One promising avenue in overcoming some of the current limitations in treatment response prediction research is the application of genetic networks that encapsulate interactions among pharmacogenes, although network tools have been rarely applied in the context of pharmacogenomic interactions.

Drug response is not a simple Mendelian trait rather involves a number of genes that interact with each other in a self-organizing manner (Zhou and Lauschke 2019). For example, the combination between *CYP2D6* and *CYP2C19* alleles reduces toxic risk in amitriptyline therapy, which thus could be used as an individualized antidepressive regimen (Steimer et al. 2005). Breastfed infants of mothers carrying CYP2D6 ultrarapid metabolizers combined with the UGT2B7*2/*2 genotype display an increased risk for central nervous system depression (Madadi et al. 2009). While multiple genes are considered, an intricate but well-orchestrated interaction network can better explain pharmacogenetic variation in drug response (Huang et al. 2013; Zhao and Iyengar 2012; McGillivray et al. 2018; Cheng et al. 2018, 2019). However, the identification of such pharmacogenetic networks is challenged by the complexity of analytical approaches.

More recently, Sun et al. (2021) have developed a functional graph theory for inferring genetic networks from SNP data in association studies. This theory is founded on the integration of functional mapping and evolutionary

DOI: 10.1201/9780429171512-8

game theory into graph theory. In a genetic system mediating pharmacodynamic reactions, each gene acts like a player in a complex game, striving to maximize its genetic impact based on its own strategy and the strategies of its interacting genes (other players) (von Neumann and Morgenstern 1944). This maximization process repeats until the Nash equilibrium is achieved, at which both interacting parties learn their optimal strategies and reach a balance (Nash 1950). As the refinement and evolutionary extension of the Nash equilibrium, evolutionarily stable strategies are introduced to model the dynamic changes of players' strategies (Maynard Smith and Price 1973). Sun et al. (2021) quantified evolutionarily stable strategies by using a Lotka-Volterra (LV) prey–predator model (Berryman 1992; Marrow et al. 1996; Abrams 2000; Cortez and Ellner 2010), establishing the mathematical foundation of functional graph theory.

Functional graph theory has been used to reconstruct genome-wide interactome networks for complex traits in GWAS (Wang et al. 2021; Yang et al. 2021; Feng et al. 2021). Compared to widely used correlation-based (including Pearson or Spearman correlation) and Bayesian networks (Vijesh et al. 2013; Wang and Huang 2014; Huynh-Thu and Sanguinetti 2019; Yaghoobi et al. 2012), the networks from functional graph theory have many favorable properties. First, they are fully informative, coded by bidirectional, signed, and weighted interactions, circumventing weighted but not causal or casual but sign-unknown limitations of existing networks (Chen et al. 2019). Second, functional networks are individualized, i.e., functional graph theory can reconstruct a network specifically for an individual sample, although current approaches can only infer an overall network from all samples. Third, individualized networks can be collapsed into context-dependent networks, providing more information for context testing than context-agnostic networks. Fourth, functional graph theory is flexible to marry with various disciplines; for example, by integrating it with developmental modularity theory and dynamic patch theory, we can reconstruct multilayer, multiscale, multispace, and multifunctional genetic network from an unlimited number of genes and other agents (Wu and Jiang 2021). In this chapter, we introduce functional graph theory to reconstruct pharmacogenetic networks as one of the very first tools for systems pharmacogenomics.

6.2 Functional Graph Theory

6.2.1 Functional Mapping

Consider a clinical trial that samples n patients to investigate the genetic control of pharmacological response to a drug. All the patients are genotyped for a panel of p SNPs. To test how they respond differently to the drug, each patient receives medical interventions at a series of ascending drug dosages. After a certain time of dosing, the patients are measured for plasma concentrations and a drug effect parameter, producing longitudinal data. Let $\mathbf{y}_i = (y_i(c_{i1}), \ldots, y_i(c_{iT_i}))$ denote T_i drug effect values measured at different plasma concentrations, which have been adjusted for all possible covariate effects. We associate each SNP with effect-concentration curve to estimate and test its genetic effect on drug response.

As described in Chapter 2, functional mapping integrates a pharmacodynamic equation, such as the E_{max} equation, to model concentration-varying drug effects for each genotype, with the covariance matrix structured by an autoregressive model (Lin et al. 2005a, b, 2007; Wu and Lin 2008). Consider SNP s ($s = 1, \ldots, p$) with two alleles A and a, whose allele frequencies are denoted as p_s and q_s, respectively. Through functional mapping, we estimate genotype-dependent effect-concentration curves, denoted as $\mu_{s2}(c)$ for genotype AA, $\mu_{s1}(c)$ for genotype Aa, and $\mu_{s0}(c)$ for genotype aa. According to quantitative genetic theory, we calculate the additive and dominant genetic effects of drug effect-concentration curves at SNP s as

$$a_s(c) = \frac{1}{2}\left(\mu_{s2}(c) - \mu_{s0}(c)\right) \tag{6.1a}$$

$$d_s(c) = \mu_{s1}(c) - \frac{1}{2}\left(\mu_{s2}(c) + \mu_{s0}(c)\right) \tag{6.1b}$$

We further calculate the genetic variances of drug effect-concentration curves at SNP s as

$$\sigma_{gs}^2(c) = 2p_s q_s \left[a_s(c) + (q_s - p_s)d_s(c)\right]^2 + \left(2p_s q_s d_s(c)\right)^2 \tag{6.2a}$$

where the additive and dominant genetic variances are

$$\sigma_{as}^2(c) = 2p_s q_s \left[a_s(c) + (q_s - p_s)d_s(c)\right]^2 \tag{6.2b}$$

$$\sigma_{ds}^2(c) = \left(2p_s q_s d_s(c)\right)^2 \tag{6.2c}$$

Functional mapping can not only estimate the genetic effects and variances of each SNP but also test the significance of each genetic effect at a given SNP through permutation tests. An estimated genetic effect, regardless of whether it is significant, represents the net effect of an SNP in the genetic system (Wang et al. 2021; Yang et al. 2021).

6.2.2 Social Decomposition of the Net Genetic Effect

To describe how the net genetic effect of an SNP is partitioned into its under-lying components due to its different actions and interactions, we introduce a real example of forest research. A survey of forest production shows that species-rich mixed forests are more productive than when species are grown in monocultures (Gamfeldt et al. 2013). This positive relationship between tree species diversity in forests and their growth performance has been confirmed by a number of subsequent studies (Liang et al. 2016; Gómez-González et al. 2022). Consider two species A and B, which are grown in mixtures (Figure 6.1a). As a control, each species is also grown in monocultures. Let u_c and u_m denote the production of species A in monocultures and co-cultures, respectively. Similarly, let v_c and v_m the production of species B in monocultures and co-cultures. We use a simple mathematics to formulate forest production in mixtures, expressed as

$$u_c = u_m + \left(u_c - u_m \right) \tag{6.3a}$$

$$v_c = v_m + \left(v_c - v_m \right) \tag{6.3b}$$

which suggests that the production of each species in mixture can be explained by two components, the production in monoculture (where the

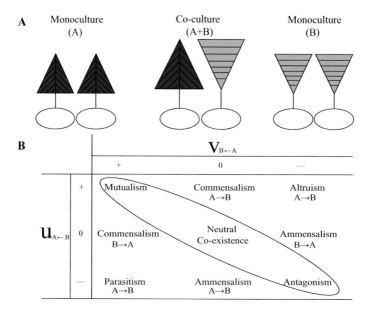

FIGURE 6.1
Ecological experiment of biological interactions. (a) Cultural experiment includes the mono-culture of two forest tree species (A and B) and their co-culture. (b) Dependent growth of two species in co-culture is due to different types of ecological interactions.

species is grown in a socially isolated environment) and the difference of production in co-cultures (where two species are grown in a socialized environment) from that in monocultures. The first component, called *independent growth*, reflects the intrinsic capacity of growth of a species, whereas the second component, called *dependent* or *social growth*, occurs due to the interaction of this species with its interactive partner (Jiang et al. 2018a, b). We rewrite equations (6.3a) and (6.3b) as

$$u_c = u_m + u_{A-B} \qquad (6.4a)$$

$$v_c = v_m + v_{B-A} \qquad (6.4b)$$

where the size and sign of $u_{A \leftarrow B}$ and $v_{B \leftarrow A}$ reflect the strength of a species-species interaction and its direction (Figure 6.1b). If both $u_{A \leftarrow B}$ and $v_{B \leftarrow A}$ are positive, then this suggests that species A and B cooperate with each other, forming a mutualistic relationship. In contrast, if both of them are negative, the two species compete against each other, by which an antagonistic relationship is produced. If $u_{A \leftarrow B}$ ($v_{B \leftarrow A}$) is positive and $v_{B \leftarrow A}$ ($u_{A \leftarrow B}$) is zero, then this suggests that species B (A) is commensalistic to species A (B). If $u_{A \leftarrow B}$ ($v_{B \leftarrow A}$) is negative and $v_{B \leftarrow A}$ ($u_{A \leftarrow B}$) is zero, this implies that species B (A) is amensalistic to species A (B). If $u_{A \leftarrow B}$ ($v_{B \leftarrow A}$) is positive but $v_{B \leftarrow A}$ ($u_{A \leftarrow B}$) is negative, this suggests that species B (A) is altruistic to species A (B), whereas species A (B) is parasitic to species B (A). As described above, if we can estimate $u_{A \leftarrow B}$ and $v_{B \leftarrow A}$, we can determine a bidirectional, signed, and weighted interaction between two species. We argue that gene-gene interactions, as a complex game system at the microecological level, obey a similar principle used by species-species interactions at the macroecological level.

6.2.3 LV Modeling of Evolutionary Game Theory

As described by equations (6.3a) and (6.3b), the overall growth of an organism in a social environment can be dissected into independent and dependent growth components. The separation of these two components can help identify the type of ecological interactions (Figure 6.1b) and estimate their strength. This separation can be made possible by culturing two interactive species in monocultures and co-cultures. However, in the situation where many species co-exist to interact with each other, such a cultural experiment can be hardly conducted. Also, in genetic studies, there is no possibility to "culture" a gene and a pair of genes to create socially isolated and socialized environments, especially when we consider thousands of genes in a cell.

Sun et al.'s (2021) functional graph theory can be used to separate independent and dependent components of a biological entity existing as a member of a society, without need to conduct cultural experiments. A statistical mechanic method developed from this theory can estimate and test independent and social expression components of biological entities that co-exist in complex communities. Functional graph theory is derived from the LV-based ODE modeling of Maynard Smith and Price's (1973) evolutionary game theory (Weibull 1995; Sandholm 2009). According to the argument by equations (6.3a) and (6.3b), we consider the net genetic variance explained by an SNP to be decomposed into its independent genetic variance component due to the own innate strategy of this SNP expressed in an isolated condition and the dependent genetic variance component arising from the accumulative influence of interactions by other SNPs. This consideration, in agreement with evolutionary game theory, can be modeled by the LV equation (Berryman 1992; Marrow et al. 1996; Abrams 2000; Cortez and Ellner 2010). Let $y_s(c) = \sigma_{gs}^2(c)$ denote the net genetic variance of SNP s estimated by equation (6.2a) through functional mapping. We build a system of nonlinear LV-based ODEs with respect to plasma concentration as follows:

$$\dot{y}_s(c) = Q_s\left(y_s(c):\Theta_s\right) + \sum_{s'=1, s' \neq s}^{m} Q_{ss'}\left(g_{s'}(c):\Theta_{ss'}\right), \; s = 1,\dots,p \qquad (6.5)$$

where $Q_s(y_s(c):\Theta_s)$ denotes the independent genetic variance of SNP s and $\Sigma\, Q_{ss'}(y_{s'}(c):\Theta_{ss'})$ denotes the accumulated dependent genetic variance of SNPs influenced by all possible other SNPs. We express the independent genetic variance of SNPs as a function of $y_s(c)$, specified by parameters Θ_s, and its dependent genetic variance as a function of $y_{s'}(c)$, specified by parameters $\Theta_{ss'}$. Next, we implement a statistical algorithm to estimate independent genetic variances and dependent genetic variances for each SNP based on the above ODEs.

6.2.4 Reconstructing Causal, Sparse, and Stable Networks

After the ODEs of equation (6.5) are solved, we code the estimates of $Q_s(y_s(c):\Theta_s)$ as nodes and those of $Q_{ss'}(y_{s'}(c):\Theta_{ss'})$ as edges into mathematical graphs as a network of gene-gene interactions. Network inference should meet three central issues: causality, sparsity, and stability (Michailidis and d'Alché-Buc 2013). The causality of networks inferred by the ODEs can be reflected by the sign of dependent genetic variance components (see Figure 6.1b). Network sparsity in living systems is a ubiquitous emergent pattern; i.e., the percentage of the active interactions (connectivity) scales inversely proportional to the system size (Busiello et al. 2017). This pattern enables the organism to better buffer against stochastic perturbations (May 1972; Allesina and Tang 2012). In network inference, sparsity implies that not all other $(m-1)$ SNPs are allowed to connect with a given SNP s ($s=1, \dots, m$) and, thus, it is essential to select a small set of the most significant SNPs that are linked to SNP s. A variable selection procedure can be implemented to do so based on a regression model derived from the integrals of ODEs in equation (6.5), i.e.,

$$y_s(c) = W_s\left(y_s(c):\Theta_s\right) + \sum_{s'=1,s'\neq s}^{m} W_{ss'}\left(g_{s'}(c):\Theta_{ss'}\right) + e_s(c), \; s = 1,\ldots,m \quad (6.6)$$

where $y_s(c)$ is the genetic effect response for SNP s at concentration c, $g_{s'}(c)$ $(s'=1,\ldots,s-1,s+1,\ldots,m)$ is a predictor of SNP s based on SNP s', $e_s(c)$ is the residual error, distributed as $N(0,\sigma_s^2)$, and $W_s()$ and $W_{ss'}(\;)$ are the integrals of $Q_s()$ and $Q_{ss'}(\;)$ in equation (6.5), respectively, which can be linearized and fitted by a nonparametric Legendre Orthogonal Polynomial (LOP) approach.

In practice, the number of SNPs as predictors is exceedingly larger than that of plasma concentrations (like samples). This "curse of dimensionality" due to big-$(m-1)$ and little-T (which is the number of concentration) can be resolved by implementing LASSO or its variants (Tibshirani 1996; Zou and Hastie 2005; Yuan and Lin 2006; Wang and Leng 2008). It is likely that the number of concentrations is not enough, as compared to the number of SNPs, to allow variable selection to function properly. In this case, we can interpolate the values of genetic variances within the concentration interval as many as needed, because concentration-varying genetic variances can be viewed as a curve. After the number of the most significant predictor SNPs (m_s) for response SNP s is determined, the fully connected ODEs in equation (6.5) are reduced to sparsely connected ones, i.e.,

$$\dot{y}_s(c) = Q_s\left(y_s(c):\Theta_s\right) + \sum_{s'=1,s'\neq s}^{m_s} Q_{ss'}\left(g_{s'}(c):\Theta_{ss'}\right), \; s = 1,\ldots,p \quad (6.7)$$

where all notations are the same as equation (6.5), except for p over the summation replaced by m_s. The reduced ODEs ensure the sparsity of network inference because each SNP is not necessarily connected with every other SNP.

Network stability is the capacity of a network to be resilient to perturbations caused from external factors other than interactions (Akinola et al. 2019). Viewing the network as an interactive game, stability refers to whether the game reaches a Nash equilibrium, a state where no player has incentive to move (Demichelis and Ritzberger 2003; Lomonosov and Sitharam 2007). The optimality of network implies the closest approach of a Nash equilibrium to optimizing the overall function of the network (Lomonosov and Sitharam 2007), which can be achieved by maximizing a likelihood, i.e., under a system of specified ODEs, the genetic data of all SNPs is most probable. That said, the maximum likelihood estimates of ODE parameters from given data can guarantee network stability.

Let $\mathbf{y}_s = (y_s(1),..., y_s(T))$ denote the estimated genetic variances of SNP s at T concentrations. It is assumed that residual errors for the same SNP follow a multivariate normal distribution with zero mean vector and autocorrelation-structured covariance matrix and that residual errors among SNPs have no interdependence. Under these assumptions, we formulate the likelihood function of the data as

$$L_m(\boldsymbol{\omega};\mathbf{y}) = \prod_{s=1}^{m} f_s(\mathbf{y}_s;\boldsymbol{\omega}_s) \qquad (6.8)$$

where the model parameters of multivariate density function $f_s(\mathbf{y}_s;\boldsymbol{\omega}_s)$ include mean vector $\boldsymbol{\mu}_s$ and covariance matrix Σ_s ($s=1, ..., m$). The mean vectors of m SNPs are expressed as

$$\left\{ \begin{array}{c} \boldsymbol{\mu}_1 = (\mu_1(1),...,\mu_1(T)) \\ \vdots \\ \boldsymbol{\mu}_m = (\mu_m(1),...,\mu_m(T)) \end{array} \right. \qquad (6.9)$$

which is fitted by the integrals of sparse LOP-built ODEs given in equation (6.7). Each covariance matrix is structured by a two-parameter (ϕ_s, v_s^2) SAD(1) model (Zhao et al. 2005a). Let $\boldsymbol{\omega} = (\boldsymbol{\omega}_1,..., \boldsymbol{\omega}_m)$, with $\boldsymbol{\omega}_s = \left(\Theta_s, (\Theta_{ss'})_{s'=1}^{m_s}; \phi_s, v_s^2\right)$. The values of the model parameters that maximize the likelihood function (6.8) over the parameter space are

$$\hat{\boldsymbol{\omega}} = \underbrace{\arg\max}_{\omega \in \Omega} \hat{L}_n(\boldsymbol{\omega};\mathbf{y}) \qquad (6.10)$$

which intuitively make the genetic variance data most probable. Note that a log-transformation may be used to assure the normality of the $\mathbf{y}$ data.

6.2.5 Bidirectional, Signed, and Weighted Formulation of Epistasis

In classic genetics, epistasis is defined as a genetic interaction where one mutation masks the effects of another mutation (Bateson 1907). Fisher (1918) generalized this concept to describe the effect that deviates from the expected summed effect of individual loci. Fisher's generalization that enables the measurement of the magnitude and sign of epistasis between different loci has been widely recognized and has played an instrumental role in quantitative genetic studies during the past century (Costanzo et al. 2016; Sackton and Hartl 2016; Domingo et al. 2019). However, this definition can only describe the overall effect of genetic interactions between two loci (Figure 6.2a), which may be due to one of many latent interaction types

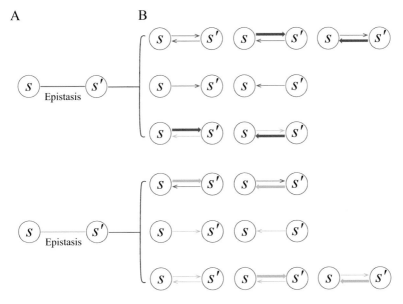

FIGURE 6.2
Observed epistasis attributed to different types of SNP-SNP interactions. Non-arrowed lines between SNP *s* and *s'* denote their non-causal epistasis, whereas arrowed lines stand for the casualty of epistasis, with the thickness of lines proportional to the strength of epistasis. Red and blue lines represent promotion and inhibition, respectively.

(Figure 6.2b). For example, classic quantitative genetic theory can only allow positive nondirectional epistasis or negative nondirectional epistasis to be estimated. Indeed, positive nondirectional epistasis estimated may be due to the mutual promotion of two loci, the unidirectional promotion of one locus for the second, or the promotion of one locus for the second although the second inhibits the first but to a lesser extent. Similarly, negative non-directional epistasis detected may arise also from one of the three possible types (Figure 6.2b).

The ODE model of equation (6.7) can leverage the definition of epistasis by capturing the full information of bidirectional, signed, and weighted gene-gene interactions, as opposed to the classic theory that can only determine the strength and sign of epistasis (Figure 6.2). Specifically, by comparing the integrals of estimated $Q_{ss'}(\cdot)$ and $Q_{s's}(\cdot)$ under ODEs of equation (6.5), denoted as $P_{ss'}(\cdot)$ and $P_{s's}(\cdot)$, respectively, we classify epistasis into different types (Table 6.1):

- *Symmetrical synergism*: Two SNPs promote each other at the same strength, in which case both $P_{ss'}(\cdot)$ and $P_{s's}(\cdot)$ are positive and equal in size;

TABLE 6.1

Qualitative Class of Epistasis and Its Quantitative Characterization by the ODE Game Model

		Quantitative Description		
No	**Qualitative Definition**	$P_{k \leftarrow k'j}\left(N_{ij}\right)$		$P_{k' \leftarrow kj}\left(N_{ij}\right)$
1	Symmetric synergism	+	=	+
2	Asymmetric synergism	+	≠	+
3	Directional synergism toward k	+		0
4	Directional synergism toward k'	0		+
5	Altruism toward k or exploitation by k	+		−
6	Altruism toward k' or exploitation by k'	−		+
7	Symmetric antagonism	−	=	−
8	Asymmetric antagonism	−	≠	−
9	Directional antagonism toward k	−		0
10	Directional antagonism toward k'	0		−
11	Coexistence	0		0

Note: $P_{k \leftarrow k'j}\left(N_{ij}\right)$ and $P_{k' \leftarrow kj}\left(N_{ij}\right)$ are the dependent expression levels of gene k by gene k' and gene k' by gene k, respectively.

- *Asymmetrical synergism*: Two SNPs promote each other but to different extents, in which case $P_{ss'}(\cdot)$ and $P_{s's}(\cdot)$ are positive but not equal in size. $P_{ss'}(\cdot) > P_{s's}(\cdot)$ implies that SNP s is more beneficial from SNP s' than the other way around;

- *Directional synergism*: One SNP (say s') promotes the other (s), but the second has no effect on the first, in which $P_{ss'}$ is positive but $P_{s's}(\cdot)$ is zero;

- *Altruism/Aggression*: One SNP promotes the other but the second inhibits the first, in which case $P_{ss'}(\cdot)$ is positive but $P_{s's}(\cdot)$ is negative, explained as the altruism of SNP s' for SNP s or the aggression of SNP s for SNP s';

- *Symmetrical antagonism*: Two SNPs inhibit each other at the same strength, in which case both $P_{ss'}(\cdot)$ and $P_{s's}(\cdot)$ are negative and equal in size;

- *Asymmetrical antagonism*: Two SNPs inhibit each other but to different extents, in which both $P_{ss'}(\cdot)$ and $P_{s's}(\cdot)$ are negative but not equal in size;

- *Directional antagonism*: One SNP inhibits the other but the second is neutral to the first, in which case, $P_{ss'}$ is negative but $P_{s's}(\cdot)$ is zero.

We encapsulate all these types of epistasis that occur among all m SNPs into an interaction network, which is regarded as being a fully informative epistatic network. Topological analysis of the network allows us to identify hub SNPs, i.e., those with more links than the average of all SNPs, which play a pivotal role in maintaining network behavior. Links of the network can be outgoing if one SNP regulates a second SNP, or incoming if one SNP is regulated by a second SNP. We call those hub SNPs having more outgoing links than incoming links a leader. While existing approaches for linkage and association mapping can only estimate the net genetic effect of an SNP, the LV-based ODE model partitions the net effect into its independent (endogenous) and dependent (exogeneous) components. Based on these two components, we can assess whether a specific SNP impacts the phenotype directly or through indirect paths involving other SNPs.

6.2.6 Pharmacokinetically and Pharmacodynamically Varying Networks

One important advantage of LV-based ODEs in equation (6.7) is that they can not only identify specific SNPs with which a given SNP interacts and the pattern in which each interaction is exerted but also monitor, track, and predict how epistatic networks change over plasma concentration. This predictive capacity results from the dependent component $P_{ss'}(\cdot)$ as a function of concentration. Meanwhile, the independent component $P_s(\cdot)$ also changes as a function of concentration, suggesting that the capacity of an SNP to exhibit its genetic effect independently of any other loci can be traced when concentration varies. By coding $P_s(\cdot)$ as nodes and $P_{ss'}(\cdot)$ as edges, we ultimately reconstruct pharmacodynamically varying genetic networks that detail the actions and interactions of all SNPs in drug response.

If pharmacogenetic studies aim to investigate the genetic control of how a drug is affected by the body, we can integrate the PK equation into functional mapping to estimate the genetic variance of plasma concentrations for each SNP at different time points (Figure 1.2a). These estimated genetic variances are used to establish a system of LV-based ODEs based on functional graph theory. Similarly, we can reconstruct pharmacokinetically varying genetic networks that cover all SNPs.

6.3 Functional Pharmacogenetic Interaction Networks: An Example

6.3.1 Estimation of Pharmacogenetic Effect Curves by Functional Mapping

We demonstrate the application of functional graph theory by analyzing a real dataset from a pharmacogenetic association study. This study includes 163 subjects differing in demographic factors, such as race, gender, age, and body mass, treated by dobutamine at increasing dose levels from 0 (baseline) to 5, 10, 20, 30, and 40 mcg/min. Dobutamine is a drug designed to improve patients' heart function when the patients cannot exercise. Heart rate, one of the physiological parameters used to assess drug response, was measured after the subjects received dobutamine at each dosage level. Five SNPs, located within three candidate genes for heart function, were genotyped, aimed to characterize quantitative trait nucleotides for dose-effect response curves. The $\beta_1 AR$ gene includes two polymorphisms located at codons 49 (with two alleles A and G) and 389 (with two alleles C and G), the $\beta_2 AR$ gene includes two polymorphisms located at codons 16 (with two alleles A and G) and 27 (with two alleles C and G), and the $\alpha_1 A$ gene includes a polymorphism located at codon 492. The heart rate data were adjusted for covariate effects due to demographic differences.

Many mathematical models have been developed to describe the pharmacodynamic response of drug-body interactions (Felmlee et al. 2012; Finlay et al. 2020). One of the simplest and most popular models is the Hill equation (Giraldo 2003; Gesztelyi et al. 2012; Reeve and Turner 2013; Meyer et al. 2019). Let E denote the effect elicited by a drug at its concentration C. The Hill equation is expressed as

$$E = E_0 + \frac{E_{\max} C^H}{E_{50}^H + C^H} \tag{6.11}$$

where E_0 is the baseline, $E_{\max}$ is the maximal effect that can be evoked by the given drug in the given system (geometrically: upper asymptote), EC_{50} is the concentration producing half maximum effect (geometrically: midpoint location), and H is the Hill coefficient (geometrically: a factor characterizing the slope of the effect-concentration curve at the midpoint). In this four-parametric (E_0, $E_{\max}$, EC_{50}, H) form of the Hill equation, the lower asymptote is implicitly the baseline.

We implement the Hill equation into functional mapping to estimate Hill coefficients for each genotype at an SNP. A log-likelihood ratio test shows that, among five SNPs studied, only codon27 from the $\beta_2 AR$ gene is statistically significant ($P<0.05$), showing that this locus participates in mediating heart rate response to dobutamine. We use the estimated Hill coefficients to draw the genotypic curves of heart rate response at each SNP, regardless of whether it is significant or not, from which the additive genetic curve and dominant genetic curves are estimated using equations (6.1a) and (6.1b) (Figure 6.3a). Based on equation (6.2a), we estimate and draw the curves of genetic variance explained by each SNP (Figure 6.3b). We find that genetic variance due to a single SNP periodically changes with concentration, despite with SNP-dependent patterns. SNP codon27 from the $\beta_2 AR$ gene displays a concentration-varying change in genetic variance in a way that is strikingly different from the other four SNPs. These SNP-dependent differences imply the occurrence of genetic interactions, which can be encapsulated into pharmacodynamically varying genetic networks using functional graph theory.

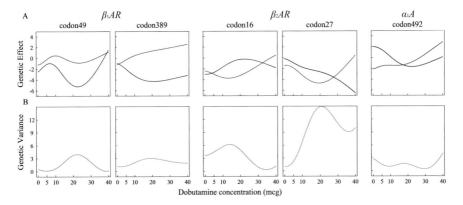

FIGURE 6.3
Functional mapping of heart rate response to dobutamine. (a) Additive genetic effect curves (red line) and dominant genetic effect curves (blue line) estimated from three genotypic values at each SNP. (b) Genetic variance curves of each SNP over different concentrations of dobutamine.

6.3.2 Reconstructing Pharmacogenetic Interaction Networks

We use the LV-based ODEs in equation (6.7) to estimate the independent and dependent components of each SNP, from which we reconstruct an overall inter-SNP interaction network for dobutamine response (Figure 6.4a). We find that SNPs vary dramatically in their intrinsic capacity to express independent genetic variances. Codon27 in the $\beta_2 AR$ gene has the largest independent genetic variance, followed by codon16 in the same gene and codon492 in gene $\alpha_1 A$.

Two SNPs in the $\beta_1 AR$ gene, especially codon389, have the lowest genetic variances, which implies that they exert a small effect on heart rate response if they are in isolation. Codon492 triggers altruistic/aggressive epistasis with all other SNPs, thought to play an important role in stabilizing the balance of the pharmacogenetic network. Codon49 exerts directionally antagonistic epistasis to codon389 from the same gene $\beta_1 AR$, while two SNPs codon16 and codon27 from gene $\beta_2 AR$ establish an asymmetrical altruistic/aggressive relationship. SNPs from different genes also interact with each other, through directional synergism (from codon49 to codon27) and altruism/aggression (between codon389 and codon16).

Functional graph theory can capture instantaneous networks over spatio-temporal gradients. We apply it to visualize and trace how pharmacogenetic networks change in interaction architecture over the concentration of dobutamine (Figure 6.4b). Such topological changes can interrogate how epistasis mediates the drug response of heart rate. There is a dramatic discrepancy between network structure pre- and post-treatment of dobutamine. Prior to the treatment, five SNPs have low independent genetic variances, which are linked with each other to a low extent. Yet, after the drug was administered,

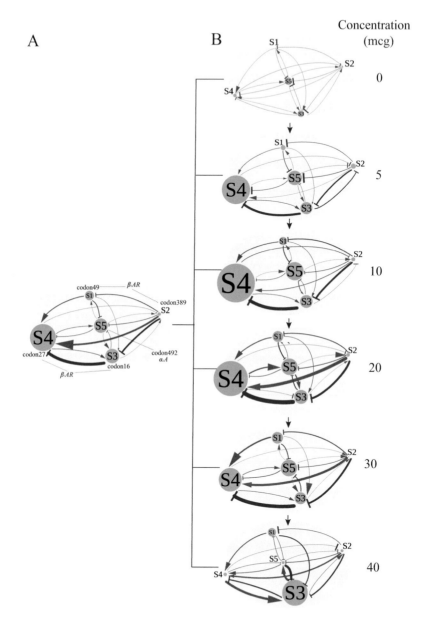

FIGURE 6.4

Pharmacogenetic networks for dose-response curves of heart rate reconstructed by functional graph theory. (a) Overall network from a series of concentration doses. (b) Concentration-specific networks showing topological changes with concentration. The nodes of networks are denoted by circles, whose size is proportional to the independent genetic variance value. The edges of networks are denoted by arrowed lines with red and blue indicating promotion and inhibition, respectively. The thickness of lines is proportional to the strength of promotion or inhibition.

the value of independent genetic variance increases strikingly for all SNPs, especially codon27 in gene $\beta_2 AR$, and, also, interaction strength and pattern produce a pronounced change. For example, directional antagonistic epistasis from codon389 to codon49 in gene $\beta_1 AR$ becomes stronger from pre- to post-treatment and further this epistasis increases with the concentration of dobutamine. Codon389 and codon16 from different genes switch their interaction pattern from altruistic/aggressive epistasis pre-treatment to asymmetric antagonistic epistasis post-treatment. We further find that while some epistasis, such as codon389-codon49 epistasis and codon27-codon49 epistasis, is consistent in strength over increasing concentration, many display change with concentration (Figure 6.4b). For example, codon16 and codon 27 from gene $\beta_2 AR$ form an altruistic/aggressive relationship, but the aggression of the latter for the former becomes much stronger as concentration increases from 5 to 20 mcg but reduces gradually after 20 mcg. Taken together, we identify two types of epistatic network change, i.e., a qualitative change in independent genetic variance and epistatic variance from no drug to drug conditions, which is switched on by the administration of dobutamine, followed by a quantitative change with an increasing dose of the drug, mediated by dose change.

We illustrate how an SNP is regulated by other SNPs to mediate drug response over dose change (Figure 6.5a). We find that SNPs are associated with heart rate response in different ways. Codon389 is the only SNP whose net genetic variance is consistent with its independent genetic variance because it receives small and also sign-opposite epistasis. The genetic variance of all other SNPs is underestimated by a marginally based functional mapping model, because for these SNPs the independent genetic variance component

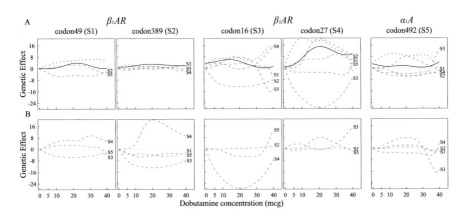

FIGURE 6.5
(a) Net genetic variance curves (solid blue line) for each SNP decomposed into independent genetic variance curve (dash blue line) due to its own capacity and dependent genetic variance curves (red line) resulting from influences of other SNPs (as regulators). (b) Dependent genetic variance curves of regulatees by each SNP.

is larger than the net genetic variance. In other words, if these SNPs were isolated from their counterparts, they could release larger genetic variance than what was observed. For example, codon49 has a relatively small net genetic variance (which is not significant by statistical testing), but its independent genetic variance is virtually large, which is not expressed due to strong negative epistasis from codon389 in the same gene $\beta_2 AR$, despite positive epistasis from codon492 in gene $\alpha_1 A$ to a lesser extent. The net genetic variance of codon27 is significant according to functional mapping, but its independent genetic variance is even larger, because of the accumulated negative epistasis from other SNPs. It is interesting to see that codon27 simultaneously receives negative epistasis from codon16 and codon492 (as negative regulators) and positive epistasis from codon389 and codon49 (as positive regulators), but after positive-negative cancelation the dependent genetic variance is negative, making the independent genetic variance of codon27 not fully expressed. By inhibiting negative regulators and activating positive regulators, the genetic variance of codon27 can be amplified on the purpose of better using this SNP for improving drug response.

We also illustrate how each SNP regulates other SNPs to mediate drug response (Figure 6.5b). We find that codon389 and codon492 each regulate all other SNPs, whereas codon49, codon16, and codon27 each mediate three of the remaining SNPs. Codon389 and codon15 are found to be a big regulator, which strikingly promote and inhibit the same SNP codon27, respectively. Taken together, codon27 is a unique SNP that can play a more critical role in mediating dobutamine-induced heart rate response than what is observed by either silencing all regulators (because of its large independent genetic variance) or activating or inhibiting strong regulators.

6.4 Fine-Grained Dissection of Pharmacogenetic Networks

6.4.1 Model

Equation (6.7) provides a general framework for reconstructing pharmacogenetic networks from genetic variances of individual SNPs estimated by functional mapping. Thus, genetic interactions estimated by functional graph theory are part of the genetic variance of an SNP influenced by other SNPs. In classic quantitative genetics, genetic interactions can also be described as genetic effects, including four types of epistatic effects, i.e., additive×additive, additive×dominant, dominant×additive, and dominant×dominant epistatic effects. We need to infer a genetic network that encapsulates each of these epistatic types.

Genetic variance at an SNP includes additive genetic variance due to additive effect and dominant genetic variance due to dominant effect. Let $a_s(c)$

and $d_s(c)$ denote the additive and dominant genetic effects of SNP s, respectively, which are estimated from equations (6.1a) and (6.1b) by functional mapping. Functional graph theory suggests that the expression of genetic effect at an SNP is determined both by this SNP intrinsic strategy and the strategies of other SNPs that co-occur in a gene community. Thus, each genetic effect is thought to include its independent component and dependent components due to its interactions with the same or different types of genetic effects at other SNPs. As can be seen from equation (6.7), we formulate this argument by a system of LV-based ODEs as

$$
\begin{bmatrix} \dot{a}(c) \\ \dot{d}(c) \end{bmatrix} = \begin{bmatrix} \dot{a}_1(c) \\ \dot{d}_1(c) \\ \vdots \\ \dot{a}_p(c) \\ \dot{d}_p(c) \end{bmatrix}
$$

$$
= \begin{bmatrix} \mathcal{A}_1\left(a_1(c):\Phi_1^a\right) + \sum_{s=2}^{m}\mathcal{A}_{a1\leftarrow s}\left(a_s(c):\Phi_{a1\leftarrow s}^a\right) + \sum_{s=2}^{m}\mathcal{A}_{d1\leftarrow s}\left(d_s(c):\Phi_{d1\leftarrow s}^a\right) \\ \mathcal{D}_1\left(d_1(c):\Phi_1^d\right) + \sum_{s=2}^{m}\mathcal{D}_{a1\leftarrow s}\left(a_s(c):\Phi_{a1\leftarrow s}^d\right) + \sum_{j'=2}^{m}\mathcal{D}_{d1\leftarrow s}\left(d_s(c):\Phi_{d1\leftarrow s}^d\right) \\ \mathcal{A}_m\left(a_m(c):\Phi_m^a\right) + \sum_{s=1}^{m-1}\mathcal{A}_{am\leftarrow s}\left(a_s(c):\Phi_{am\leftarrow s}^a\right) + \sum_{s=1}^{m-1}\mathcal{A}_{dm\leftarrow s}\left(d_s(c):\Phi_{dm\leftarrow s}^a\right) \\ \mathcal{D}_m\left(a_m(c):\Phi_m^d\right) + \sum_{j'=1}^{m-1}\mathcal{D}_{am\leftarrow s}\left(a_s(c):\Phi_{am\leftarrow s}^d\right) + \sum_{s=1}^{m-1}\mathcal{D}_{dm\leftarrow s}\left(d_s(c):\Phi_{dm\leftarrow s}^d\right) \end{bmatrix} \quad (6.12)
$$

where the first term of the right side is an independent (*endogenous*) effect, determined by this SNP's own strategy and the sum of the second and third terms of the right side is a dependent (*exogenous*) effect, determined by the strategies of other SNPs. We coin the following concepts:

- The *endogenous additive effect* of SNP s, denoted as $\mathcal{A}_s(\cdot)$, reflects its capacity to exert an additive effect when this SNP is assumed to be in isolation;
- The *endogenous dominant effect* of SNP s, denoted as $\mathcal{D}_s(\cdot)$, reflects its capacity to exert a dominant effect when this SNP is assumed to be in isolation;
- The *exogenous additive × additive effect* of SNP s, denoted as $\mathcal{A}_{as\leftarrow s'}(\cdot)$ $(s' = 1, ..., s-1, s+1, ..., m)$, is the effect of the accumulated additive effects of other SNPs on the additive effect of that SNP;

- The *exogenous dominant × additive effect* of SNP s, $\mathcal{A}_{ds\leftarrow s'}(\bullet)$, is the effect of the accumulated dominant effects of other SNPs on the additive effect of that SNP;
- The *exogenous additive × dominant effect* of SNP s, denoted as $\mathcal{D}_{as\leftarrow s'}(\bullet)$, is the effect of the accumulated additive effects of other SNPs on the dominant effect of that SNP;
- The *exogenous dominant × dominant effect* of SNP s, denoted as $\mathcal{D}_{ds\leftarrow s'}(\bullet)$, is the effect of the accumulated dominant effects of other SNPs on the dominant effect of that SNP.

We note that the terms $\mathcal{A}_{s\leftarrow s'}(\bullet)$ and $\mathcal{D}_{s\leftarrow s'}(\bullet)$ form the community interaction functions in classical population dynamics or the payoff functions in ordinary evolutionary game theory. Because explicit forms of these terms do not exist, we implement a nonparametric smoothing approach, such as LOP, to model their dynamic behaviors.

Equation (6.12) is a full model that allows all possible entities to be fully interconnected, but a highly dense network does not assure the living system to be robust to stochastic errors. We implement variable selection to choose a small set of the most significant entities that are linked with a given SNP. Let m_{saa} and m_{sad} denote the numbers of the most significant additive and dominant effects from different SNPs which are associated with the additive effect of SNP s and m_{sda} and m_{sdd} denote the numbers of the most significant additive and dominant effects from different SNPs associated with the dominant effect of SNP s, respectively. With these numbers, a system of ODEs in equation (6.12) reduces to its sparse form:

$$
\begin{bmatrix} \dot{a}_s(c) \\ \dot{d}_s(c) \end{bmatrix}
$$

$$
\begin{bmatrix} \mathcal{A}_s\left(a_s(c):\Phi_s^a\right)+ \displaystyle\sum_{s'=1,s'\neq s}^{m_{saa}} \mathcal{A}_{as\leftarrow s'}\left(a_{s'}(c):\Phi_{as\leftarrow s'}^a\right)+ \displaystyle\sum_{s'=1,s'\neq s}^{m_{sad}} \mathcal{A}_{ds\leftarrow s'}\left(d_{s'}(c):\Phi_{ds\leftarrow s'}^a\right) \\ \mathcal{D}_s\left(d_s(c):\Phi_s^d\right)+ \displaystyle\sum_{s'=1,s'\neq s}^{m_{sda}} \mathcal{D}_{as\leftarrow s'}\left(a_{s'}(c):\Phi_{as\leftarrow s'}^d\right)+ \displaystyle\sum_{s'=1,s'\neq s}^{m_{sdd}} \mathcal{D}_{ds\leftarrow s'}\left(d_{s'}(c):\Phi_{ds\leftarrow s'}^d\right) \end{bmatrix} \quad (6.13)
$$

We formulate a likelihood approach for solving these sparse ODEs and use the estimated independent and dependent genetic effect components to reconstruct pharmacodynamical genetic networks that code all possible epistatic types. These networks provide a tool to study the fine-grained genetic architecture of drug response by modeling detailed additive and dominant effects of each SNP.

6.4.2 Effect-Based Pharmacogenetic Networks

We analyze the same dataset from the pharmacogenetic association study as described in Section 6.3. We use functional mapping to estimate the additive and dominant genetic effect curves for each SNP (Figure 6.3a). There is considerable SNP-dependent variability in these two types of genetic effect, implying the possibility of reconstructing genetic interaction networks. We formulate a likelihood function of genetic effect data for all SNPs, implemented by a set of ODEs in equation (6.13) and SAD(1)-structuring covariance matrix. Using the estimated ODE parameters, we reconstruct effect-based pharmacogenetic interaction networks at the additive×additive (aa), additive×dominant (ad), dominant×additive (da), and dominant×dominant (dd) epistatic levels (Figure 6.6). The aa and ad networks are defined as the networks in which the additive genetic effects of SNPs (additive regulatees) are regulated by the additive and dominant effects of other SNPs (regulators), respectively, whereas da and dd networks are those in which the dominant genetic effects of SNPs (dominant regulates) are regulated by the additive and dominant effects of other SNPs (regulators), respectively. We find that these four types of interaction networks have different topological structures in terms of the number, strength, and pattern of SNP-SNP links.

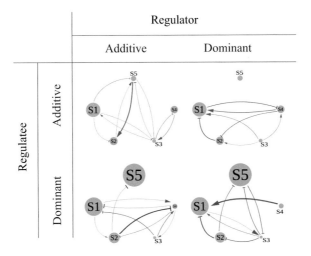

FIGURE 6.6
Effect-based pharmacogenetic networks for heart rate response to dobutamine in terms of additive × additive, additive × dominant, dominant × additive, and dominant × dominant epistatic effects. The nodes of networks are the independent genetic effects of SNPs as regulatees, denoted by circles with size proportional to the magnitude of the independent genetic effects. The edges of networks represent the dependent genetic effects of regulatees affected by regulators, denoted by arrowed red and bluelines indicating promotion and inhibition, respectively. The thickness of lines is proportional to the strength of promotion or inhibition.

As seen in Figure 6.4a, the SNPs studied were expressed differently if they were in isolation. We find that codon49, codon389, and codon492 display strong overdominant inheritance, with the dominant effect of codon492 being strikingly larger than its additive effect, when they were isolated from other SNPs. By comparing the aa and ad networks, we find that additive regulatees are regulated by the additive effects of regulators in a different way from that used by their dominant effects. For example, the additive effect of codon492 in gene $\alpha_1 A$ receives additive directional antagonistic epistasis from codon49 and establishes asymmetric synergistic epistasis with the additive effect of codon389 and asymmetric antagonistic epistasis with the additive effect of codon16 (aa network), but the additive effect of codon492 is not influenced by the dominant effects of any other SNPs (ad network). We also find pronounced differences in the da and dd networks, suggesting that the dominant effects of SNPs are affected differently by the additive and dominant effects of regulators.

Figure 6.7 illustrates how the additive and dominant genetic effects of each SNP on heart rate response are affected by the additive and dominant effects of other SNPs over different concentrations of dobutamine. The additive effect of codon49 is very low, but its independent additive effect component is virtually large, which is canceled out by regulators of different signs. Similarly, we find that the dominant effects of codon389 and codon492 each have a large independent dominant effect component, which is counteracted by regulators. The net additive effect of codon27 has a different sign from its independent additive effect, because it receives epistasis from codon49 and codon16 in different signs. Taken together, the observed additive and dominant effect of an SNP is the consequence of its intrinsic capacity and the epistatic influence of other SNPs. It is possible that the genetic effect of an SNP can be amplified by activating or inhibiting the expression of the genetic effects of its strong regulators.

6.5 Modularity Theory and Dunbar's Law

6.5.1 Genome-Wide Network Validation of Omnigenic Theory

As a complex trait, drug response is thought to be polygenic; i.e., there is a large number of genes (each with minor effects) involved in mediating pharmacological reactions to medical interventions (Koido et al. 2020; Babb de Villiers et al. 2020; Reay et al. 2020; Johnson et al. 2022). Yet, uncertainty on the exact number of genes has long been part of the debate on quantitative inheritance since quantitative genetics emerged as a discipline over one century ago (Fisher 1918; Lange 1997; Crouch and Bodmer 2020). More recently, omnigenic theory has been postulated to explain quantitative inheritance

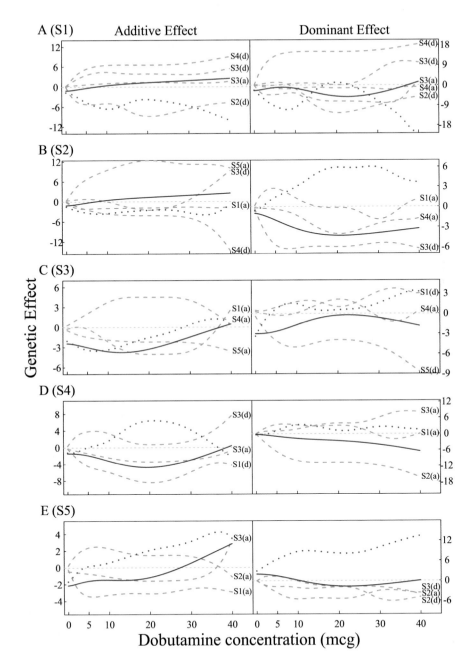

FIGURE 6.7
Net additive and dominant genetic variance curves (solid blue line) for each SNP decomposed into independent genetic variance curve (dash blue line) due to its own capacity and dependent genetic variance curves resulting from additive (red line) or dominant influences (green line) of other SNPs (as regulators). Codon49 (a) and codon389 from $\beta_1 AR$ (b), codon16 (c) and codon27 from $\beta_2 AR$ (d), and codon492 from $\alpha_1 A$ (e).

(Boyle et al. 2017), stating that genetic architecture is constituted by a complete set of genes. According to this theory, each and every gene participates in the genetic control of a complex disease or trait in a variety of ways. Some genes directly affect the trait, whereas many others do so indirectly through other genes. Indirect pathways form a complex network in which information flows from one node (gene) to the next. Functional graph theory is equipped with a capacity to trace and visualize the information flow of all genes involved in the network. Despite this, the algorithm described above is only focused on the network modeling of a limited number of genes, which is far away from the theme of omnigenic theory.

GWAS aim to identify all possible significant genetic loci for drug response from a high- or even ultrahigh-dimensional pool of SNPs throughout the whole genome (Daly 2010; Motsinger-Reif et al. 2013; McInnes et al. 2021). Thus, GWAS provide a powerful fuel to test and validate the omnigenic theory of drug response, but encapsulating all genes into a network is challenged because exponentially increasing complexity due to an increasing number of SNPs can quickly prevent efficient and effective computation of LV-based ODEs. Even without computational burden, reconstructing genome-wide, fully interconnected interactome networks as an essential tool for the omnigenic test is not biologically justified, given that such highly dense systems may be vulnerable to environmental perturbations (Landi et al. 2018; Yonatan et al. 2022; Goyal 2022). The molecular interpretation of this notion is that each SNP is unlikely to interact with every other SNP in a cell. As such, how to reconstruct sparse pharmacogenetic networks that cover all SNPs is a matter of great importance in comprehending the genetic architecture of drug response.

6.5.2 Developmental Modularity Theory Meets Dunbar's Law

The early ecological theory suggested that complex systems are more stable than simple ones (Odum 1953; MacArthur 1955; Elton 1958). This empirical viewpoint was challenged by May's (1972, 1973) analytical solution. Using rigorous mathematical modeling, May's investigation complemented Gardner and Ashby's (1970) finding via computer simulation, stating that large complex systems may be stable up to a certain critical level of connectance, followed by a sudden interrupt as this critical level increases. In community ecology research, May's idea has established a widely accepted foundation to study complexity-stability relationships (Yonatan et al. 2022; Goyal 2022). We introduce this idea into functional graph theory, which can be upgraded to test omnigenic theory.

To make this introduction possible in computation, we incorporate developmental modularity theory and Dunbar's law. In biology, different entities display functional similarities and differences and, therefore, are organized into distinct modules within each of which entities are more functionally correlated with each other than with those from other modules (Callebaut and Rasskin-Gutman 2005; Wagner et al. 2007). In our case, some SNPs may change their genetic effects over time in a similar pattern, which are thus coalesced into the same communities of networks in which SNPs (nodes) are more closely interconnected than those from other network communities. SNPs with different patterns of genetic effect change are located in different network communities. Thus, by clustering all SNPs into different modules, we determine the number and size of network communities. In the end, we dissolve a big network into a set of multiple communities, each representing a subnetwork. This process has two advantages: first, this is a sparse network, which may be more stable than a full network, second, the number of SNPs within a community reduces so that computational efficiency increases.

After an optimal number of modules is determined, we take the means (or fit the mean curves) of genetic variances of all SNPs from the same module and use these means to reconstruct a module-module interaction network using a system of LV-based ODEs in equation (6.7). According to parsimony theory, an interaction network needs to be reconstructed only based on a set of key pathways that forms the network. The detection of these key pathways can be made possible by several well-established variable selection approaches, such as LASSO (Tibshirani 1996), adaptive LASSO (Zou and Hastie 2005; Yuan and Lin 2006), and adaptive group LASSO (Wang and Leng 2008). While the module network is reconstructed, SNP-SNP interaction networks for each module can also be inferred. This leads to the reconstruction of a two-layer network, on whose top is the community network and at whose bottom is multiple SNP networks nested within the community network (Figure 6.8).

As mentioned above, the number of SNPs in a module reduces, but this number may still be so large that it prevents the reconstruction of SNP network under this module. In this case, we further cluster this module into its distinct submodule in each of which the number of SNPs reduces again. If a submodule is still too large, we cluster it into its distinct sub-submodule. This clustering procedure may continue until the number of SNP within a unit reaches a tractable level for network reconstruction. This tractable number can be Dunbar's number. In modeling social networks, Dunbar (1992) found that there is a limit to the number of relationships within a network an individual can stably maintain. However, this limit is directly proportional to the network dimension (Harré and Prokopenko 2016). The integration of developmental modularity theory and Dunbar's law makes it possible to reconstruct a multiscale (between and within modules), community-delimited, sparse epistatic network.

6.5.3 Functional Clustering Algorithms

There are several statistical approaches available for clustering longitudinal data. Here, we introduce a mixture-based likelihood approach for clustering different genes into distinct modules based on the similarity of their genetic

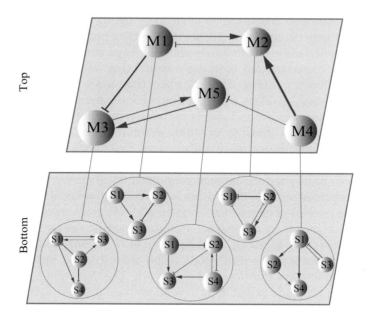

FIGURE 6.8

Diagram of a two-layer network reconstructed from functional graph theory implemented with developmental modularity theory. Functional clustering classifies all SNPs' distinct modules M1–M5 that link with each other to form a top network, with SNPs within each module forming a bottom network. The arrowed red and blue lines represent promotion and inhibition one SNP exerts for the next, with line thickness being proportional to the strength of promotion or inhibition.

variance change patterns over concentration. This algorithm, called functional clustering, proposed by Kim et al. (2008), incorporates a parametric or nonparametric function of concentration-varying genetic variances into the likelihood. Let $\mathbf{y}_s = (y_s(1), \ldots, y_s(T))$ denote the genetic variances of SNP s ($s=1, \ldots, m$) estimated at T concentrations by functional mapping. Assume that m genes can be clustered into K modules. The mixture likelihood function of the genetic variance data is formulated as

$$L(\mathbf{y}) = \prod_{s=1}^{m} \sum_{k=1}^{K} \left[\pi_k f_k (\mathbf{y}_s : \mu_k, \Sigma) \right] \qquad (6.14)$$

where π_k is the mixture proportion of module k (also called prior probability), $f_k(\mathbf{y}_s : \mu_k, \Sigma)$ is a multivariate normal distribution function with mean vector μ_k and covariance matrix Σ. We incorporate a nonparametric approach – LOP to model the mean vector and SAD(1) to model the structure of covariance matrix. Thus, LOP parameters and SAD(1) parameters that specify the normal distribution should be estimated by maximizing the likelihood function in equation (6.14).

We implement a hybrid of the EM algorithm and the simplex algorithm to solve the likelihood. The simplex algorithm is nested within the EM algorithm. The EM algorithm includes two steps, expectation (E) and maximization (M). In the E step, we calculate the (posterior) probability of gene s that belongs to module k by using

$$\Pi_{k|s} = \frac{\pi_k f_k(\mathbf{y}_s : \boldsymbol{\mu}_k, \Sigma)}{\sum_{k'=1}^{K} \left[\pi_{k'} f_{k'}(\mathbf{y}_s : \boldsymbol{\mu}_{k'}, \Sigma) \right]} \tag{6.15}$$

In the M step, we calculate the mixture proportion of module k by

$$\pi_k = \frac{1}{n} \sum_{s=1}^{m} \Pi_{k|s} \tag{6.16}$$

and LOP and SAD(1) parameters by the simplex algorithm. The E and M steps are iterated until the estimates of the parameters converge into stable values. Note that SAD(1)-structure matrix has closed forms for its determinant and inverse, which can enhance computational efficiency.

By calculating the likelihood values by assuming different numbers of modules starting from 2, we estimate an information criterion, such as AIC or BIC, in each case, from which an optimal number of modules, say K_o, is determined. We then calculate the posterior probability of each gene assigned to a module and then use these probabilities to determine the most likely module to which this gene belong. Ultimately, we determine how many genes are in each module and which gene belongs to a module. We then fit the mean curve of all genes within a module by LOP and further use these mean curves to reconstruct the module-module interaction network.

If we want to cluster all genes into distinct modules based on the similarity of their genetic additive and dominant effects, we implement a bivariate functional clustering model (Wang et al. 2012). Let $(\mathbf{y}_{as}; \mathbf{y}_{ds}) = (y_{as}(1), ..., y_{as}(T); y_{ds}(1), ..., y_{ds}(T))$ denote the additive and dominant genetic variances of SNP s ($s=1, ..., m$), respectively, estimated at T concentrations by functional mapping. A bivariate mixture likelihood function of the data is written as

$$L(\mathbf{y}; \mathbf{z}) = \prod_{s=1}^{m} \sum_{k=1}^{K} \left[\pi_k f_k(\mathbf{y}_{as}; \mathbf{y}_{ds} : \boldsymbol{\mu}_{ak}; \boldsymbol{\mu}_{dk}, \Sigma) \right] \tag{6.17}$$

where π_k is defined as above, $f_k(\mathbf{y}_{as}; \mathbf{y}_{ds} : \boldsymbol{\mu}_{ak}; \boldsymbol{\mu}_{dk}, \Sigma)$ is a bivariate longitudinal normal distribution function with additive and dominant effect mean vector $(\boldsymbol{\mu}_{ak}; \boldsymbol{\mu}_{dk})$ (fitted by LOP) and covariance matrix Σ, expressed as

$$\Sigma = \begin{pmatrix} \Sigma_a & \Sigma_{ad} \\ \Sigma_{da} & \Sigma_d \end{pmatrix} \tag{6.18}$$

with Σ_a and Σ_d are the residual covariance matrices for additive and dominant effects and $\Sigma_{ad} = \Sigma_{da}$ is the residual covariance matrices between additive and dominant effects. The structure of Σ can be modeled by bivariate SAD(1) (Zhao et al. 2005b).

The hybrid algorithm as described above can be used to solve the likelihood in equation (6.17) and estimate the LOP and SAD(1) parameters. Likewise, AIC or BIC is used to determine an optimal number of modules among m genes. Module-module interaction networks in terms of additive and dominant effects can be reconstructed.

6.6 Concluding Remarks

Interindividual variability in drug response presents a pressing need to develop precision medicine. It has been increasingly clear that the genetic factors involved in this variability cannot be sufficiently understood at individual levels, rather through epistatic modeling of different genetic entities (Zhao and Iyengar 2012; Huang et al. 2013; Hicks et al. 2017; Zhou and Lauschke 2019). Although systems pharmacogenomics has emerged as a discipline (Cheng et al. 2018, 2019), there is serious scarceness of computational tools for network modeling. Existing approaches borrowed from other fields, such as physical, engineering, and social sciences, are powerful for network inference, but their applications may be limited because their networks fail to capture all features of gene-gene interactions, including epistatic strength, causality, and directed sign. Also, current approaches lack a capacity to coalesce a high-dimensional pool of genome-wide genes into pharmacogenetic networks, making it difficult to chart a complete picture of genetic architecture for drug response.

In this chapter, we introduce a new theory – functional graph theory to pharmacogenetic network modeling. This theory – the combination of functional mapping, evolutionary game theory, and LV predator-prey theory (Sun et al. 2021) – has proven to be powerful for reconstructing bidirectional, signed, and weighted interaction networks using GWAS data (Wang et al. 2021; Yang et al. 2021). Functional mapping incorporates pharmacokinetic and pharmacodynamic equations to estimate how genetic effects or variances due to single SNPs change over time and drug concentration, whereas evolutionary game theory decomposes such net effects or variances of each SNP into two underlying components through a system of LV-based ODEs, the independent component due to the intrinsic capacity of this SNP and the dependent component resulting from the regulation of other SNPs on this SNP. The independent and dependent components, coded as nodes and edges, respectively, are coalesced into mathematical graphs. The sign and magnitude of dependent components between different SNPs capture and record the full features of genetic interactions (epistasis), bidirectional, signed, and weighted. This capacity of functional graph theory to dissect epistasis into its underlying formation mechanisms overcome the limitation of originally defined epistasis by early geneticists (Bateson 1907; Fisher 1918) and leverages the precision application of this concept in clinical practice.

We apply functional graph theory to analyze a candidate-gene association study aimed at testing how heart rate responds to dobutamine. Although this study was conducted on a small scale, it can well demonstrate the application of functional graph theory. Among five SNPs genotyped from three candidate genes, $\beta_1 AR$, $\beta_2 AR$, and $\alpha_1 A$, for cardiovascular function (Graham et al. 1996; Woo et al. 2015), only codon27 in gene $\beta_2 AR$ is significantly associated with dose-dependent heart rate based on functional mapping. However, functional graph theory provides new insight into the genetic control mechanisms of all SNPs including those insignificant ones. First, codon49, codon16, and codon492 are found to be insignificant because they receive inhibition from other SNPs (Figure 6.5a). Virtually, those SNPs have a remarkable intrinsic capacity, i.e., they could be expressed at a high level if they were separated from their negative regulators. The most notable example is codon492 whose large independent component is not expressed because it is largely canceled out by inhibition it receives from codon389, codon27, and codon16. Thus, by blocking the expression of these negative regulators, codon492's genetic variance can increase to its independent value, which can be better used in practical medicine.

Second, codon27 is a significant SNP, but its impact can be amplified for two reasons. The first reason is that it has a large independent genetic variance component, thus by blocking the expression of regulators, codon27 can fully release its independent variance (Figure 6.5a). The second reason is that among these regulators, codon16 is a big negative regulator. By blocking the expression of this regulator, the net genetic variance of codon27 can be even larger than its independent genetic variance. In practice, because of its clear links with other SNPs, codon27 can be readily manipulated to maximize its impact on drug response.

Functional graph theory is a dynamic model that can trace topological changes of pharmacogenetic networks over dose gradients (Figure 6.4b). Based on the dynamic change, one can determine how epistasis between a specific pair of SNP changes from one dose level to the next and also the dose level at which epistasis is maximally or minimally expressed. This information can help medical doctors design an optimal dose based on the size and pattern of epistasis between certain SNPs. Functional graph theory can be extended to infer any context-specific pharmacogenetic networks; for example, males and females may respond to the same drug in different ways, and networks can be reconstructed separately for two genders. By comparing sex-specific networks, we can characterize genetic epistatic mechanisms underlying sex differences in drug response. Also, the same drug may be efficacious or toxic, determined by its underlying genetic architecture. Functional graph theory can be modified to reconstruct efficacy- and toxicity-specific genetic networks, used as critical information for designing drugs with maximum benefits and minimum side-effects.

Functional graph theory can reconstruct genetic networks based on additive and dominant effects of SNPs, providing an alternative approach for understanding the genetic architecture of drug response. In correspondence to genetic variance-based networks named the random genetic networks, we call genetic effect-based networks the fixed genetic networks. Both random and fixed genetic networks can visualize and trace how different SNPs interact with each other to mediate drug response, but they may provide different information. A random genetic network can quantify the contribution of epistasis to the overall genetic variance, which can be used as a criterion to assess its importance and significance for translational medicine, whereas a fixed genetic network can design a practical scheme on how to utilize epistasis. For example, the additive effect specifies the difference between two homozygotes, whereas the dominant effect describes the difference of the heterozygote from the mean of the two homozygotes. Thus, by characterizing how the additive and dominant effects of regulators affect the additive and dominant effect of a regulate (leading to additive × additive, additive × dominant, dominant × additive, and dominant × dominant epistasis), we can precisely alter genetic effects of the regulator that are directly relevant to phenotypic values of complex traits, i.e., heart rate in our example. As such, fixed networks provide more precise information about the genetic architecture of drug response and its translation into practical clinics.

To address a major challenge in inferring a high-dimensional network involving a complete set of genome-wide SNPs, functional graph theory introduces developmental modularity theory and Dunbar's law. By clustering all genes into distinct modules, submodules, and sub-submodules all the way to units containing a tractable number of SNPs, functional graph theory can reconstruct multilayer, multiplex, multiscale, and multifunctional networks. Using such networks, one can trace the roadmap of how each SNP mediated drug response directly or through a cascade of indirect pathways. From this information flow, one can determine and choose which SNPs can readily be used to improve drug response and which optimal manipulating strategy is designed to best use a particular SNP.

7

Learning Individualized Pharmacogenetic Networks

7.1 Introduction

Drug response is expressed as a multifactorial trait, similar in many ways to a complex disease, such as type-2 diabetes, schizophrenia, and cancer, as well as a quantitative trait like body height, blood pressure, or serum lipid levels (Evans and Johnson 2001; Zhang and Nebert 2017). Different from a simple definition of disease or trait variation, interindividual variability in drug response can be expressed by various effect types (efficacy, adverse, and toxic) among different patients receiving the same drug, varying efficacies among different patients administered the same drug dose, or a range of doses that produce the same efficacy for all patients (Brunton et al. 2006; Giacomini et al. 2017; Özdemir et al. 2018). Thus, to better study the genetic variation of drug response, it is sorely needed to incorporate the mechanisms of how the body absorbs, distributes, and eventually eliminates a drug over time (referred to as pharmacokinetics or PK) and how a drug affects the body at different concentrations (referred to as pharmacodynamics or PD), which mediate drug efficacy or drug toxicity.

A series of statistical models have been proposed to map drug response as a function-valued trait by integrating the mathematical aspects of PK and PD into the context of genetic association studies (Lin et al. 2005a, b, 2007; Wu and Lin 2008; Wang et al. 2015a). This so-called functional mapping can not only provide a clinically more meaningful interpretation of pharmacogenetic variation but also increase the statistical power of pharmacogene detection. For example, augmented sample sizes are required for traditional static association approaches to achieve the same power by functional mapping (Wang et al. 2021). While functional mapping can identify key individual genetic variants for drug response, it has become clear that most pharmacological traits are influenced by numerous small-effect variants, together with environmental factors, acting to form complicated networks of gene-gene interactions (i.e., epistasis) and gene-environment interactions (Zhou and Pearson 2013; Klengel and Binder 2013;

Chhibber et al. 2014; Marderstein et al. 2021; McInnes et al. 2021). Thus far, we are still unclear about a complete picture of the genetic architecture underlying drug response.

Current GWAS for complex traits have developed to a point at which all genetic variants genotyped through the whole genome can be coalesced into intricate but well-orchestrated interactome networks to comprehend genetic architecture (Sun et al. 2021). This task is realized by functional graph theory – the combination theory of functional mapping and graph theory through evolutionary game theory (Wu and Jiang et al. 2021; Dong et al. 2021; Feng et al. 2021). Functional graph theory decomposes the net genetic effect of each gene (estimated by marginally based functional mapping) into its independent component (occurring in an assumed isolated condition) and dependent component (due to the influence of other genes on it). The comparison of independent and dependent components allows us to assess and chart the roadmap of how each gene affects a complex phenotype, directly or through an indirect path.

It is straightforward to apply functional graph theory to infer pharmacogenetic networks for drug response in pharmacological GWAS. Such networks reflect an overall property of genetic interactions inferred from all sampled subjects, but failing to capture population heterogeneity in interaction architecture. For some certain subjects, the combination of two genes produces a mutualistic effect on drug efficacy, but for others this combination becomes antagonistic. Apart from this variability in interaction types, interindividual changes may occur in the strength of the same interaction types. For example, in some subjects, one gene displays a week aggression toward the second, whereas this aggression is particularly strong in other subjects. The central theme of individualized or precision medicine is to tailor the right medications for the right persons, administered at a right dose and timing, which, thereby, requires precise information about individualized genetics in drug response.

In this chapter, we extend functional graph theory to reconstruct individualized pharmacogenetic interaction networks from PK- and PD-embedded GWAS data. We estimate genotypic mean curves for drug response at each SNP using functional mapping and assign these curves to individual subjects based on their genotype at a specific SNP. A system of non-linear Lotka-Volterra (LV)-based ordinary differential equations (ODEs) are built to dissect genotypic curves at an SNP into their independent components assumed to form in an isolation and dependent components due to influences of the genotypes at other loci. We perform computer simulation to validate the statistical behavior of functional graph theory and justify its utility by analyzing a real data set for a pharmacogenetic association study.

7.2 A Framework for Network Inference

7.2.1 Pharmacogenetic Mapping

We design a pharmacogenetic GWAS setting in which n subjects are sampled from a natural population. To assess their variability in drug response, these subjects are administered at a series of drug doses. A therapeutic variable that reflects drug response (drug efficacy, adverse effect, or toxic effect) is measured for each subject prior to drug administration (baseline) and following the administration of the drug at each dose. Considering differences in administration schedule, let $(c_{i0}, c_{i1}, ..., c_{iT_i})$ denote different dosage concentrations for a specific subject i (where $c_{i0}=0$) $(i=1, ..., n)$ and $(y_i(c_{i0}), y_i(c_{i1}), ..., y_i(c_{iT_i}))$ denote the observed values of drug response of this subject. All these subjects are genotyped at a panel of m genome-wide distributed SNP loci. In the subsequent analysis, we use adjusted phenotypic data of drug response that are corrected for all possible covariates including population structure detected using all m SNPs. The data structure for association studies is illustrated in Figure 7.1a.

Consider SNP s $(s=1, ..., m)$ with three genotypes AA, Aa, and aa, whose observations are denoted as n_{sAA}, n_{sAa}, and n_{saa}, respectively. Functional mapping is built on the likelihood function of observed phenotypic data at a given SNP, expressed as

$$L_s\left(\mathbf{y}\right)=\prod_{i=1}^{n_{sAA}}f_{sAA}\left(y_i\,;\mu_{sAA|i}\,,\Sigma_{si}\right)\prod_{i=1}^{n_{sAa}}f_{sAa}\left(y_i\,;\mu_{sAa|i}\,,\Sigma_{si}\right)\prod_{i=1}^{n_{saa}}f_{saa}\left(y_i\,;\mu_{saa|i}\,,\Sigma_{si}\right) \quad (7.1)$$

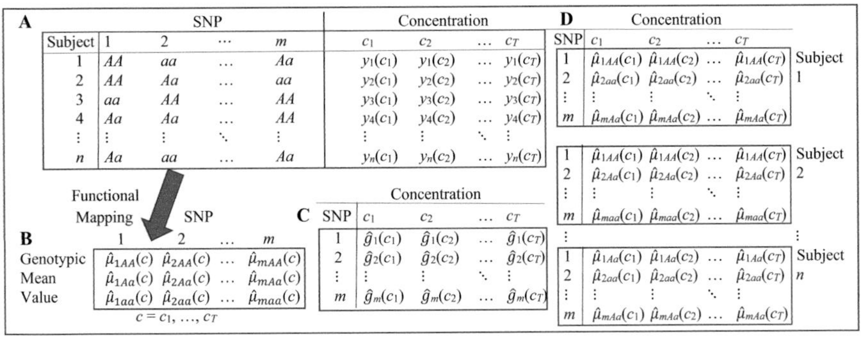

FIGURE 7.1
Data structure of a pharmacogenetic study. (a) Original data including m SNPs and drug response measurements at c_T concentrations for n subjects. (b) Concentration-varying mean values for each of three genotypes at each SNP estimated by functional mapping. (c) Concentration-varying genetic values or genetic effects estimated from mean genotypic values. (d) Concentration-varying genotypic values at each SNP expressed in individual subjects.

where $f_{sj}\left(\mathbf{y}_i;\mathbf{\mu}_{sj|i},\Sigma_{si}\right)$ is the multivariate normal probability density function of drug response data for subject i carrying genotype j ($j=1$ for AA, 2 for Aa, 3 for aa) at SNP s, with genotype-dependent mean vector $\mathbf{\mu}_{sj|i}$ and covariance matrix Σ_{si}.

Functional mapping conducts statistical modeling of joint mean-covariance structure based on the biological or biomedical questions. In pharmacological studies, we model mean vector $\mathbf{\mu}_{sj|i}=\left(\mu_{sj|i}\left(c_{i0}\right),\mu_{sj|i}\left(c_{i1}\right),\ldots,\mu_{sj|i}\left(c_{iT_i}\right)\right)$ by the commonly used the E_{max} equation (Goutelle et al. 2008). In general, the genotypic mean value at a given dose is expressed as

$$\mu_{sj|i}\left(c_{i\tau}\right)=E_{0sj}+\frac{E_{maxsj}c_{i\tau}^{H_{sj}}}{EC_{50sj}^{H_{sj}}+c_{i\tau}^{H_{sj}}} \tag{7.2}$$

where parameters $\Theta_{sj}=(E_{0sj},E_{maxsj},EC_{50sj},H_{sj})$ are the baseline, the asymptotic drug effect, the drug concentration at a half of E_{maxsj}, and the slope of drug response for genotype j at SNP s. In addition, functional mapping implements an autoregressive model, such as the first-order structured antedependence (SAD(1)) model to fit the structure of covariance matrix.

By maximizing the likelihood (7.1), functional mapping obtains the maximum likelihood estimates (MLEs) of model parameters including Θ_{sj} and uses $\hat{\Theta}_{sj}$ to estimate the MLEs of genotypic mean curves, generally denoted as $\hat{\mu}_{sj}(c)$ ($s=1,\ldots,m;j=1,2,3$) (Figure 7.1b), using equation (7.2). By testing whether these curves significantly differ among genotypes, functional mapping identifies a set of significant SNPs for drug response. Further bioinformatics analysis of these significant SNPs helps interpret their biological and biochemical functions.

7.2.2 LV-Based ODE Modeling of Epistatic Networks

According to quantitative genetic theory, we calculate the additive and dominant genetic effect curves based on genotypic curves $\hat{\mu}_{sj}(c)$ and further use the MLEs of these effect curves, combined with allele frequencies at an SNP, to obtain the MLEs of genetic variance curves. Wang et al. (2021) used the genetic standard deviation curves of each SNP as its overall genetic effect curves. These function-valued genetic effect data at each SNP (Figure 7.1c) serve as the basic data for inferring the overall network of SNP-SNP interactions over all subjects.

As described above, functional mapping estimates the genotypic mean values of each genotype at SNP s, $\hat{\mu}_{sj}(c)$, over a series of dose levels (Figure 7.1b). We assign $\hat{\mu}_{sj}(c)$ to subject i carrying genotype j to reflect its concentration-varying genotypic values at SNP s. Considering all SNPs, this assignment produces an ($m\times c_T$) matrix of genotypic values for subject i (Figure 7.1d). This subject-dependent data can be used to infer individualized genetic networks by implementing functional graph theory.

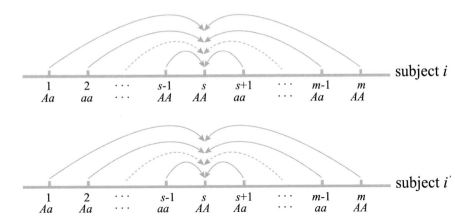

FIGURE 7.2
Diagram showing how epistasis changes from subject to subject. Subjects i and i' have the same genotype AA at a typical SNP s, but the influence this genotype receives from other loci varies between two subjects. For example, genotype AA at SNP s is affected by genotype AA in subject i but aa in subject i' at SNP s–1, by genotype aa in subject i but Aa in subject i' at SNP s+1, etc. We argue that the difference of subject i from subject i' is not only due to genotypic differences at different loci, but also due to epistasis expressed at the genotype level, both causes of which can be characterized by functional graph theory.

To show how epistasis is subject-dependent, we draw a diagram where two subjects i and i' carry different combinations of genotypes over m SNPs (Figure 7.2). Consider SNP s, whose genotype is AA for both subjects. This genotype is affected by genotype AA at SNP s–1, aa at SNP s+1, etc. for subject i, but affected by genotype aa at SNP s–1, Aa at SNP s+1, etc. for subject i'. Such a difference may make two subjects different in drug response.

Let $z_s(c) = \hat{\mu}_{sj}(c)$ denote the concentration-varying genotypic value of genotype j (j=1, 2, 3) at SNP s estimated for a given subject (note that the genotype of the subject at an SNP is fixed so that subscript j can be omitted). According to functional graph theory, the genotypic value of a subject at an SNP includes two components, independent component that is expressed when this SNP is assumed to be in isolation and dependent component that results from the influence of other SNPs on this SNP, which is characterized by a system of nonlinear LV-based ODEs. Thus, the $z_s(c)$ value at SNP s is expressed as

$$\dot{z}_s(c) = Q_s(z_s(c)) + \sum_{s'=1, s' \neq s}^{m} Q_{ss'}(z_{s'}(c)) + \epsilon_s(c) \tag{7.3}$$

where $Q_s(\cdot)$ is the independent component, determined by SNP s' own genotypic value $z_s(c)$, $Q_{ss'}(\cdot)$ is the dependent component, determined by the genotypic value $z_{s'}(c)$ of SNP s', and $\epsilon_s(c)$ is the residual error, distributed as $N\left(0, \sigma_s^2(c)\right)$. Since there is no explicit form for $Q_s(\cdot)$ and $Q_{ss'}(\cdot)$, we implement a nonparametric smoothing approach, such as Legendre Orthogonal Polynomials (LOP), to model their dynamic changes (Zhao et al. 2005a, b). The residual error may be antedependent; i.e., the error at a drug dose is influenced by those at its previous dose. Thus, we implement an autoregressive approach, such as the SAD(1), to model the residual covariance structure.

Equation (7.3) is a full ODE model that allows each SNP to be linked with all other m–1 SNPs. However, such a full interconnection does not occur in living systems because it is vulnerable to stochastic perturbations (May 1972; Gross et al. 1972; Allesina and Tang 2012). A stable system should be structurally sparse; i.e., the percentage of the active interactions scales inversely proportional to the system size (Liu et al. 2011; Suweis et al. 2013; Busiello et al. 2017; Espinosa-Soto 2018). System sparsity suggests that each entity in the network may receive influences from a limited number of its co-existing entities. To choose a small set of the most significant SNPs linked with a given SNP, we build a nonlinear regression model based on equation (7.3), where the genotypic value at a given SNP as a response is regressed on those at all other SNPs as predictors across concentration levels. This nonlinear regression can be linearized because its predictor terms are fitted by a nonparametric approach. We implement a variable selection approach, such as regularization-based LASSO and its variants (Tibshirani 1996; Zou and Hastie 2005; Yuan and Lin 2006; Wang and Leng 2008), to choose the most important predictors (say m_s). After variable selection for SNP s, we replace the summation of links over m–1 SNPs in equation (7.3) by the summation of links over the m_s most significant SNPs, by which a full ODE model reduces to a sparse ODE model. In pharmacogenetic studies, the number of concentration levels is so much lower than that of SNPs that variable selection cannot work properly. To circumvent this issue, we may interpolate as many as genetic values on genotypic curves within the full range of concentration levels.

Sun et al. (2021) formulated a likelihood approach for solving the sparse ODEs implemented with the fourth-order Runge-Kutta algorithm and estimating the parameters that structure the covariance matrix using the simplex algorithm. We code $Q_s\left(z_s(c)\right)$'s integrals, $P_s(c)$, as nodes, and $Q_{ss'}\left(z_{s'}(c)\right)$'s integrals, $P_{ss'}(c)$, as edges into networks that cover all possible gene-gene interactions. Such networks are sparse, in which the SNPs are not fully interconnected, and also, stable because their inference is based on the optimization technique of maximizing the likelihood of equation (7.1). The causality property of the networks is discussed below.

7.2.3 Bidirectional, Signed, and Weighted Epistasis

Bateson (1907) first defined epistasis as the masking of the effect of allelic substitution at one locus by the allelic state at a second locus This definition was generalized by Fisher (1918) to describe the effect of nonadditive interaction between two or more genes on a phenotype, often identified with the interaction term in the analysis of variance (Costanzo et al. 2016, 2019). The original definition can be readily translated into clinical trials through direct comparison and selection on genotypes, but its detection is relied on mutation characterization, whose widespread use, thus, is impossible. The generalized definition facilitates epistatic detection for a range of species, including outbred humans, yet it is somewhat an abstract concept, with a particular difficulty in being translated into concrete genotypes, making it of limited use.

Functional graph theory can combine the advantages of each definition, overcome their disadvantages, and produces new advantages both definitions do not own. First, epistasis refers to the overall effect of genetic dependence or interaction between two loci (Figure 6.2a), failing to characterize its causality and the sign of the casualty. For example, positive (nondirectional) epistasis detected from current quantitative genetic theory may derive from the mutual promotion of two loci, the unidirectional promotion of one locus for the second, or the promotion of one locus for the second although the second inhibits the first but to a lesser extent (Figure 6.2b). Similarly, negative nondirectional epistasis detected may arise also from one of the three possible types as shown in Figure 6.2b.

We can leverage the definition of epistasis by capturing the full information of bidirectional, signed, and weighted gene-gene interactions (Figure 6.2). Specifically, by comparing $P_{ss'}(c)$ and $P_{s's}(c)$, respectively, we classify epistasis into different types (Table 6.1):

- *Symmetrical synergism*: Two SNPs promote each other at the same strength, in which case both $P_{ss'}(c)$ and $P_{s's}(c)$ are positive and equal in size.

- *Asymmetrical synergism*: Two SNPs promote each other but to different extents, in which case $P_{ss'}(c\bullet)$ and $P_{s's}(c)$ are positive but not equal in size. $P_{ss'}(c) > P_{s's}(c)$ implies that SNP s is more beneficial from SNP s' than the other way around.

- *Directional synergism*: One SNP (say s') promotes the other (s), but the second has no effect on the first, in which $P_{ss'}$ is positive but $P_{s's}(c)$ is zero.

- *Altruism/aggression*: One SNP promotes the other but the second inhibits the first, in which case $P_{ss'}(c)$ is positive but $P_{s's}(c)$ is negative, explained as the altruism of SNP s' for SNP s or the aggression of SNP s for SNP s'.

- *Symmetrical antagonism*: Two SNPs inhibit each other at the same strength, in which case both $P_{ss'}(c)$ and $P_{s's}(c)$ are negative and equal in size.

- *Asymmetrical antagonism*: Two SNPs inhibit each other but to different extents, in which both $P_{ss'}(c)$ and $P_{s's}(c)$ are negative but not equal in size.
- *Directional antagonism*: One SNP inhibits the other but the second is neutral to the first, in which case, $P_{ss'}$ is negative but $P_{s's}(c)$ is zero.

Second, classic definitions and approaches consider epistasis between two loci at a time. We encapsulate epistasis that occurs among all m SNPs into an interaction network, which is regarded as being a fully informative epistatic network. Topological analysis of the network allows us to identify hub SNPs, i.e., those with more links than the average of all SNPs, which play a pivotal role in maintaining network behavior. Links of the network can be outgoing if one SNP regulates a second SNP, or incoming if one SNP is regulated by a second SNP. We call those hub SNPs having more outgoing links than incoming links a leader. While existing approaches for linkage and association mapping can only estimate the net genetic effect of an SNP, the LV-based ODE model partitions the net effect into its independent (endogenous) and dependent (exogeneous) components. Based on these two components, we can assess whether a specific SNP impacts the phenotype directly or through indirect pathways involving other SNPs.

Third, current approaches estimate epistasis as a population parameter using a large number of samples, but it is possible that the magnitude and pattern of how different loci depend on each other vary from subject to subject. Understanding the individualization of epistasis can provide rich information about clinical translation and precision medicine. Moreover, as a function of dose concentration, time, or environmental regime, $P_{ss'}(c)$ and $P_{s's}(c)$ allow signal-dependent and context-typical epistatic networks to be reconstructed for each subject, shedding light on the genetic architecture of drug response and its biological etiology.

7.2.4 Example for Individualized Networks Mediating Drug Response

Revisit Example 2.1: A pharmacogenetic study includes 163 patients differing in age, gender, race, body height, and body mass index, aimed at investigating the medical effect of dobutamine (Lin et al. 2005a, b). Dobutamine is a drug designed to improve the heart function of patients who cannot pursue any physical exercise. The patients received dobutamine at an increasing dose from 0 (baseline) to 5, 10, 20, 30, and 40 mcg/min. Heart rate was measured repeatedly 5 minutes after the drug was injected at each dose. We find that the change of heart rate with dose concentration for each patient can well be fitted by the E_{max} equation, as shown in equation (7.2).

β-Adrenergic receptor (βAR) stimulation occurs in peripheral blood circulation, metabolic regulation, muscle contraction, and central neural activities (Woo et al. 2015). Two subtypes of βAR, $\beta_1 AR$ and $\beta_2 AR$, are found to regulate cardiac structure and function, although they play different even opposite functional roles. The subtype of α_1-adrenergic receptor, $\alpha_1 A$, is an important mediator of sympathetic nervous system responses involved in cardiovascular homeostasis (Graham et al. 1996). To test whether and how these receptors as candidate genes mediate dobutamine response, common polymorphisms were genotyped for patients within each gene. Two polymorphisms were genotyped at codons 49 (with two alleles A and G) and 389 (with two alleles C and G) for the $\beta_1 AR$ gene, at codons 16 (with two alleles A and G) and 27 (with two alleles C and G) for the $\beta_2 AR$ gene, and at codon 492 for the $\alpha_1 A$ gene.

We implement the E_{max} equation (7.2) into functional mapping to test how each SNP is associated with the dose-response curve of patients. Using the MLEs of E_{max} equation parameters (E_0, E_{max}, H, and EC_{50}) for each genotype at an SNP estimated by functional mapping, we chart the dose-response curves of genotypic value at each SNP (Figure 7.3a). Through permutation tests, we only detect SNP codon389 from the $\beta_1 AR$ gene that is significantly associated with heart rate curves. Regardless of the significance of an SNP, we assign its genotype-specific curves to each subject based on his/her genotype. For example, if a subject carries AA at codon49, CC at codon389, GG at codon16, CG at codon27, and CT at codon492, then this subject is assigned an

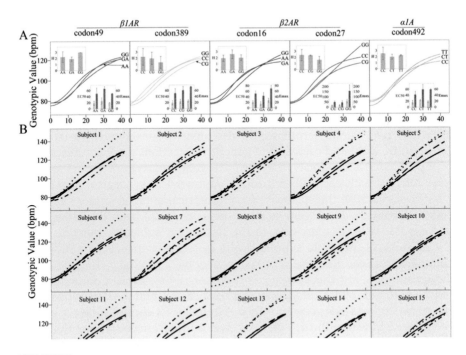

FIGURE 7.3
Genotypic dose-response curves fitted by the E_{max} equation through functional mapping. (a) The pattern of three different genotypes' heart rate response to a series of dobutamine doses at each of five SNPs. In each plot, the estimates of E_{max} equation parameters, E_{max}, H, and EC_{20}, are shown for each genotype. (b) Genotypic values of 15 randomly chosen subjects at five SNPs. Curve colors are SNP-dependent, green for codon49, blue for codon389, red for codon16, purple for codon27, and yellow for codon492.

AA-CC-GG-CG-CT curve across five SNPs. Figure 7.3b illustrates genotypic curves of response to dobutamine for 15 randomly chosen subjects at 5 SNPs. As expected, subjects with the same genotype at an SNP share the same genotypic dose-response curve, but when 5 SNPs are viewed as a whole, substantial interindividual variability is found in the pattern of how genotypes respond to the drug. For example, the genotypic value at codon49 is larger than those at the four other SNPs for subjects 1, 6, 9, 11, and 14 but this difference does not occur for some subjects, such as subjects 2 and 3. For subjects 8 and 10, the genotypic value at codon49 is even smaller than those at the other SNPs. While no huge discrepancy in SNP-typical genotypic curves is detected for subject 2, and 3, genotypic curves differ dramatically among five SNPs for subject 12. Taken together, genotype-specific differences at different SNPs for the same subject imply that there exist substantial epistatic interactions that impact the subject's drug response, whereas subject-specific differences in the pattern of genotype-specific difference indicate that the strength, sign, and direction of epistasis change from subject to subject (Figure 7.4).

Based on five genotype-dependent dose-response curves for each subject, we apply functional graph theory to reconstruct a five-node subject-specific pharmacogenetic network. To demonstrate such individualized networks, we choose five subjects for topological comparison (Figure 7.5). Looking at how five SNPs affect drug response, we find that their interaction networks are not fully interconnected for all subjects, accounting for 40%–50% of all possible pairwise links among 5 nodes. Also, two SNPs from the same gene display consistent interactions for all chosen subjects, except for subject 4 with no interaction between two SNPs from the β_2AR gene. Interactions also occur between SNPs from different genes in all subjects. Despite the similarity in network architecture, we do also identify considerable variation in the strength, sign, and causality of genetic interactions among subjects. For example, two SNPs, codon49 from the β_1AR gene and codon27 from the β_2AR gene, interact with each other through symmetrical synergism for subject 2, but they establish the epistasis of asymmetrical antagonism for subject 1. Codon16 from the β_2AR gene is altruistic to codon27 from the same gene, whereas the latter is repressive to the former for subject 1, but this parasitic epistasis is shifted to symmetrically synergistic epistasis for subject 2. Codon492 from the α_1A gene is linked by codon49 from the β_1AR gene for all chosen subjects, but this epistatic is directionally synergistic for subjects 1 and 2 and directionally antagonistic for subjects 3, 4, and 5. There is no direct link between the β_2AR gene and the α_1A gene for all chosen subjects, except for subject 5 in whom the α_1A gene receives a link from codon16 of the β_2AR gene. In general, five SNPs are positively regulated by each other to govern heart rate curves in response to dobutamine for subject 2, but different degrees of negative regulation are detected for all other subjects.

Based on ODE equations (7.3), we divide the net dose-response curve of a genotype at an SNP into its independent and dependent curves. By comparing the independent and dependent dose-response curves, we can better

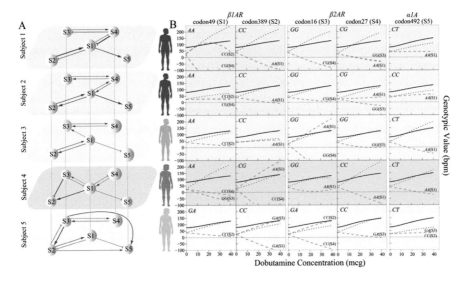

FIGURE 7.4
Subject-specific genetic networks reconstructed by functional graph theory. (a) Five-node inter-action networks underlying heart rate response to dobutamine for five randomly chosen sub-jects from a panel of candidate gene association study population, in which nodes represent the independent genotypic values of each SNP, with circle size proportional to the value, and edges represent directed epistasis from one SNP to next, with line thickness proportional to the strength of epistasis. Red and blue arrowed lines denote promotion and inhibition, respec-tively. (b) Decomposition of net genotypic dose-response curve at each SNP (blue line) into its independent genotypic curve (red line) and dependent genotypic curve (green line) for five randomly chosen subjects. Five SNPs, codon49, codon389, codon16, codon27, and codon492, are denoted as S1–S5 in order.

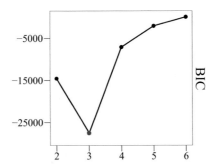

FIGURE 7.5
BIC plot over the number of categories detected by penta-variate functional clustering.

characterize the role of each SNP in mediating drug response for a specific subject (Figure 7.5). We find that relative differences among the net, indepen-dent, and dependent curves are SNP- and subject-specific. For subject 1, the slope of the independent curve of genotype AA at codon49 is greater than the net curve at codon49, codon 389, codon16, and codon27, because these SNPs receive marked negative regulation from other SNPs. In other words, if codon49 was isolated from other SNPs, it was supposed to display a greater expression of drug response in subject 1 than what was observed in a socialized condition. Thus, to improve the heart rate of subject 1 by dobutamine, we need to genetically manipulate the interactive relationship of codon49 with its regulators. If the increase of heart rate with increasing doses of the drug is too fast for subject 1, we may activate the expression of negative regulators so that the role of codon49 in mediating drug response can be augmented. Note that the genotypic value of codon49 for subject 1 is up- and down-regulated by codon389 and codon27, respectively, but because down-regulation is larger than up-regulation, the net genotypic value of codon49 is smaller than its independent value.

For the same subject 1, his/her genotype (CT) at codon492 is promoted by the genotype (AA) at codon49, making its net genotypic value beyond its independent value (Figure 7.5b). Thus, if this subject needs to reduce his/her heart rate, we can design a specific drug to silence strengthen the activity of codon492. Similarly, based on three types of genotypic curves at each SNP, we can make the corresponding therapies to improve the heart rate of subject 2. It is interesting to see that the genotype (GG) of subject 3 at codon16 receives an almost equally large amount of up-regulation (by genotype AA at codon49) and down-regulation (by genotype GG at codon27). The cancelation of up- and down-regulation makes the net genotypic value of this subject at codon16 similar to its independent genotypic value. In practice, the heart rate of subject 3 can be increased or decreased through codon16 by promoting or inhibiting the genotypic expression of codon49 and codon27, respectively. However, the heart rate of this subject cannot be improved through codon27 from the same β_2AR gene, because his/her genotype at coodn27 received little regulation from codon16, which may not add adequately large dependent genotypic value to net value. Taken together, from the decomposition of net genotypic values for individual SNPs, we can not only understand the genetic mechanisms underlying drug response but also are provided with information useful for designing effective therapies to improve drug efficacy for specific patients.

7.3 Coalescing Individualized Networks into Stratification-Specific Networks

7.3.1 Functional Clustering

Epistasis may vary among subjects. Functional graph theory has shown its capacity to reconstruct subject-dependent epistatic networks. These individualized networks can provide key information for personalized medicine that tailors unique disease treatments and preventions for each person by taking into account his or her genes, environment, and lifestyle. Compared to personalized medicine, precision medicine is more practical in clinics because it focuses on professional judgment for risk stratification that goes beyond the individual. In order for genetic networks to be used in precision medicine, we need to characterize the general rule that governs the network structure of patients from the same stratification.

We provide a clustering procedure for combining individualized networks into stratification-specific networks. Let $\mathbf{z}_{isj_s} = \left(z_{isj_s}(c_1), ..., z_{isj_s}(c_T) \right)$ denote the vector containing the concentration-varying mean values of drug effect for genotype j_s at SNP s for subject i. Let $\mathbf{z}_i = (\mathbf{z}_{i1j_1}, ..., \mathbf{z}_{imj_m})$ denote the genotypic values at all m SNPs for subject i. Based on $\mathbf{z}_i$, we implement functional clustering algorithms (Kim et al. 2008; Wang et al. 2012) to classify all subjects into K distinct groups. Any subject i may and only may belong to a particular group, which can be characterized by formulating a mixture-based likelihood, expressed as

$$L(z) = \prod_{i=1}^{n} \left[\pi_1 f_1 \left(\mathbf{z}_i : \mu_1, \Sigma \right) + ... + \pi_K f_K \left(\mathbf{z}_i : \mu_K, \Sigma \right) \right]$$

where $f_k \left(\mathbf{z}_i : \mu_k, \Sigma \right)$ is a multivariate normal density probability function of genotypic values at all SNPs for group k ($k=1, ..., K$) with mean vector μ_k and covariance matrix Σ and π_k is the proportion (prior probability) of group k to all subjects (prior probability). Because genotypic values of m genes can be assumed to be independent, the above likelihood can be rewritten as

$$L(\mathbf{z}) = \prod_{i=1}^{n} \left[\pi_1 \prod_{s=1}^{m} f_{1s} \left(\mathbf{z}_{isj} : \mu_{1s}, \Sigma_s \right) + ... + \pi_K \prod_{s=1}^{m} f_{Ks} \left(\mathbf{z}_{isj} : \mu_{Ks}, \Sigma_s \right) \right] \quad (7.4)$$

where $f_{ks} \left(\mathbf{z}_{isj} : \mu_{ks}, \Sigma_s \right)$ is a multivariate normal density probability function of genotypic values at SNP s for group k ($k=1, ..., K$) with mean vectors μ_{ks} (modeled by the E_{max} equation) and covariance matrix Σ_s (modeled by SAD(1)).

We implement the simplex algorithm into the EM algorithm to obtain the MLEs of model parameters including the group proportion, group- and SNP-specific PD parameters, and SNP-specific SAD(1) parameters. In the E step, we calculate the posterior probability of subject i that belongs to group k, using the equation:

$$\Pi_{k|i} = \frac{\pi_k \prod_{s=1}^{m} f_{ks} \left(\mathbf{z}_{isj} : \mu_{ks}, \Sigma_s \right)}{\pi_1 \prod_{s=1}^{m} f_{1s} \left(\mathbf{z}_{isj} : \mu_{1s}, \Sigma_s \right) + ... + \pi_K \prod_{s=1}^{m} f_{Ks} \left(\mathbf{z}_{isj} : \mu_{Ks}, \Sigma_s \right)} \quad (7.5)$$

In the M step, we use the following equation to estimate the proportion of group k:

$$\pi_k = \frac{1}{n}\sum_{i=1}^{n}\Pi_{k|i} \tag{7.6}$$

and use the simplex algorithm to estimate parameters involved in mean vectors $\mu_k = (\mu_{k1}, \ldots, \mu_{ks}, \ldots, \mu_{km})$ and covariance matrix $(\Sigma_1, \ldots, \Sigma_s, \ldots, \Sigma_m)$. The E and M steps are iterated until the estimates of all parameters converge into stable values. The values at convergence are the MLEs of the model parameters.

The optimal number of groups ($\tilde{L}$) can be determined according to information criteria, such as AIC and BIC. After this number is determined, we calculate the posterior probability of subject i to a specific group using equation (7.5). A subject is attributed to a specific group k, if $\Pi_{k|i}$ for this subject is the largest among $\tilde{L}$ posterior probabilities. Thus, we stratify all subjects into $\tilde{L}$ groups.

Using the estimated concentration-varying mean values of drug effect for each group, $\hat{\mu}_k$ ($k=1, \ldots, \dot{K}$), under the likelihood (7.4), we implement functional graph theory to reconstruct $\dot{K}$ group-specific genetic networks. Subjects within the same group have similar interaction architecture, which is different from that of different groups. These networks provide key information for precision medicine that tailors disease treatments for individual groups.

7.3.2 Example for Stratification-Specific Networks

Based on the genotypic dose-response curves of five SNPs (see Figure 7.3b for an example), we use five-dimensional functional clustering to class 142 subjects into different categories, in each of which subjects are more similar to each other in drug response than to those from other categories. As shown by the AIC plot (Figure 7.6), the optimal number of categories is three, each with a proportion of 0.718 (102), 0.014 (2), and 0.268 (38), suggesting that subjects are extremely unevenly allotted into categories. There are very few subjects in category 2, whose drug response is under genetic control in a way that is different from the majority of the association panel. In general, the joint mean dose-response curve of five SNPs differs dramatically among three categories (Figure 7.6), but such a difference is SNP-dependent. At two SNPs with the $\beta_2 AR$ gene, three categories have a small discrepancy but display a tremendous variability at codon492 of the $\alpha_1 A$ gene. The genotypic dose-response curves of the same category differ among five SNPs, implying the occurrence of remarkable genetic interactions within the category (Figure 7.6).

We reconstruct five-node pharmacogenetic networks for each category using its mean genotypic curves (Figure 7.7a). We find that interaction

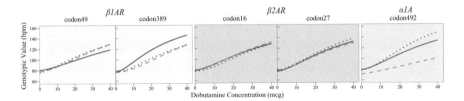

FIGURE 7.6
Population stratification by five-variate functional clustering. The AIC plot suggests that a total of 142 subjects can be parsimoniously classified into three categories based on their similarity of genotypic dose-response curves to dobutamine. The mean genotypic curves of each category are charted for each SNP, with different line colors denoting different categories (blue for category 1, red for category 2, and green for category 3).

architecture differs dramatically among categories, suggesting that the genetic mechanisms underlying drug response are category-dependent. Subjects from the same category initiate a similar genetic mechanism to mediate their response to dobutamine, whereas those from different categories use different mechanisms. For subjects from categories 1 and 3, codon49 from the β_1AR gene promotes codon16 from the β_2AR gene whereas the latter inhibits the former, but this altruistic/parasitic relationship does not take place in category 2. In category 1, codon49 inhibits codon492 from the α_1A gene, but this asymmetrical antagonism does not occur in categories 2 and 3. Codon389 from the β_1AR gene establishes symmetric antagonism with codon16 from the β_2AR gene in category 3 but with codon492 from the α_1A gene in category 2. Many other differences can be observed between categories.

We further decompose the net genotypic curve of each category at each SNP into its independent and dependent components (Figure 7.7b), from which a clearer picture of the role of genetic interactions in modulating drug response can be charted. We find that interaction architecture related to each SNP differs remarkably among categories. For example, codon49 from the β_1AR gene has a greater genotypic independent value of drug effect, with a greater slope of drug response, than its net genotypic value in categories 1 and 3, which is due to negative regulation from codon16 from the β_2AR gene. Because of small positive regulation received from codon492 of the α_1A gene, the net genotypic value of codon49 from the β_1AR gene is not much different from its independent value. For categories 1 and 3, heart rate can be improved through codon49 from the β_1AR gene by altering the activity of codon16 from the β_2AR gene. Yet, this strategy may not be effective for category 2, which needs a different one.

For category 1, codon389 from the β_1AR gene receives up-regulation from codon49 from the β_1AR gene and down-regulation from codon16 from the β_2AR gene to a similar extent, and the cancelation of these types of regulation makes no difference between the independent and net genotypic values

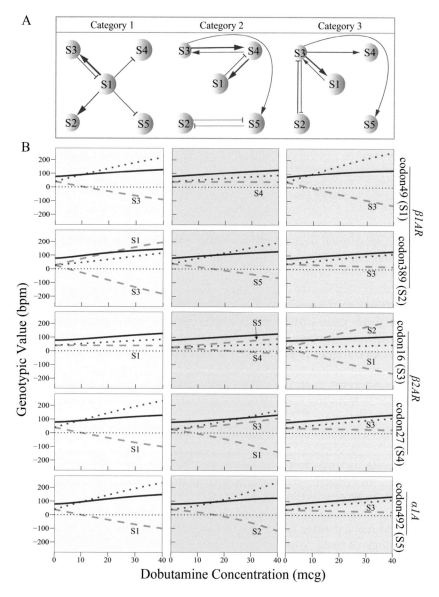

FIGURE 7.7
Category-specific genetic networks by functional graph theory. (a) Five-node interaction networks underlying heart rate response to dobutamine for three categories, in which nodes represent the independent genotypic values of each SNP, with circle size proportional to the value, and edges represent directed epistasis from one SNP to next, with line thickness proportional to the strength of epistasis. Red and blue arrowed lines denote promotion and inhibition, respectively. (b) Decomposition of net genotypic dose-response curve at each SNP (blue line) into its independent genotypic curve (red line) and dependent genotypic curve (green line) for three categories. Five SNPs, codon49, codon389, codon16, codon27, and codon492, are denoted as S1–S5 in order.

of codon389. Thus, by altering the expression of codon49 and codon16, heart rate can be improved through codon389 for category 1. In category 2, codon389 is negatively regulated by codon492, leading the independent genotypic value of the former to be smaller than its net value. By altering the expression of codon492, the heart rate of category 2 can be improved through codon389. By closely looking at curve differences among net, independent, and dependent genotypic values at each SNP for each category, we can design an optimal strategy to improve the heart rate of patients from specific categories.

7.4 Computer Simulation

We perform Monte Carlo simulation to examine the statistical properties of functional graph theory used for reconstructing personalized networks. We assume a set of five SNPs S1–S5, which interact with each other in a manner consistent to subject 5, including altruism/parasitism between S1 and S2 as well as between S2 and S3, asymmetrical synergism between S3 and S4, directional synergism between S3 and S4, and directional antagonism between S1 and S5 (Figure 7.4a). We use the estimated genotypic values at each SNP for this subject, along with SAD(1)-structuring covariance matrix, to simulate longitudinal phenotypic data at 6 and 100 dose levels. Note that genotypic curves estimated by functional mapping allow any number of dose levels to be interpolated over a dose-response curve. Residual variances in the covariance matrix are adjusted by different ratios of residual standard deviations to genotypic values at a middle dose level, 0.03, 0.05, and 0.10. A larger ratio is related to lower precision of genotypic value estimation by functional mapping.

By repeating simulations 1000 times, we use the functional graph model to estimate the mean net genotypic curve and mean independent and dependent genotypic curves and the standard deviations of these curves. Figure 7.8 illustrates the estimation of three types of genotypic curves, in a comparison with their corresponding true curves, under different simulation scenarios. In general, the accuracy and precision of each type of curve are reasonably good, even under the worst condition with a small number of doses and a relatively large residual error. The estimates of curves can be much improved with decreasing residual errors and increasing dose numbers (Figure 7.8a, b). It appears that the improvement of curve estimation can be made by increasing the dose number when the residual error is large. This may inform us of increasing curve estimation accuracy by interpolating genotypic values at as many as dose points over dose-response curves. Residual errors are derived from functional mapping, whose size can be controlled by increasing sample size. Wang et al. (2021) demonstrated that functional mapping can

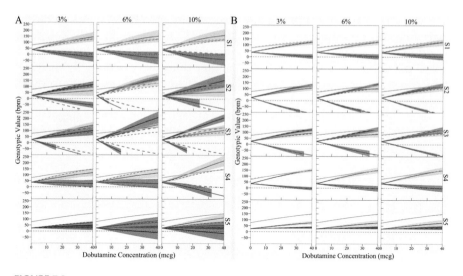

FIGURE 7.8
The estimated net genotypic dose-response curve, estimated independent component curve, and dependent component curve (solid lines), in comparison to the corresponding true curves (slashed lines), under $C=6$ (a) and 100 (b) dosage levels. Residual errors are assumed to be 3%, 6%, and 10%. Grey areas represent confidence intervals of estimated curves.

remarkably increase mapping precision, relative to traditional static mapping approaches, at the same sample size.

We further conduct a simulation study to assess the power of interaction detection and its false positive rate (FPR). Again, we use estimates of genotypic values for subject 1 (Figure 7.4a) to simulate a subject-specific network data from which the genetic network is inferred by formulating and maximizing a likelihood. To solve this likelihood, we assume that none of the four interactions in subject 1 exist (the null hypothesis) and at least one interaction exists (the alternative hypothesis). Under each hypothesis, we estimate ODE and covariance-structuring parameters and plug in these estimates into the likelihood to estimate the likelihood values. Log-likelihood ratios are then calculated as a test statistic to be compared against the critical threshold determined from permutation tests. The power of global interaction detection is calculated under different simulation scenarios (Figure 7.9a). In general, the functional graph model has a modest power for interaction detection (0.40) with a small number of doses (6) and a relatively large residual error (10%), but the power increases to>0.90 at the same residual error when dose number increases to 100. Reducing residual error can tremendously increase the power of interaction detection. We also calculate the power of detecting individual interactions, which follows a similar trend to the global test (Figure 7.9b).

To calculate FPR, we simulate the genotypic value data at five SNPs with no interaction. FPR is a proportion of simulations, in which significant

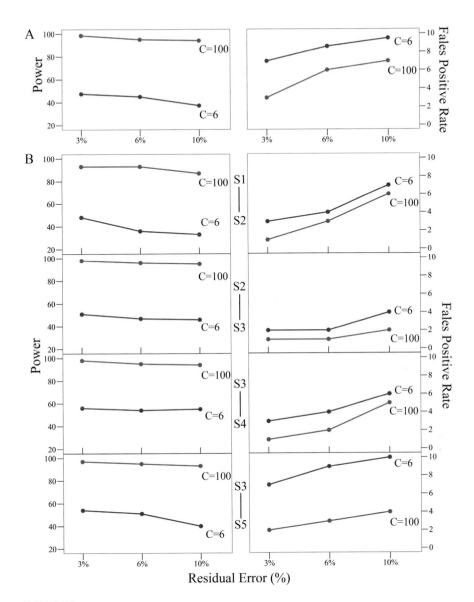

FIGURE 7.9
Power (left panel) and false positive rate (right panel) of epistatic detection in the overall network (a) and for individual SNP pairs (b) under different residual errors and under $C=6$ and 100 dosage levels.

interactions are detected from the interaction-absent simulation data to all simulations. We find that PFR is quite low for global interaction detection (< 10%) and for individual interaction detection (< 3 – 8%) under all simulation scenarios (Figure 7.9).

7.5 Reconstructing Multilayer Genetic Networks

It has been aware from GWAS that genetic variants associated with complex traits or diseases are distributed widely across the whole genome (Boyle et al. 2017). A recent genetic theory, called omnigenic theory, formulated from GWAS analyses of three diseases suggests that essentially all genes throughout the genome contribute to phenotypic variation through regulatory networks (Boyle et al. 2017). Although this publication of this theory has immediately sparked controversy, it can offer a rational interpretation on why significant genes detected by so many GWAS can only account for a small proportion of the heritability. If omnigenic theory is reasonably correct, how can we validate it and capitalize on it to understand the genetic architecture of complex traits.

One way to validate this theory is to combine all SNPs from a GWAS into a well-organized interaction network, in which the roadmap of how each SNP acts and interacts with any pother SNPs to affect the phenotype can be characterized and visualized (Sun et al. 2021). However, a GWAS often involves thousands of thousands of SNPs on a limited number of samples, making it statistically impossible to reconstruct a large-scale interactome network using an entire set of SNPs. Furthermore, a large, densely interconnected network does not comply with general principles of stability and robustness, because it is vulnerable to environmental intervention (Contreras and Fagiolo 2014; Heeren and McNally 2016). Increasing evidence shows that the robustness of complex biological systems can be benefited from the coupling between different layers of interaction (Liu et al. 2020; Panditrao et al. 2022) and the modularity of networks (Girvan and Newman 2002; Alcalá-Corona et al. 2021). All this encourages us to reconstruct a multilayer, multimodule, and multiplex genetic networks from a high-dimensional PGx GWAS data.

We implement functional clustering to class all SNPs into their distinct modules based on their similarity of genotypic dose-response curves, due to the high probability that SNPs within modules are functionally, but not necessarily directly, related to each other. Each module includes a certain number of SNPs that are interdependent more heavily on each other than on those from other modules. Thus, modules form multiple relatively less densely interconnected network communities. For a subject who carries one of three genotypes at SNP s ($s=1$, ..., m), let $\mathbf{z}_s = (z_s(1),...,z_c(C))$ denote the concentration-varying genotypic value of this subject over a series of concentrations $(1, ..., c, ..., C)$ at this SNP. Assuming that m SNPs can be categorized into L modules, the mixture-based likelihood of genotypic values over all SNPs is formulated as

$$L(\mathbf{z}) = \prod_{s=1}^{m} \left[\phi_1 f_1(\mathbf{z}_s; \mu_1, \Sigma) + ... + \phi_L f_L(\mathbf{z}_s; \mu_L, \Sigma) \right] \qquad (7.7)$$

where ϕ_l $(l = 1,\ldots, L)$ the (prior) probability of mixture component l, i.e., a probability by which a specific SNP s belongs to module l and $f_l(\mathbf{z}_s; \boldsymbol{\mu}_l, \boldsymbol{\Sigma})$ is a multivariate normal probability density function of genotypic value at SNP s, with mean vector $\boldsymbol{\mu}_l$ and covariance matrix $\boldsymbol{\Sigma}$. The mean vectors can be modeled by module-specific E_{max} equations, whereas the covariance matrix is modeled by a SAD(1) approach.

We implement a hybrid of the EM algorithm and simplex algorithm to estimate E_{max} parameters for each module and the structure parameters that model the covariance matrix. Specifically, in the E step, we estimate the (posterior) probabilities of SNP s that belongs to module l given genotypic values at this SNP, expressed as

$$\Phi_{l|s} = \frac{\phi_l f_l(\mathbf{z}_s; \boldsymbol{\mu}_l, \boldsymbol{\Sigma})}{\phi_1 f_1(\mathbf{z}_s; \boldsymbol{\mu}_1, \boldsymbol{\Sigma}) + \ldots + \phi_L f_L(\mathbf{z}_s; \boldsymbol{\mu}_L, \boldsymbol{\Sigma})} \tag{7.8}$$

In the M step, we calculate the posterior probability of SNP s that is attributed to module l as

$$\phi_s = \frac{1}{m} \sum_{s=1}^{m} \Phi_{l|s} \tag{7.9}$$

and estimate module-specific E_{max} parameters within $\boldsymbol{\mu}_l$ and covariance-structuring parameters using the simplex algorithm. The E and M steps are alternatively iterated until all parameters converge into stable values as the MLEs of the parameters. We use an information criterion, such as AIC, to determine an optimal number of modules, denoted as $\tilde{L}$. An SNP is assigned to module l, if $\Phi_{k|i}$ for this gene is the largest among $\tilde{L}$ posterior probabilities calculated by equation (7.8).

Using the estimated mean genotypic values of different modules, $\hat{\boldsymbol{\mu}}_l$ ($l=1, \ldots, \tilde{L}$), we use functional graph theory to reconstruct an $\tilde{L}$-node module-module interaction network. Each module can be viewed as a network community in which SNPs are more tightly interlinked with each other than with those from other communities. Next, we reconstruct genetic networks at the SNP level for each module, forming a bottom network, above which the genetic network at the module level serves as the first-layer (top) network. If the number of SNPs within a module is too large to effectively reconstruct a network, we further classify this module into its distinct submodules and then reconstruct genetic network at the submodule level as the second-layer network. If the number of SNPs within a submodule is still too large, we classify it into sub-submodules and reconstruct their networks as the third-layer networks. This procedure continues until the number of SNPs within a unit reaches Dunbar's number at which SNPs within a community can communicate with each other, like a living system, following the parsimony theory (Dunbar 1992; Coelho et al. 2019). The networks reconstructed from individual SNPs are regarded as bottom networks. Taken together, using a number of SNPs from a GWAS project, we reconstruct a multilayer, multimodule, and multiplex interaction network. The advantage of this network lies in its capacity to cover all possible genome-wide SNPs and their possible epistasis, thus providing a powerful tool to test and validate omnigenic theory and, ultimately, better chart the complete portrait of the genetic architecture underlying drug response. From a biological perspective, such multilayer and multiplex networks can better buffer against stochastic perturbations (Liu et al. 2020; Girvan and Newman 2002; Alcalá-Corona et al. 2021).

7.6 Concluding Remarks

Networks are central features of complex systems. The genetic architecture of drug response can be viewed as a system in which a number of genes, perhaps all genome-wide genes, as predicted by omnigenic theory (Boyle et al. 2017), act and interact with each other in a complicated way (Mani et al. 2008; Weigelt and Reis-Filho 2014; Biswas et al. 2019; Lozovsky et al. 2021; Magaña et al. 2020). As such, reconstructing pharmacogenetic networks to disentangle the genetic machineries of how patients respond to medications opens up a new gateway to pharmacogenomic research as a core of precision medicine. There have been several attempts to identify genetic networks for drug response (Costanzo et al. 2016; Lee et al. 2020b; Park et al. 2021), but these attempts may be limited when they are applied in practice. Their main disadvantages include that the networks reconstructed by existing approaches are not informative in terms of network architecture. Widely used correlation-based and information-theoretic approaches identify undirected networks and, hence, lack causality (Steuer et al. 2002; Bansal et al. 2007). Bayesian networks can recover causality (Darwiche 2009), but they can only handle directed graphs, failing to accommodate cycles and feedback motifs that are common in genetic regulatory networks. When the network is modeled by a system of differential equations, both causality and feedback motifs can be inferred (Gardner et al. 2003; Sontag et al. 2004; Srividhy et al. 2007; Wu et al. 2014; Chen et al. 2017). However, these dynamic approaches still cannot capture the systematical characterization of how each gene is expressed independently and interacts with every other gene and, also, may have a limited application because they rely on high-density time series data, which are difficult to generate. Furthermore, all the above-mentioned approaches were developed for network reconstruction from the abundance data of genes, proteins, or microbes and have no power to infer genetic networks from joint SNP and phenotype data sets.

We develop functional graph theory to overcome the limitation of existing network models (Sun et al. 2021; Wu and Jiang 2021). Functional graph theory combines elements of multiple disciplines into a unified context. In statistical genetics, functional mapping has been proposed to map the developmental pattern of genetic effects exerted by individual genes (Ma et al. 2002; Wu and Lin 2006, 2008; Lin et al. 2005a, b; Wang et al. 2015a). Functional graph theory integrates functional mapping, evolutionary game theory, and the LV prey-predator model into mathematical graphs, in which nodes represent the independent genetic effects of genes when assumed to be in isolation and edges denote directional, signed, and weighted interactions between pairs of genes. Functional graph theory has been applied to reconstruct genetic interactome networks mediating growth traits in Euphrates poplar (Wang et al. 2021; Feng et al. 2021) and microbial resistance to antibiotics (Yang et al. 2021) from a number of samples, but it lacks a capacity to characterize sample-specific genetic networks.

In this chapter, we modify functional graph theory to disentangle this limitation by assigning genotypic values of each SNP to each subject that carries that genotype. Thus, for each subject, the net genotypic value of each SNP can be decomposed into its two components through a system of ODEs for each subject. The first component is the independent genotypic value of a given SNP that is expressed in a condition where it is assumed to be in isolation, and the second component is the dependent genotypic value that results from the epistasis of the genotype of other SNPs on this SNP. We code independent components of each SNP as nodes and its dependent component as edges linking it to other SNPs, reconstructing fully informative networks that capture all fundamental features of epistatic interactions for individual subjects.

Epistasis is traditionally defined as a population concept, but our model can assign epistasis into individual members. Furthermore, we can discern which genotype at one locus epistatically promotes or inhibits the expression of the genotype at the other locus for each subject, rather than measure epistasis as a genetic variance. Such individualized networks are expected to have an immediate implication for designing personalized medicine. From genetic networks of a specific subject, we can more precisely alter the activity of certain genotypes toward maximizing drug efficacy.

In practice, compared to personalized medicine, precision medicine that designs the right therapies for a group of patients with similar genetic blueprints is more reasonable and economically efficient. We implement high-dimensional statistical models to stratify all subjects into different categories. Interaction architecture is more similar for subjects within the same category than for those from different categories. Based on genetic networks for each category, we can design specific drugs that are supposed to work for all subjects within this category. Functional graph theory is used to reconstruct category-specific genetic networks that record the causal dependence of the net genotypic dose-response curves of individual genes. These category-specific genetic networks provide a clue for precision medicine designed for a group of genetically similar subjects.

The application of functional graph theory to analyze a candidate-gene PGx association study produces several genetic results that cannot be characterized by existing mapping approaches. For a given subject, the genetic effects of an SNP on heart rate response to dobutamine can be classified into three types. In the first type, the genotype of the SNP displays a strong independent drug response on its merit, although it receives positive or negative regulation by other SNPs; for example, in subject 1, strong independent values of genotype AA at codon49 and genotype CC at codon389 from the β_1 AR gene are inhibited by a negative regulator, respectively (Figure 7.5b). This information can be directly used to improve the heart rate of subject 1's heart rate response to dobutamine through codon49 by implementing gene editing to alter the expression of certain genotypes at its negative regulator. In the second type, the small independent genotypic value of an SNP is augmented by the genotypes at positive regulators; e.g., genotype CT at the $\alpha_1 A$ gene is promoted by genotype AA at codon49 to produce a larger net genotypic value. In the third type, a genotype at a locus has a very small independent value, but it is largely regulated by positive and negative regulators to a similar extent, whose cancelation makes the net genotypic value of this locus similar to its independent value. This type includes genotype GG of codon16 from the $\beta_2 AR$ gene in subject 3 and genotype CC at codon389 from the β_1 AR gene in subject 4, etc. By silencing its negative regulators, SNPs that are observed to be less significant can still potentially trigger their impacts on increasing drug efficacy.

The advent of next-generation sequencing techniques has made it possible to generate thousands of thousands of SNPs for a PGx GWAS in a cost-effective way. We integrate modularity theory to classify all SNPs into different modules. Each module represents a network community in which SNPs are more tightly interconnected with each other than those from different communities. Depending on the number of SNPs, we can determine whether a network community should be divided up into network subcommunities. In the end, we can reconstruct multilayer, multimodule, and multiplex networks from an unlimited number of SNPs. Such networks not only can detail how each SNP acts and interacts with every other SNPs to mediate drug response, but also they are biologically robust to external and internal random errors.

8

A Game-Theoretic Model of Cell Crosstalk in Drug Response

8.1 Introduction

Multicellular development relies on how well cells coordinate with each other through cell-cell interactions or communications across an organism's diverse cell types and tissues (Rouault and Hakim 2012; Bonnans et al. 2014; Zhou et al. 2018; Armingol et al. 2021). Genomic studies of cell-cell interactions have facilitated our understanding of signals mediating cellular differentiation, homeostasis, and immune responses (Armingol et al. 2021). Increasing evidence shows that the ability of therapeutic cells to interact directly or indirectly with other cells influences their efficacy (Weinstein et al. 2018; Wang et al. 2020; Pemovska et al. 2021). It has been believed that cell-based therapies, emerging as a valuable tool in tissue engineering, regenerative medicine, and cancer immunotherapy (Yamamoto et al. 2019; De Luca et al. 2019), can improve through regulating and engineering cell-cell interactions (Custódio and Mano 2016; Rothbauer et al. 2018; Irvine and Dane 2020). For example, because of the role of cell-cell communication in the propagation of hepatotoxicity, targeting connexin 32, one of the key gap junction proteins connecting different cells in the liver, is an effective strategy for ameliorating drug toxicity both during and after exposure (Naiki-Ito et al. 2012; Patel et al. 2012).

Cells communicate with each other through cell signaling pathways, which can be categorized into four types (Armingol et al. 2021): (1) autocrine signaling, by which a signal secreted from the cell acts as a ligand and binds to the receptors present on the same cells, (2) paracrine cell-cell communication, i.e., the cell signals travel a shorter distance to reach the receptors present on the neighboring cell surface, (3) juxtacrine, by which two cells communicate with each other through gap junctions, and (4) endocrine cell-cell communication, i.e., the signals travel to distant cells to reach the target cell receptors through the circulatory system, i.e., the blood plasma. Each of these types is mediated

DOI: 10.1201/9780429171512-10

by the signaling process of chemical modules, i.e., hormones and cytokines, which are determined by the coordinated expression of the cognate genes from ligand-receptor pairs (Armingol et al. 2021).

Several statistical methods have been developed to infer intercellular communication. Based on mathematical models used for identifying ligand-receptor interactions, these methods can be grouped into one of four categories: (1) differential combination, by characterizing significantly differentially expressed genes between ligand and receptor pairs, including iTALK (Wang et al. 2019d), CellTalker (Cillo et al. 2020), and PyMINEr (Tyler et al. 2019), (2) network modeling, aimed to build a network of ligand-receptor relationships and downstream component expression, including CCCExplorer (Choi et al. 2015), NicheNet (Browaeys et al. 2020), SoptSC (Wang et al. 2019b), and SpaOTsc (Cang and Nie 2020), (3) expression permutation, by computing a communication score for each ligand-receptor pair and evaluating its significance either through cluster label permutation, nonparametric tests, or through empirical methods, including CellPhoneDB (Vento-Tormo et al. 2018; Efremova et al. 2020), CellChat (Jin et al. 2021), ICELLNET (Noël et al. 2021), and SingleCellSignalR (Cabello-Aguilar et al. 2020), and (4) tensor, which explicitly models ligand-receptor interactions using a tensor, including scTensor (Tsuyuzaki et al. 2019). Armingol et al. (2021) provided a detailed review of each of these methods and their features including their strengths and weaknesses.

The use of these methods is impaired by their several limitations. First, they cannot capture all features of cell-cell interactions, including bidirectionality, sign, and magnitude, making it difficult to understand the biological relevance of cellular communication. Second, these methods can only infer an overall relationship between cells using a large number of samples, failing to characterizing sample-to-sample heterogeneity. Third, no high-dimensional statistical models have been implemented and, thus, it is difficult for them to reconstruct cell-cell interaction networks from a dimensional data of gene expression.

In this section, we describe a game-theoretic model that overcomes the limitations of the existing methods. It disentangles how genes induce cells to crosstalk across different tissues or organs and how different cells interact with each other to form an intricate but well-orchestrated network through genes and proteins. This model, named GameTalker, is founded on evolutionary game theory by which cell signaling makes each cell aware of its neighboring cells and all cells work according to these signals. We incorporate allometric scaling theory to convert static expression data into their quasi-dynamic representation, making this model a generic approach for learning cell-cell interactions from a broader domain of data. The model provides a new avenue for understanding the role of cell-cell interactions in shaping multiple physiological and pathophysiological processes as well as drug sensitivity vs. resistance.

8.2 GameTalker: A Crosstalk Model of Tumor-Microenvironment Interactions

8.2.1 Modeling Inter-, Intra-, and Extratumoral Heterogeneities

To articulate the principle of GameTalker, we focus on the modeling issue of cell-cell interactions across tumor and microenvironment. It has been recognized that cancer is extremely difficult to treat largely because the tumor is highly heterogeneous. Intertumoral heterogeneity refers to the diversity of tumors among different patients, while intratumoral heterogeneity describes genomic and phenotypic variation from cell to cell within a tumor lesion (Rodriguez-Meira et al. 2019; Lawson et al. 2018; Losic et al. 2020; Wagner et al. 2019; Jacob et al. 2020; Grzywa et al. 2017; Sang et al. 2019a). Indeed, a tumor mass consists not only of a heterogeneous population of cancer cells but also a variety of resident and infiltrating nontumor cells known as the extratumoral microenvironment (TME) (Román-Pérez et al. 2012). Intertwined relationships of intra-, extra-, and intertumoral heterogeneities underly the complexity of cancer, making it less effective and efficient to use existing cancer therapies only based on overall disease symptoms (Grzywa et al. 2017; Chang et al. 2019; Liu et al. 2018; Dzobo et al. 2018). A wide agreement has now been reached that an improved cancer treatment can be made by targeting both specific cancer cells and TME components for individual patients (Venkatesan and Swanton 2016; Galon and Bruni 2020; Ramón et al. 2020; El-Deiry et al. 2017; de Lartigue 2018).

Cancer cells do not divide, proliferate, and metastasize in isolation, rather they perform these functions through cooperation and coordination with other cells and with the microenvironment where they reside (Ramón et al. 2020; Witz 2008; Najafi et al. 2019). These intra- and extra-tumoral interactions are increasingly being recognized as a contributor to both tumor progression and treatment resistance (de Looff et al. 2019; Najafi et al. 2019; Lim et al. 2018). However, the complexity of interactions among tumor cells and their microenvironment, established through reciprocal paracrine exchanges, is extremely high. Resolving this complexity can help to chart a detailed atlas of cell-cell interactions of utmost importance and utility for determining the critical roadmap for understanding tumor progression but is impossible without sophisticated approaches.

GameTalker overcomes this challenge by combining elements from multiple disciplines. Since Nowell (1976) pioneered the view of cancer as an evolutionary process of interactive cells, a rich body of literature has supported the usefulness of ecological and evolutionary principles to dissect tumor heterogeneity (Tabassum and Polyak 2015; Gatenby and Gillies 2008; Korolev et al. 2014; Nawaz and Yuan 2016). More recently, game theory, which originated from economic research in the 1940s, has emerged as a new way of studying cancer etiology (Basanta et al. 2011; Orlando et al. 2012; Pacheco et al. 2014; Basanta and Anderson 2013; Archetti et al. 2015). GameTalker integrates ecology theory and evolutionary game theory into a unified framework that can not only reconstruct cell-cell interaction networks but also unravel the mechanistic details of the network formation. GameTalker classifies all possibly existing interactions into biologically meaningful patterns, quantifies the strength of each interaction, and tracks their patient- and tumor-specific changes across spatiotemporal gradients. From a methodological perspective, reconstructing fully informative networks of bidirectional, signed, and weighted interactions critically relies on temporal data that are difficult to generate in practice. GameTalker integrates allometric scaling laws that can interpret physical and biological phenomena, making it possible to infer fully informative interaction networks from static data.

8.2.2 Methodological Foundation of GameTalker

Evolutionary game theory: Tumor cells interact with their surrounding microenvironment in a way that can be interpreted through the lens of game theory in which each player strives to maximize its payoff based on its own strategy and the strategy of its interactive partners. Tumor cells are capable of regulating and altering gene expression in nontumor cells residing in or infiltrating into the microenvironment. Conversely, microenvironmental components regulate gene expression in tumor cells. These interactions reciprocally exert selective pressures on each of the two types of cells, thereby simultaneously shaping the phenotype of nontumor cells and directing the tumor into certain molecular evolution pathways leading to metastasis (Grzywa et al. 2017; Liu et al. 2018). Both the tumor and its microenvironment should be recognized as contributors to tumor progression and treatment resistance (de Looff et al. 2019), but they form complex bidirectional paracrine interactions and communication.

   Quasi-dynamic modeling of evolutionary game theory through allometric scaling laws: Dynamic modeling is a prerequisite for evolutionary game theory to be applied. However, it is difficult or even impossible to collect dynamic data. We address this issue by integrating allometric scaling laws. Consider n patients who are monitored for the expression profiles of m genes in cells from both tumors and their TME. These genes shape the pattern of how these two types of cells communicate and crosstalk to determine tumor progression. Tumor cells and their TME can be viewed as a functional complex in which these two compartments interact with each other like players in a game. Let y_{Tij} and y_{Mij} denote the expression value of gene j ($j=1, ..., m$) in a tumor and its TME from patient i ($i=1, ..., n$), respectively. We define the sum

$$E_{ij} = y_{Tij} + y_{Mij} \tag{8.1}$$

as the expression index (EI) of the tumor-microenvironment complex in terms of gene j for parent i (Wang et al. 2013b). Thus, y_{Tij} and y_{Mij} establish a part-whole relationship with E_{ij} across patients, which is thought to follow a physical law – the allometric scaling law, which can be described by a power equation:

$$y_{Tj}\left(E_{ij}\right) = \alpha_{Tj}E_{ij}^{\beta_{Tj}} \tag{8.1a}$$

$$y_{Mj}\left(E_{ij}\right) = \alpha_{Mj}E_{ij}^{\beta_{Mj}} \tag{8.1b}$$

where α_{Tj}, α_{Mj} and β_{Tj}, β_{Mj} are the proportionality coefficients and allometric exponents of the power equation for gene j expressed in tumor and TME, respectively. By expressing y_{Tij} and y_{Mij} as a function of E_{ij} (an independent variable similar to time), the power equation coverts gene expression data collected in discrete patients into a continuous representation in a quasi-dynamic form.

As a game-like system composed of the tumor-microenvironment complex, we formulate the two coupling quasi-dynamic ordinary differential equations (qdODEs) to model their reciprocal interactions between two compartments, the tumor and TME, expressed as

$$\dot{\mathbf{y}}_{j}\left(E_{ij}\right) = \begin{bmatrix} \dot{y}_{Tj}\left(E_{ij}\right) \\ \dot{y}_{Mj}\left(E_{ij}\right) \end{bmatrix}$$

$$= \begin{bmatrix} Q_{Tj}\left(\hat{y}_{Tj}\left(E_{ij}\right):\psi_{Tj}\right) + Q_{T\leftarrow Mj}\left(\hat{y}_{Mj}\left(E_{ij}\right):\psi_{T\leftarrow Mj}\right) \\ Q_{Mj}\left(\hat{y}_{Mj}\left(E_{ij}\right):\psi_{Mj}\right) + Q_{M\leftarrow Tj}\left(\hat{y}_{Tj}\left(E_{ij}\right):\psi_{T\leftarrow Tj}\right) \end{bmatrix} + \begin{bmatrix} \varepsilon_{Tj}\left(E_{ij}\right) \\ \varepsilon_{Mj}\left(E_{ij}\right) \end{bmatrix}$$

$$\tag{8.2}$$

where the overall expression value of each compartment is decomposed into an independent expression component that describes component behavior in isolation, i.e., $Q_{Tj}\left(\hat{y}_{Tj}\left(E_{ij}\right):\psi_{Tj}\right)$ or $Q_{Mj}\left(\hat{y}_{Mj}\left(E_{ij}\right):\psi_{Mj}\right)$, and a dependent expression component that models the influence of one partner on the other, i.e., $Q_{T\leftarrow Mj}\left(\hat{y}_{Mj}\left(E_{ij}\right):\psi_{T\leftarrow Mj}\right)$ or $Q_{M\leftarrow Tj}\left(\hat{y}_{Tj}\left(E_{ij}\right):\psi_{T\leftarrow Tj}\right)$, and $\varepsilon_{Tj}\left(E_{ij}\right)$ and $\varepsilon_{Mj}\left(E_{ij}\right)$ are normally distributed residual errors. Note that $\hat{y}_{Tj}\left(E_{ij}\right)$ and $\hat{y}_{Mj}\left(E_{ij}\right)$ are the EI-dependent fitted expression values of the tumor and TME by a power equation in (8.1a) and (8.1b). Both independent and dependent expression components are fitted by a nonparametric function with basis parameters given in ψ' s, respectively. Equation (8.2) represents a generalized standard evolutionary game theoretic formalism.

Interaction estimation and test: Let $\mathbf{y}_{j}=[\mathbf{y}_{Tj};\ \mathbf{y}_{Mj}]^{T}=[y_{Tj}(E_{1j}),\ \dots,\ y_{Tj}(E_{nj});$ $y_{Mj}(E_{1j}),\ \dots,\ y_{Mj}(E_{nj})]^{T}$ denote expression values of gene j in the tumor and TME over n patients. The likelihood of $\mathbf{y}_{j}$ is formulated as

$$L_j\left(\mathbf{y}_j\right) = f_j\left(\mathbf{y}_{Tj}; \mathbf{y}_{Mj} : \boldsymbol{\mu}_{Tj}; \boldsymbol{\mu}_{Mj}, \boldsymbol{\Sigma}_j\right) \tag{8.3}$$

where the bivariate longitudinal normal density probability function $f_j(\cdot)$ contains the mean vector

$$\begin{bmatrix} \boldsymbol{\mu}_{Tj} \\ \boldsymbol{\mu}_{Mj} \end{bmatrix} = \begin{bmatrix} \mu_{Tj}\left(E_{1j}\right), \ldots, \mu_{Tj}\left(E_{nj}\right) \\ \mu_{Tj}\left(E_{nj}\right), \ldots, \mu_{Mj}\left(E_{nj}\right) \end{bmatrix}$$

$$= \begin{bmatrix} Q_{Tj}\left(\hat{y}_{Tj}\left(E_{1j}\right): \psi_{Tj}\right) + Q_{T \leftarrow Mj}\left(\hat{y}_{Mj}\left(E_{1j}\right): \psi_{T \leftarrow Mj}\right), \ldots, \\ Q_{Tj}\left(\hat{y}_{Tj}\left(E_{nj}\right): \psi_{Tj}\right) + Q_{T \leftarrow Mj}\left(\hat{y}_{Mj}\left(E_{nj}\right): \psi_{T \leftarrow Mj}\right) \\ Q_{Mj}\left(\hat{y}_{Mj}\left(E_{1j}\right): \psi_{Mj}\right) + Q_{M \leftarrow Tj}\left(\hat{y}_{Mj}\left(E_{1j}\right): \psi_{M \leftarrow Tj}\right), \ldots, \\ Q_{Mj}\left(\hat{y}_{Mj}\left(E_{1j}\right): \psi_{Mj}\right) + Q_{M \leftarrow Tj}\left(\hat{y}_{Mj}\left(E_{nj}\right): \psi_{M \leftarrow Tj}\right) \end{bmatrix} \tag{8.4}$$

and covariance matrix

$$\boldsymbol{\Sigma}_j = \begin{pmatrix} \boldsymbol{\Sigma}_{Tj} & \boldsymbol{\Sigma}_{TMj} \\ \boldsymbol{\Sigma}_{MTj} & \boldsymbol{\Sigma}_{Mj} \end{pmatrix}. \tag{8.5}$$

We use qdODEs in equation (8.2) to model the mean vector in equation (8.4) and SAD(1) to model $\boldsymbol{\Sigma}_j$. By implementing a hybrid of the fourth-order Runge-Kutta algorithm and simplex (Nelder-Mead) algorithm under the maximum likelihood, we obtain the maximum likelihood estimates (MLEs) of qdODE parameters $(\psi_{Tj}, \psi_{Mj}, \psi_{T \leftarrow Mj}, \psi_{M \leftarrow Tj})$ and SAD(1) parameters.

Equation (8.4) contains bidirectional tumor-TME interactions, called the full model. To test whether there exists a significant tumor-TME interaction, we formulate three new likelihoods, in which the mean vector is, respectively, replaced by the following partial models:

$$\begin{bmatrix} \mu_{Tj}\left(E_{ij}\right) \\ \mu_{Mj}\left(E_{ij}\right) \end{bmatrix} = \begin{bmatrix} Q_{Tj}\left(\hat{y}_{Tj}\left(E_{ij}\right): \psi_{Tj}\right) \\ Q_{Mj}\left(\hat{y}_{Mj}\left(E_{ij}\right): \psi_{Mj}\right) \end{bmatrix}, \tag{8.6}$$

where neither the effect of tumor on TME nor the effect of TME on tumor exists,

$$\begin{bmatrix} \mu_{Tj}\left(E_{ij}\right) \\ \mu_{Mj}\left(E_{ij}\right) \end{bmatrix} = \begin{bmatrix} Q_{Tj}\left(\hat{y}_{Tj}\left(E_{ij}\right): \psi_{Tj}\right) + Q_{T \leftarrow Mj}\left(\hat{y}_{Mj}\left(E_{ij}\right): \psi_{T \leftarrow Mj}\right) \\ Q_{Mj}\left(\hat{y}_{Mj}\left(E_{ij}\right): \psi_{Mj}\right) \end{bmatrix}, \tag{8.7}$$

where only the effect of TME on tumor exists,

$$
\begin{bmatrix} \mu_{Tj}(E_{ij}) \\ \mu_{Mj}(E_{ij}) \end{bmatrix} = \begin{bmatrix} Q_{Tj}\left(\hat{y}_{Tj}(E_{ij}):\psi_{Tj}\right) \\ Q_{Mj}\left(\hat{y}_{Mj}(E_{ij}):\psi_{Mj}\right) + Q_{M \leftarrow Tj}\left(\hat{y}_{Mj}(E_{ij}):\psi_{M \leftarrow Tj}\right) \end{bmatrix}, \quad (8.8)
$$

where only the effect of tumor on TME exists.

We re-estimate qdODEs and SAD(1) parameters under each new likelihood and calculate likelihood values, denoted as L_{00}, L_{10}, and L_{01} in order. Let L_{11} denote the likelihood value calculated under the full model fitted by equation (8.4). We calculate the following log-likelihood ratios (LRs):

$$
LR_{11|00} = -2\left(\log L_{00} - \log L_{11}\right) \quad (8.9a)
$$

$$
LR_{11|10} = -2\left(\log L_{10} - \log L_{11}\right) \quad (8.9b)
$$

$$
LR_{11|01} = -2\left(\log L_{01} - \log L_{11}\right) \quad (8.9c)
$$

$$
LR_{10|00} = -2\left(\log L_{00} - \log L_{10}\right) \quad (8.9d)
$$

$$
LR_{01|00} = -2\left(\log L_{00} - \log L_{01}\right) \quad (8.9e)
$$

These test statistics are compared with the critical thresholds determined from permutation tests. If $LR_{11|00}$, $LR_{11|10}$, and $LR_{11|01}$ are all insignificant, then we can claim that no tumor-TME interaction exists. If $LR_{11|00}$ is significant, then this means that at least a unidirectional interaction exists. If $LR_{11|00}$ and $LR_{11|10}$ are both significant but $LR_{11|01}$ is not significant, then this implies that there only exists a unidirectional interaction from TME to tumor. If $LR_{11|00}$ and $LR_{11|01}$ are both significant but $LR_{11|10}$ is not significant, then this implies that there only exists a unidirectional interaction from tumor to TME. The significance of the influence of TME on tumor or tumor on TME can also be tested by comparing $LR_{10|00}$ and $LR_{01|00}$, respectively. In summary, these LR tests allow us to assess not only the strength of tumor-TME interaction but also its direction.

8.2.3 Transcriptomic Atlas of Tumor-Microenvironment Interactions

The likelihood tests based on equations (8.9a–e), along with the MLEs of independent and dependent expression components, can be used to classify and quantify the patterns of tumor-TME interaction. These patterns include *synergism* (both compartments promote each other), *antagonism*

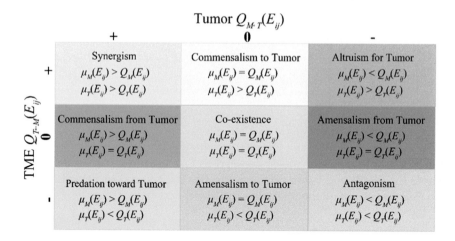

FIGURE 8.1

Qualitative classifications and quantitative descriptors of tumor-microenvironment interactions driven by gene j from the qdODE mage model. The independent and dependent expression components are expressed as a function of E_{ij}.

(both compartments inhibit each other), *commensalism* (one compartment promotes the other while the second is neutral to the first), *amensalism* (one compartment inhibits the other while the second is neutral to the first), and *altruism/predation* (one compartment promotes the other but the second inhibits the first) (Figure 8.1). As a function of EI, these MLEs allow us to chart a spatiotemporal change of tumor-TME interaction from one patient to the next and from pre-intervention to post-intervention for the same patient and incorporate the impact of various demographical factors into this interaction.

We use GameTalker to individually analyze all m genes. Thus, we can illuminate the detailed atlas of the role each gene plays in mediating tumor-TME crosstalk. This atlas is mapped to individual patients, from which one can characterize which genes drive the cooperation or competition between the tumor and its microenvironment and how these interactions influence the patients' tumorigenesis. Ultimately, this atlas provides scientific guidance on delivery strategies of anticancer drugs.

8.2.4 Mapping Tumor-TME Interactions for Liver Cancer

Allometric scaling of gene expression across the tumor and microenvironment: Losic et al. (2020) collected RNA-seq data of 49,722 genes based on bulk samples at 2–5 intratumoral regions of liver cancer and at 1–4 TME regions for 12 patients (Figure 8.2). Of these genes, we choose 27,290 genes that occur in >15% samples for tumor-TME interaction modeling. Differences in gene expression among different regions within and outside tumors reflect strong

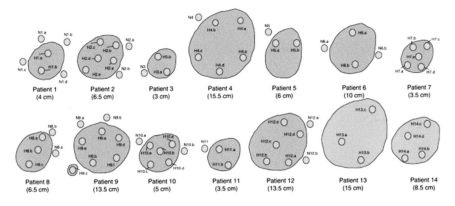

FIGURE 8.2
Multiregional sampling strategies from different geographic distributions of the liver tumor (H – tumor sample; N – nontumoral adjacent environment; Orange – samples bulk sequenced; Green – samples single-cell sequenced). (Adapted from Losic et al. 2020.)

cellular heterogeneity. Cell-cell crosstalk may occur between the tumor and TME for the same patient. GameTalker can unveil how individual genes mediate humor-TME crosstalk and communications. We average the expression value of a gene over all regions within each compartment, tumor, and TME, for each patient, forming two-variate (tumor and TME) longitudinal data across patients. Patient #7 is excluded from subsequent modeling because they have no TME data.

We calculate the sum of averaged gene expression values between the tumor and TME for each patient as the EI of the patient. From the scatterplots of the expression value of each gene on each compartment against EI, we find that the EI-varying gene expression value for each compartment can be fitted by the power equation (8.1a and b) ($P<0.01$) (Figure 8.3). Yet, the shape of the curves differs from gene to gene and between two compartments. For example, gene *TSPAN6* has a lower expression level on the tumor than on the TME for patients with a lower EI, but its more dramatic EI-dependent increase on the tumor than TME leads the expression level of this gene on the tumor to reversely surpass that on the TME for patients with a higher EI. Although the expression level of *CYP3A43* is similar in the two compartments for EI-low patients, its expression is strikingly higher on the TME than the humor for EI-high patients because of a greater slope of increase on the former than on the latter. Some genes, such as *SLC66A1* and *GINM1*, display a similar shape of EI-dependent increase curve on the tumor and TME. In summary, there is considerable variability in the pattern of EI-varying change of gene expression between different compartments and among different genes, also displaying marked gene-compartment interactions.

Gene-induced cell crosstalk: Using GameTalker, we chart a detailed atlas of how each gene plays a role in regulating tumor-TME interactions (Figure 8.4).

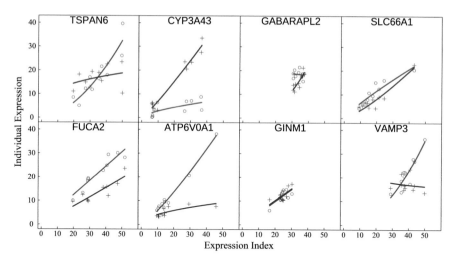

FIGURE 8.3

Expression changes of eight selected genes in the tumor (blue line) and TME (red line) over EI, fitted by the power equation. The dots represent mean intra- and extratumoral expression values of the genes for ten patients. Note that the range of EI varies from gene to gene. (Data from Losic et al. 2020.)

In some situation, the expression of genes on the TME promotes the expression of the same genes on the tumor. Among these genes, some (e.g., *NFYA*) activate synergistic tumor-TME interactions, i.e., their expression on the TME also promotes the expression on the tumor, some (e.g., *TRIP4*) induce commensalistic interactions, in which the tumor has no effect on the expression on the TME, and the other (e.g., *NOTCH3*) mediates altruistic relationships where the tumor has an adverse effect on the expression on the TME. In some situation, the expression of genes on the tumor has no effect on their expression on the TME, including tumor-induced commensalistic genes, e.g., *FLT4*, (whose expression on the tumor promotes that on the TME), tumor-TME coexisting genes, e.g., *IGHJ2* (whose expression on the tumor is neutral to that on the TME), and tumor-induced amensalistic genes, e.g., *UBE2A* (whose expression on the tumor inhibit their expression on the TME). In the other situation, the expression of genes on the tumor represses the expression of the same genes on the TME. This type of genes includes TME-predating genes, e.g., *CASP10* (in which the expression on the tumor promotes that on the TME), TME-induced amensalistic genes, e.g., *LAMTOR3* (where the expression on the tumor is neutral to that on the TME), and antagonistic genes, e.g., *ANKIB1* (in which the expression on the tumor also inhibits that on the TME).

Figure 8.5 illustrates the frequencies of genes that participate in mediating different types of tumor-TME crosstalk. Among all, 27,290 genes with adequate information for interaction modeling, only less than 10% have

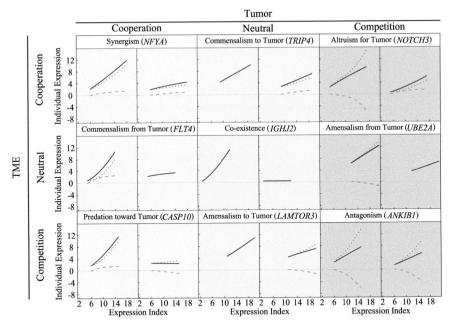

FIGURE 8.4
Nine types of tumor-TME interactions induced by genes. For each interaction type, the influences of TME on the tumor and of the tumor on TME are shown in the left and right plots, respectively, where the solid line represents the net expression change of a gene in a compartment, which is decomposed into its independent expression component (dotted line) and dependent expression component affected by gene expression in the other compartment (broken line). Note that the range of EI varies from gene to gene. (Data from Losic et al. 2020.)

nothing to do with tumor-TME interactions. More than 90% of the genes mediate the crosstalk of cells from the tumor and its microenvironment, revealing the multifactorial feature of tumor-TME interactions. We find that 84% of these active genes mediate bidirectional interactions (mutualism, antagonism, and altruism/predation), whereas only 16% mediate directional interactions (commensalism and amensalism). In general, the TME uses a higher percentage of these active genes to repress the tumor than to promote the tumor (52% vs. 33%), whereas similar percentages are detected for the tumor to repress vs. promote the TME (46% vs. 41%). This finding, in conjunction with more genes detected to be involved in tumor-TME antagonism (32%) than in tumor-TME synergism (18%), suggests that both intimate cooperation and competition shape the co-evolution of tumor cells and microenvironmental cells, but competition plays a more important role than cooperation. This information, recorded in a detailed encyclopedia of how each gene mediates tumor-TME crosstalk, can be helpful for designing specific drugs to control the tumor by jointly targeting the tumor and its microenvironment.

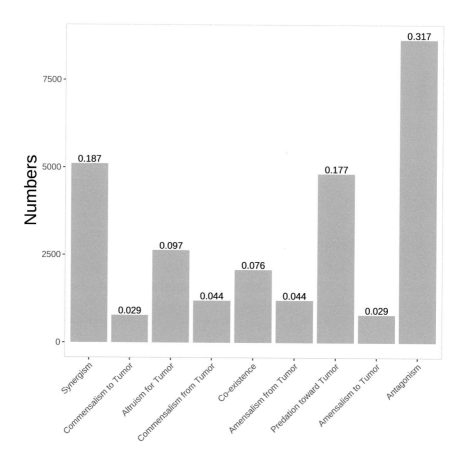

FIGURE 8.5
Frequency of genes that mediate nine types of tumor-microenvironment interactions.

8.3 Modeling Personalized Cell-Cell Interaction Networks

8.3.1 A Generic Formulism of Intratumoral and Extratumoral Internal Workings

GameTalker can test and quantify the tumor-TME interaction induced by a gene. It can be extended to reconstruct interaction networks constituted by many cells. Intratumoral heterogeneity refers to the existence of distinct cells or cell types varying in transcriptomic profiles within a single tumor, whereas extratumoral heterogeneity means that similar but functionally different cellular variation occurs in the microenvironment around this tumor. All the intra- and extratumoral cells build a complex web of reciprocal interactions, whose internal workings can be understood through cellular networks. Consider a tumor and its surrounding microenvironment. We assume that n_T geographically varying intratumoral cells and n_E extratumoral cells at different positions from the peritumor are sampled and profiled for m genes. Let $n = n_T + n_E$ and let y_{ji} denote the abundance level of gene i ($i=1, \ldots, m$) in cell j ($j=1, \ldots, n$). Similar to equation (8.1), we define $E_i = \sum_{j=1}^{n} y_{ji}$ as the EI of gene i in the entire tumor-TME system. It can be seen that y_{ji}, now denoted as $y_j(E_i)$, and E_i establish a part-whole relationship, which can be physically modeled by the power equation, like equation (8.1a and b). Let $\hat{y}_j(E_i)$ denote the fitted value of $y_j(E_i)$ across genes by the power equation.

A tumor and its surroundings are jointly considered as a complex game system, in which different cells are its interactive elements or players. We integrate evolutionary game theory and prey-predator theory to build a system of generalized nonlinear qdODEs to characterize the internal working of this system. These qdODEs for the tumor-TME system are expressed as

$$\dot{y}_j(E_i) = Q_j\big(\hat{y}_j(E_i):\psi_j\big) + \sum_{j'=1, j'=j}^{n} Q_{j \leftarrow j'}\big(\hat{y}_{j'}(E_i):\psi_{j \leftarrow j'}\big) + \varepsilon_j(E_i) \qquad (8.10)$$

where $Q_j\big(\hat{y}_j(E_i):\psi_j\big)$ is the independent abundance of gene i expressed in cell j that occurs when the cell is assumed to be in isolation, $Q_{j \leftarrow j'}\big(\hat{y}_{j'}(E_i):\psi_{j \leftarrow j'}\big)$ is the dependent abundance of gene i in cell j that results from the influence of the same gene expressed in a different cell j' ($j'=1, \ldots, j-1, j+1, \ldots, m$) on it, and $\varepsilon_j(E_i)$ is the residual error, distributed as $N(0, \sigma_j^2(E_i))$. The independent abundance of cell j is a function of its own gene expression level, fitted by a nonparametric approach with parameter ψ_j, whereas the dependent abundance of cell j is a nonparametric function of the gene expression level of cell j' with parameters $\psi_{j \leftarrow j'}$. Equation (8.10) builds a general framework for characterizing cell-cell interaction networks mediated by m genes.

In general, living systems are not densely filled by element-element links, because sparse interconnections are more robust to buffer against stochastic errors than full interconnections (May 1972; Gross et al. 1972; Allesina and Tang 2012). As such, we should identify the most significant links that constitute the system. This can be done by selecting a small subset of the most important cells that link with a given cell through the implementation of variable selection. We build a nonparametric regression model based on equation (8.10); i.e., the gene expression level of a cell (as a response) is a function of expression levels of all other cells (as predictors) across genes. There are several basic approaches for variable selection acting on this regression model, including sequential methods (e.g., backward elimination, forward selection, and stepwise regression) and penalized methods, also known as shrinkage or regularization methods (including LASSO and elastic net).

After variable selection, m summations of the dependent components for cell j, as shown by equation (8.1), reduce to m_j ($m_j < m$) summations because as the number of cell j's most significant links, m_j is part of m. A reduced qdODE model is used to estimate the qdODE parameters from gene expression data of cells. We formulate a likelihood and solve it by integrating the qdODE equations and covariance matrix-structuring SAD(1). The estimated qdODE parameters ($\hat{\psi}_j$ and $\hat{\psi}_{j \leftarrow j'}$) are used to obtain the MLEs of the independent abundance levels and dependent abundance levels for individual cells.

8.3.2 Reconstructing Bidirectional, Signed, and Weighted Cell-Cell Interaction Networks

We code the MLEs of $\hat{Q}_j\left(\hat{y}_j(E_i):\hat{\psi}_j\right)$ as nodes and the MLEs of $\hat{Q}_{j \leftarrow j'}\left(\hat{y}_{j'}(E_i):\hat{\psi}_{j \leftarrow j'}\right)$ as edges into mathematical graphs. These graphs meet three important network requirements, stability (network reconstruction via a maximum likelihood-based optimal technique), causality (the direction of network edges determined by the sign of the dependent expression component), and sparsity (the most important edges chosen by variable selection).

8.3.3 Detection of Personalized Intra- and Extratumoral Cell-Cell Interactions

In Losic et al.'s (2020) liver-sequencing study, 12 patients, carrying different sizes of tumor, were bulk sequenced for intra- and extratumoral regions. We choose three tumor size-different patients (#1, #2, and #9; Figure 8.6a) to reconstruct cell-cell crosstalk networks (CCCN). Multiple intra- and extratumoral cell types were identified for each patient, with two vs. four for patient #1, five vs. two for patient #2, and 6 vs. 2 for patient #9. For each patient, we calculate the EI of each gene expressed in the intratumoral-intertumoral system and plot the gene expression of each cell type against the EI across genes, which can well be fitted by the power equation ($P<0.01$) (Figure 8.6b). In general, extratumoral cells display a greater slope of EI-varying change than do intratumoral cells, regardless of tumor size, suggesting that the TME contributes more substantially to the intratumoral-intertumoral system than the tumor. There is also considerable variability in the slope of EI-varying change among different regions from the same compartment.

We use GameTalker to reconstruct 6-node, 7-node, and 8-node CCCN for parent #1, #2, and #9, respectively (Figure 8.7a). The pattern of cellular links within compartments and across compartments is patient-dependent, but there are some patient-common trends, i.e., cell interactions within (tumor and TME) compartments are generally synergistic or commensalistic, and intratumoral cells exert unidirectional outgoing impacts on cells in the TME. In patient #9, even cells from two separate subtumors have strong commensalistic relationships. In patient #1, one intratumoral region (H1a) is amensalistic to all TME cell types (N1a, N1b, and N1d). In patient #2, one intratumoral

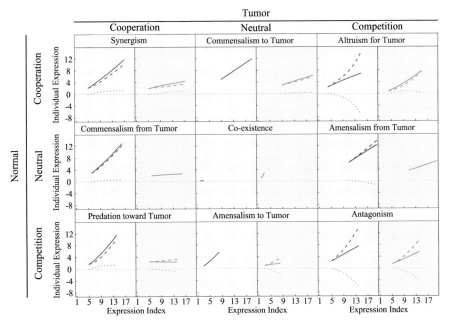

FIGURE 8.6
Nine types of tumor-TME interactions induced by genes. For each interaction type, the influences of the TME on the tumor and of the tumor on the TME are shown in the left and right plots, respectively, where the sold line represents the net expression change of a gene in a compartment, which is decomposed into its independent expression component (broken line) and dependent expression component affected by gene expression in the other compartment (dotted line). Note that the range of expression index varies from gene to gene. Data is taken from Losic et al. (2020).

region (H2e) is amensalistic to a TME cell type (N2a) and commensalistic to a second TME cell type (N2a). In patient #9, tumor cell types, H9c and H9b, commensalistic to TMEs cell types N9a and N9b, respectively. It is interesting to see that the ratio of positive (synergistic and commensalistic) interactions to negative (parasitic and amensalistic) interactions is proportional to the size of tumor; for example, only positive interactions occur for big-size tumor patient #9, only a few negative interactions for small-size tumor patient #2, and many negative interactions for intermediate-size tumor patient #1. Also, it appears that the strength of positive interactions is positively associated with tumor size.

By decomposing the EI-varying gene abundance change curve of each cell type into its independent abundance and dependent abundance curves (Figure 8.7b), we can characterize how cell interactions are mediated by genes. We find that intratumoral cells are positively regulated by each other, making their observed expression level larger than the independent abundance due to their intrinsic capacity. The TME cells are regulated by tumor cells, although the latter is not regulated by the former. Taken together, to inhibit the activity of tumor cells, an effective strategy for controlling tumor growth should be based on uncoupling cell-cell cooperation within tumors.

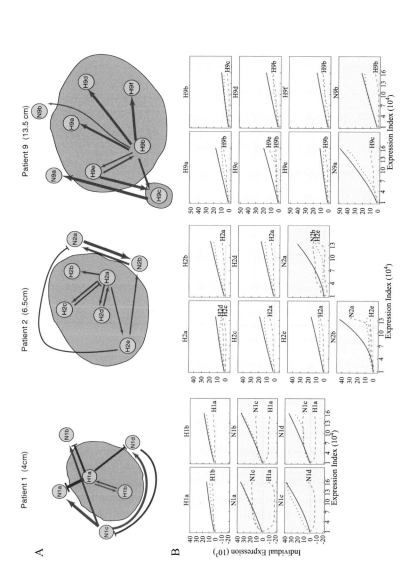

FIGURE 8.7

(a) Cell-cell interaction networks inferred by functional graph theory. Arrowed red and blue lines represent promotion and inhibition, respectively, with line thickness proportional to the strength of interaction. (b) Gene expression profiles of different intra- and extratumoral regions (solid blue line) decomposed into independent components (slashed blue line) and dependent components (solid red line) due to influence by other cell regions.

8.4 Reconstructing Multilayer Gene Regulatory Networks of Tumor-TME Interactions

8.4.1 Allometric Scaling Law of Intra- and Extratumoral Heterogeneities

Tumor cells differ from each other and also differ from their surrounding cells in transcriptomic profiles. While most cancer genomic studies pursue to detect such transcriptomic differences, few can consider gene regulatory networks (GRNs) as a predictor of tumor-TME interactions. Here, we extend GameTalker to reconstruct such networks. Consider n patients sampled from a diseased population, whose intra- and extratumoral cells are profiled for the same set of m genes. Let U_k and V_k denote the numbers of tumor regions and TME regions sampled for patient k ($k=1, \ldots, n$). Let y_{juk} and z_{jvk} denote the expression levels of gene j ($j=1, \ldots, m$) in intratumoral cell region u_k and extratumoral region v_k, respectively, from the same patient i. Each profiled region represents a sample and, thus, there are $n_T = \sum_{k=1}^{n} U_k$ intratumoral samples and $n_E = \sum_{k=1}^{n} V_k$ extratumoral samples. Now, we use y_{ji} and z_{ji} to denote the intra- and extratumoral expression levels of gene j from sample i, respectively. We define $T_i = \sum_{j=1}^{m} y_{ji}$ and $E_i = \sum_{j=1}^{m} z_{ji}$ as the EIs of intra- and extratumoral sample i, respectively. Thus, we denote y_{ji} and z_{ji} by $y_j(T_i)$ and $z_j(E_i)$, which establishes a part-whole relationship with T_i and E_i, respectively. Allometric scaling law suggests that this relationship can be fitted by the power equation.

We use Losic et al.'s (2020) region-specific RNA-seq data containing 27,290 genes in tumors and TME profiled by bulk sequencing for 12 liver cancer patients. We calculate the EI of each sample and plot the expression profile of each gene against EI across samples to produce 27,290 scatterplots for each compartment. In each case, the power equation can reasonably well fit the pattern of how individual genes are expressed over EI. Figure 8.8 provides such fitting examples for eight representative genes. Some genes, such as *FGR*, *CASP10*, and *HS3ST1*, increase their expression levels with EI, despite different slopes of increase. The slope of increase also depends on the compartment; for example, *FGR* is strongly positively associated with EI in both the tumor and TME, *CASP10* has a greater slope of increase in the tumor than TME, and *HS3ST1* has a greater slope of increase in the TME than tumor. Some genes display EI-varying decreases in their expression, with the slope of decrease depending on the gene and compartment for the same gene. Taken together, different genes display different patterns of EI-varying change pattern and also the same gene has various change patterns, which suggest that different genetic regulatory mechanisms shape these two different types of cell types.

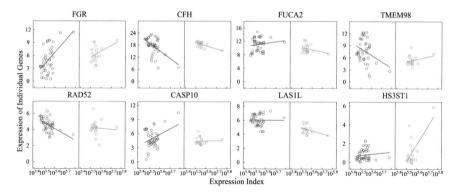

FIGURE 8.8

Expression curves of nine randomly chosen genes in different intra- (left plot, red) and extratumoral regions (right plot, green) for ten patients as a function of EI, fitted by the power equation.

8.4.2 Identifying Network Communities

We argue that the tumor and its surrounding microenvironment form a complex system, which contains intra- and extratumoral subsystems or compartments. Each compartment runs under its specific GRN covered by m genes. To completely characterize the complete genomic signature of tumor-TME interactions, we need to profile a large number of genes (m), which may reach tens of thousands. Reconstructing a network with such high-dimensional nodes is computationally challenging and statistically not well justified. This issue has been overcome by integrating developmental modularity theory (Wu and Jiang 2021). This theory states that a large complex system may be divided into a certain number of distinct smaller subsystems or modules in which components are developmentally more tightly linked with each other than with those from other subsystems (Melo et al. 2016; Alcalá-Corona et al. 2021). In living systems, the delimitation of subsystems may help the organism to better adapt to new environments (Kashtan and Alon 2005; Kashtan et al. 2007; Clune et al. 2013), avoiding the vulnerability of a large-scale network to random perturbations (May 1972, 1973). For example, the modularity of metabolic networks in bacteria is related to the frequency of environmental change (Parter et al. 2007). Thus, the decomposition of a large-scale network into its distinct modules or network communities is not only biologically justifiable but also can alleviate a computational burden.

Network communities are usually identified based on top-down decomposition. This approach recognizes the modular structure of the network by decomposing it with basic informational events. Alternatively, we propose a bottom-up decomposition approach by which we identify basic components that represent common features. Among these m genes, some display a more similar pattern of EI-varying expression changes, compared to others, which suggests that m genes can be classified into distinct modules based on their expression change similarity. Since EI-varying expression changes found the fundamental principle of GameTalker, different modules can represent distinct network communities. We implement a bivariate functional clustering approach (Kim et al. 2008; Wang et al. 2012) to cluster m genes into different modules. Let $\mathbf{y}_j = (y_j(T_1), \ldots, y_j(T_{n_T}))$ and $\mathbf{z}_j = (z_j(E_1), \ldots, z_j(E_{n_E}))$ denote the expression values of gene j across n_T intratumoral samples and n_E intertumoral samples. We formulate the mixture-based likelihood of these data as

$$L(\mathbf{y}, \mathbf{z}) = \prod_{j=1}^{m} \left[\pi_1 f_1(\mathbf{y}_j, \mathbf{z}_j) + \ldots + \pi_C f_C(\mathbf{y}_j, \mathbf{z}_j) \right] \tag{8.11}$$

which has C mixture components or clusters, each with proportion π_c ($c = 1$, ..., C) and two-variate longitudinal normal distribution function $f_c(\mathbf{y}_j, \mathbf{z}_j)$. This distribution function has mean vectors which can be fitted by the power equations, i.e.,

$$\boldsymbol{\mu}_j^T = \left(\mu_j^T(T_1), \ldots, \mu_j^T(T_{n_T}) \right) = \left(\alpha_{Tj} T_1^{\beta_{Tj}}, \ldots, \alpha_{Tj} T_{n_T}^{\beta_{Tj}} \right) \tag{8.12a}$$

$$\boldsymbol{\mu}_j^E = \left(\mu_j^E(E_1), \ldots, \mu_j^E(E_{n_E}) \right) = \left(\alpha_{Ej} E_1^{\beta_{Ej}}, \ldots, \alpha_{Ej} E_{n_E}^{\beta_{Ej}} \right) \tag{8.12b}$$

where α_{Tj}, β_{Tj} and α_{Ej}, β_{Ej} are the intercept and exponent coefficients of the power equations for EI-varying expression change of cluster c across n_T intratumoral samples and n_E intertumoral samples, respectively. The distribution function has a $(n_T + n_E)$-dimensional covariance matrix, expressed as

$$\Sigma = \begin{pmatrix} \Sigma_T & \Sigma_{TE} \\ \Sigma_{ET} & \Sigma_E \end{pmatrix} \tag{8.13}$$

where is split into four submatrices, Σ_T and Σ_E denoting the covariance matrices of n_T intratumoral samples and n_E intertumoral samples, and $\Sigma_{TE} = \Sigma_{ET}$ representing the covariance matrix between two types of samples. We use a bivariate first-order structured antedependence (2SAD(1)) model to fit the matrix structure of Σ (Zhao et al. 2005b).

We implement a hybrid of the EM algorithm and the simplex algorithm to estimate cluster-specific power equation coefficients and 2SAD(1) parameters for a given number of clusters. We use information criterion AIC to determine the optimal number of clusters that explain variation among all genes. After such a number is determined, we calculate the posterior probability with which a specific gene j belongs to a cluster c, expressed as

$$\Pi_{c|j} = \frac{\pi_c f_c(\mathbf{y}_j, \mathbf{z}_j)}{\pi_1 f_1(\mathbf{y}_j, \mathbf{z}_j) + \ldots + \pi_C f_C(\mathbf{y}_j, \mathbf{z}_j)} \tag{8.14}$$

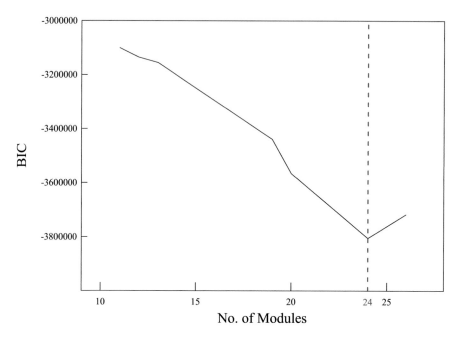

FIGURE 8.9
BIC curves over the number of modules, identifying an optimal number of modules as 24.

Gene j is assigned to a cluster c, if its posterior probability in this cluster is the largest among C clusters. Thus, gene j is involved in network community c whose total number of genes is denoted as m_c ($m_c < m$).

We cluster Losic et al.'s (2020) compartment-specific expression profiles of 27,290 genes into different modules. The optimal number of modules is 24, named M1–M24, as shown by an AIC plot (Figure 8.9). Each module not only contains a different number of genes but also displays different patterns of EI-varying expression change (Figure 8.10). Some modules, such as M2 and M10, have a low amount of expression over a range of EI, whereas some modules, such as M22 and M26, are consistently substantially expressed over EI. Some modules increase their expression levels with increasing EI, but the expression levels of other modules display EI-varying decrease. The pattern of EI-varying change may vary between the tumor and TME, with the extent of such compartment-specific variation depending on module. It is interesting to note that module 24 contains only one gene, *ALB*, which is substantially expressed over a range of EI.

We perform gene enrichment analysis of the 24 modules, with the result suggesting that modules vary in gene function (Figure 8.11). Although some different modules may perform a similar particular function, the overall function of genes from a module is largely module-dependent.

The number of genes within a module is not associated with its overall function. For example, M2 and M10 contain 6,340 and 4,400 genes, respectively,

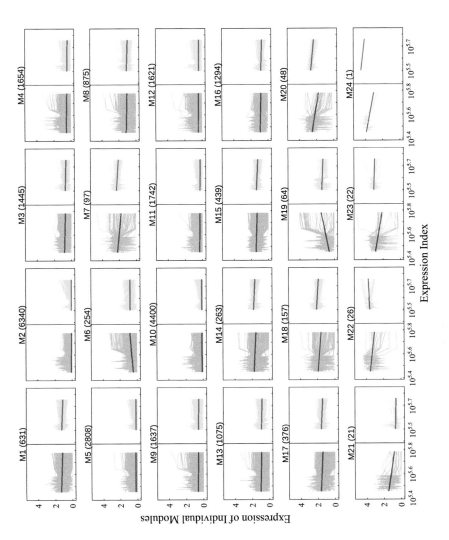

FIGURE 8.10
Expression curves of 24 modules over intra- (left plot) and extratumoral regions (right plot) classified from 28,051 genes by bivariate functional clustering.

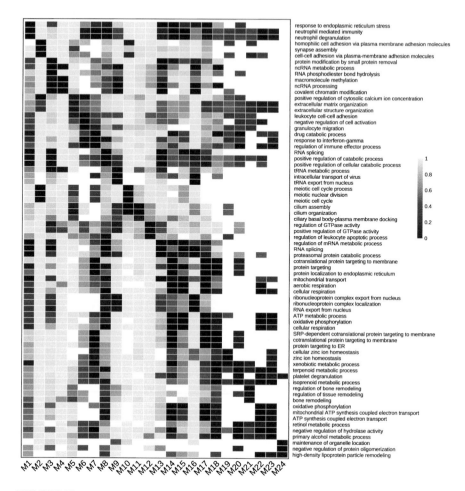

response to endoplasmic reticulum stress
neutrophil mediated immunity
neutrophil degranulation
homophilic cell adhesion via plasma membrane adhesion molecules
synapse assembly
cell-cell adhesion via plasma-membrane adhesion molecules
protein modification by small protein removal
ncRNA metabolic process
RNA phosphodiester bond hydrolysis
macromolecule methylation
ncRNA processing
covalent chromatin modification
positive regulation of cytosolic calcium ion concentration
extracellular matrix organization
extracellular structure organization
leukocyte cell-cell adhesion
negative regulation of cell activation
granulocyte migration
drug catabolic process
response to interferon-gamma
regulation of immune effector process
RNA splicing
positive regulation of catabolic process
positive regulation of cellular catabolic process
tRNA metabolic process
intracellular transport of virus
tRNA export from nucleus
meiotic cell cycle process
meiotic nuclear division
meiotic cell cycle
cilium assembly
cilium organization
ciliary basal body-plasma membrane docking
regulation of GTPase activity
positive regulation of GTPase activity
regulation of leukocyte apoptotic process
regulation of mRNA metabolic process
RNA splicing
proteasomal protein catabolic process
cotranslational protein targeting to membrane
protein targeting
protein localization to endoplasmic reticulum
mitochondrial transport
aerobic respiration
cellular respiration
ribonucleoprotein complex export from nucleus
ribonucleoprotein complex localization
RNA export from nucleus
ATP metabolic process
oxidative phosphorylation
cellular respiration
SRP-dependent cotranslational protein targeting to membrane
cotranslational protein targeting to membrane
protein targeting to ER
cellular zinc ion homeostasis
zinc ion homeostasis
xenobiotic metabolic process
terpenoid metabolic process
platelet degranulation
isoprenoid metabolic process
regulation of bone remodeling
regulation of tissue remodeling
bone remodeling
oxidative phosphorylation
mitochondrial ATP synthesis coupled electron transport
ATP synthesis coupled electron transport
retinol metabolic process
negative regulation of hydrolase activity
primary alcohol metabolic process
maintenance of organelle location
negative regulation of protein oligomerization
high-density lipoprotein particle remodeling

FIGURE 8.11
Gene enrichment analysis of 24 modules M1–M24.

but they perform a limited number of functions. On the other hand, a wide range of functions can be observed from gene-scarce M22 (26 genes) and M23 (22 genes). Taken together, 27,290 genes are distributed in different modules according to their function executed to mediate tumor-TME interactions.

8.4.3 Reconstructing Multilayer GRNs

We first reconstruct a module-module GRN at the top of networks using the mean expression level of each module. Let $\hat{y}_c(T_i)$ and $\hat{z}_c(E_i)$ denote the fitted values of module means for intra- and extratumoral compartments across samples, respectively, by the power equation. We integrate evolutionary game theory and prey-predator theory to build a system of generalized nonlinear qdODEs to characterize the community-community interactions of genes for each compartment. These qdODEs are expressed as

$$\dot{y}_c(T_i) = Q_{Tc}\left(\hat{y}_c(T_i) : \psi_{Tc}\right) + \sum_{c'=1, c' \neq c}^{C} Q_{Tc \leftarrow c'}\left(\hat{y}_{c'}(T_i) : \psi_{Tc \leftarrow c'}\right) + \varepsilon_{Tc}(T_i) \quad (8.15a)$$

$$\dot{z}_c(E_i) = Q_{Ec}\left(\hat{z}_c(E_i) : \psi_{Ec}\right) + \sum_{c'=1, c' \neq c}^{C} Q_{Ec \leftarrow c'}\left(\hat{z}_{c'}(E_i) : \psi_{Ec \leftarrow c'}\right) + \varepsilon_{Ec}(E_i) \quad (8.15b)$$

where $Q_{Tc}\left(\hat{y}_c(T_i) : \psi_{Tc}\right)$ and $Q_{Ec}\left(\hat{z}_c(E_i) : \psi_{Ec}\right)$ are the independent expression component of module c in intra- and extratumoral samples, respectively, which is assumed to occur when the module is in isolation, $Q_{Tc \leftarrow c'}\left(\hat{y}_{c'}(T_i) : \psi_{Tc \leftarrow c'}\right)$ and $Q_{Ec \leftarrow c'}\left(\hat{z}_{c'}(E_i) : \psi_{Ec \leftarrow c'}\right)$ are the dependent expression component of module c in intra- and extratumoral samples, respectively, which results from the influence of a different module c' ($c' = 1, \ldots, c - 1, c+1, \ldots, C$) on it, and $\varepsilon_{Tc}(T_i)$ and $\varepsilon_{Ec}(E_i)$ are the residual errors, distributed as $N(0, \sigma_{Tc}^2(T_i))$ and $N(0, \sigma_{Ec}^2(E_i))$. The independent expression component of module c is a function of its own expression level, fitted by a nonparametric approach with parameters ψ_{Tc} and ψ_{Ec}, whereas the dependent expression component of module c is a nonparametric function of the expression level of module c' with parameters $\psi_{Tc \leftarrow c'}$ and $\psi_{Ec \leftarrow c'}$.

To select a small set of the most significant modules that are linked with a given module, we implement a variable selection procedure. In practice, the number of modules may be exceedingly larger than the number of samples and, thus, regularization-based LASSO and its variants (Tibshirani 1996; Zou and Hastie 2005; Yuan and Lin 2006; Wang and Leng 2008) can be better used to resolve this "curse of dimensionality" issue. Through variable selection, we reduce C summations of the dependent components for module c, as shown by equations (8.15a) and (8.15b), to C_c ($C_c \ll C$) summations. To estimate the qdODE parameters constituting equation (8.15a and b) from gene expression data of the tumor and TME, we formulate a likelihood that is integrated by these qdODEs and covariance matrix-structuring SAD(1) parameters.

As discussed above, functional clustering classifies all genes into distinct modules, each with a reduced number of genes. If the gene number of a specific module is still too large to prevent the proper reconstruction of networks, we further classify this module into distinct submodules and classify a submodule into sub-submodule composed of a tractable number of genes. We call module-module networks the first-layer network at the top, submodule-submodule networks the second-layer network. We may have the third-layer network, fourth-layer network, and so on, until the gene-gene network at the bottom. Ultimately, based on functional clustering-based bottom-up decomposition, we can reconstruct multiplayer, multiplex, and multiscale GRNs for tumor-TME interactions.

8.4.4 Compartment-Specific GRNs

We use the mean expression levels of each module to reconstruct the top network of genes at the module level expressed in two different compartments, the tumor and TME (Figure 8.12a). Each module containing different numbers of genes represents a different gene community that is linked with other communities in the top network. We find that the two compartment-specific inter-community networks have some similarity; for example, the number of links for each module in both cases exhibits a power distribution, but the rank of the modules in link number differs between the two networks, suggesting that topological structure obeys a similar rule but topological organization is compartment-specific. The tumor network is slightly more densely connected than the TME network. We find that both M5 and M10 serve as hubs, each exerting many more links (mostly inhibition) to other modules than average, in the tumor, but only M5 is a hub in the TME. M5 contains genes that regulate cytosolic calcium ion concentration, extracellular matrix and structural organization, and leukocyte cell-cell adhesion (Figure 8.11). Genes in M10 are related to meiotic cell cycles, meiotic nuclear division, cilium assembly, and cilium organization.

Although the top network can explain compartment-dependent differences, a more detailed atlas of how the tumor differs from its microenvironment can be visualized from genetic networks at lower layers, especially those composed of genes at the bottom layer. We cluster each module into its distinct submodules and further cluster each submodule from each module into its distinct sub-submodules. This process allows us to reconstruct a multilayer genetic network from the top to bottom at a large scale. Figure 8.12 illustrates part of such a multilayer network composed of a 10-node submodule network at the second layer from module M10 (B) and a 6-node gene network at the bottom layer from submodule SM10 of M10 (C). We attribute compartment-dependent differences to interactions among individual genes. We find that although most genes are expressed in a similar way for the two compartments, the mechanisms underlying this similarity differ between the tumor and TME (Figure 8.12d). For example, *NMRAL2P* is observed to have a similar pattern of gene expression between the two compartments, but its independent expression level is much higher than the observed expression level in the tumor but lower than the observed expression level in the TME. The reason for the former is that *NMRAL2P* is negatively regulated by *P115* and *H3C10*, making its independent expression canceled out, and the reason for the latter is due to its positive regulation by P115, although it simultaneously receives negative regulation by *SMPX*, but to a lesser extent. In practice, by altering the expression levels of *P115* and/ or *SMPX*, we can modify the expression level of *NMRAL2P*.

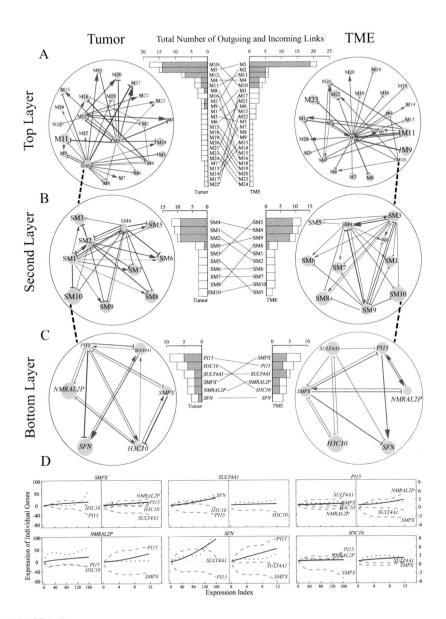

FIGURE 8.12
A multilayer genetic network expressed in the tumor and TME. (a) Top-layer networks among
24 modules M1–M24. (b) Second-layer networks among ten submodules SM1–SM10 from M10. (c)
Bottom-layer networks among six named genes from SM10 of M10. Arrowed and T-shaped lines
represent promotion and inhibition, respectively, with line thickness proportional to the strength
of interaction. In the middle between the tumor and TME networks is the distribution of the total
numbers of outgoing (striped bar) and incoming links (open bar) for each node in the network. (d)
Observed expression curves of different genes (solid line) over intra- (left plot) and extratumoral
regions (right plot) decomposed into independent components (dotted line) and dependent components (broken line) due to regulation by other genes (names shown) for SM10 networks.

8.5 Predictive Network Model for Cancer Growth

8.5.1 Normalized Allometric Scaling Laws

In the preceding sections, we have described models for reconstructing cell-cell crosstalk and cell-cell interaction networks, and GRNs. These models provide a mechanistic understanding of how these interactions at different levels mediate intra- and extratumoral heterogeneities. One additional, even more important, issue is how to predict the outcome of cancer growth based on these interactions and networks. Here, we describe mechanistically-based predictive models of cancer growth. Suppose there are n patients for each of whom we measure tumor size and the expression profiles of m genes in tumors and their TME. Let g_i denote the tumor size of patient i and let y_i and z_i denote the expression value of a gene in the tumor and TME of patient i, respectively. The tumor and its internal and external gene form a system, which can be modeled by functional graph theory. However, tumor size and gene expression have different measurement units, thus for these variables to be properly modeled as components of the system, we normalize their units as

$$G_i = 1 + \frac{g_i - g_{min}}{g_{max} - g_{min}} \quad \text{for tumor size} \tag{8.16a}$$

$$Y_i = 1 + \frac{y_i - y_{min}}{y_{max} - y_{min}} \quad \text{for tumor gene expression} \tag{8.16b}$$

$$Z_i = 1 + \frac{z_i - z_{min}}{z_{max} - z_{min}} \quad \text{for TME gene expression} \tag{8.16c}$$

where subscripts min and max represent the minimum and maximum values of a variable. We calculate the sum $E_i = G_i + Y_i + Z_i$ as the EI of patient i ($i=1, ..., n$) in terms of the gene and tumor size. Thus, as a function of EI, G_i and Y_i and Z_i are written as $G(E_i)$, $Y(E_i)$, and $Z(E_i)$, respectively, which establish a part-whole relationship with E_i. This relationship is thought to obey the allometric scaling law described by the power equation.

Losic et al. (2020) reported a liver-sequencing study including 12 patients bulk sequenced for intra- and extratumoral regions (Figure 8.1). They measured the size of the tumor (diameter in cm), carried by each patient, and profiled transcriptomic expression for multiple locations within and outside the tumor. For each gene, we calculate its mean expression value over the sampled locations, separately for intra- and extratumoral regions. After data normalization, we calculate E_i for each patient i and plot the normalized $G(E_i)$, $Y(E_i)$, and $Z(E_i)$ values against EI. We find that for all genes, the normalized values of each variable as a component of the system scales with EI in an exponential fashion. Figure 8.13 demonstrates four such examples from a pool of 28,051 genes. In each case, the scatters of component values over EI can well be fitted by the power equation, although the slope of the power curve varies from gene to gene and among three components for the same gene. Because of inter-patient variation in gene expression values, the distribution of tumor size over the EI changes from gene to gene. Overall, the goodness-of-fit by the power equation provides a basis for implementing functional graph theory.

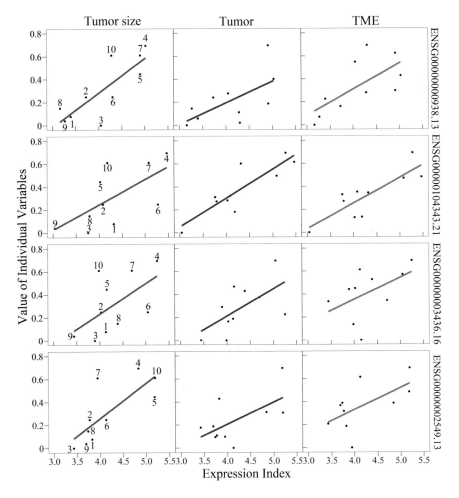

FIGURE 8.13
Power fitting of normalized values of three variables (tumor size, gene expression in the tumor, and gene expression in TME) that constitute a dynamic system across EI at four representative genes (with names given at the right *y*-axis). (Patient No. is shown in the plot of tumor size.)

8.5.2 Causal Inference of Tumor Growth from Intra- and Extratumoral Transcription

Let $\hat{G}(E_i)$, $\hat{Y}(E_i)$, and $\hat{Z}(E_i)$ denote the fitted values of EI-varying changes in tumor size, the expression level of the tumor, and TME for a given gene, respectively, by the power equation. According to functional graph theory, we formulate a causal qdODE that specifies the EI-varying dynamics of tumor size, expressed as

$$\dot{G}(E_i) = Q\left(\hat{G}(E_i):\psi_G\right) + Q_T\left(\hat{Y}(E_i):\psi_T\right) + Q_M\left(\hat{Z}(E_i):\psi_M\right) \qquad (8.17)$$

where tumor size is decomposed into its independent component $Q_j\left(\hat{G}(E_i):\psi_G\right)$ (occurring when tumor growth is independent from the expression of the gene), dependence component $+ Q_T\left(\hat{Y}(E_i):\psi_T\right)$ due to the expression level of the gene in the tumor, and $Q_M\left(\hat{Z}(E_i):\psi_M\right)$ dependence component due to the expression level of the gene in TME. There are no explicit forms of independent and dependent components, thus, a general nonparametric function is used to smooth the three components, specified by parameters ψ_G, ψ_T, and ψ_M, respectively. A likelihood approach is implemented to estimate qdODE parameters ψ_G, ψ_T, and ψ_M, from which we can further estimate the contributions of each of the three components to tumor size.

Using Losic et al.'s (2020) data, we characterize how tumor size is determined by the transcriptional activity of a gene expressed within and outside the tumor. According to the pattern of their impact on tumor size, we classify all genes into nine categories:

1. Joint T-TME promotion – genes expressed both within and outside the tumor promote tumor growth

2. T promotion-TME neutrality – the intratumoral activity of genes promotes tumor growth but their extratumoral activity has no influence on tumor growth

3. T promotion-TME inhibition – the intratumoral activity of genes promotes tumor growth but their extratumoral activity inhibits tumor growth

4. T neutrality-TME promotion – the intratumoral activity of genes is neutral to tumor growth but their extratumoral activity promotes tumor growth

5. T-TME neutrality – both the intra- and extratumoral activities of genes are neutral to tumor growth

6. T neutrality-TME inhibition – the intratumoral activity of genes is neutral to tumor growth but their extratumoral activity inhibits tumor growth

7. T inhibition-TME promotion – the intratumoral activity of genes inhibits tumor growth but their extratumoral activity promotes tumor growth

8. T inhibition-TME neutrality – the intratumoral activity of genes inhibits tumor growth but their extratumoral activity is neutral to tumor growth

9. Joint T-TME inhibition – genes expressed both within and outside the tumor inhibit tumor growth

Figure 8.14 illustrates the representative examples from each category. In general, genes are not equally allocated to nine categories. Of the 28,051 genes studied, the whelming majority promote tumor growth by their expression

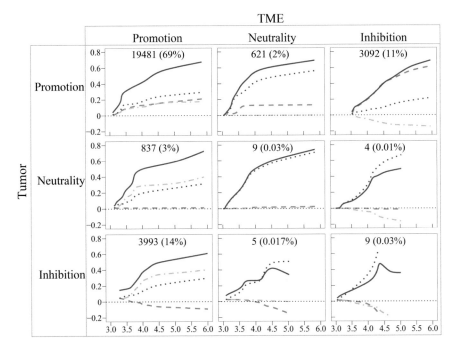

FIGURE 8.14

Nine categories of causal relationships between tumor growth and genes expressed in the tumor and TME. The observed growth curve of a tumor (solid line) decomposed into its independent growth curve (dotted line), dependent growth curve (broken line) due to the expression of a representative gene from each category in the tumor, and dependent growth curve (broken-dotted line) due to the expression of the representative gene in the TME. Representative genes are ENSG00000000005.6 for joint T-TME promotion, ENSG00000096006.12 for T promotion-TME neutrality, ENSG00000171227.7 for T promotion-TME inhibition, ENSG00000071991.9 for T neutrality-TME promotion, ENSG00000160221.18 T-TME neutrality, ENSG00000124205.18 for T neutrality-TME inhibition, ENSG00000156049.7 for T inhibition-TME promotion, ENSG00000180071.20 for T inhibition-TME neutrality, and ENSG00000284648.1 for joint T-TME inhibition. The distribution of 28,051 genes that belong to these nine categories is shown in each plot.

either in the tumor or in its microenvironment, or both. For example, tumor growth is promoted by the expression of 23,194 genes (83%) in the tumor and by the expression of 24,311 genes (87%) in the microenvironment. There are as many as 19,481 genes (69%) that promote tumor growth through their joint intra- and extratumoral expression. Very few genes inhibit tumor growth or are neutral to tumor growth. These findings suggest that by inhibiting the expression level of most genes within and/or outside the tumor, we are in a good shape to control tumor growth.

8.5.3 Causal Inference of Tumor Growth from Tumor-TME Crosstalk

As shown above, tumor growth is affected by gene expression in the tumor itself and its microenvironment. Also, we identify the frequent occurrence of gene-induced cell crosstalk across the tumor and microenvironment. A question naturally arises about whether such cell crosstalk affects tumor growth. We extend functional graph theory to address this issue. We postulate that tumor size is not only determined by the expression levels of gene j in intra- and extratumoral cells, but also through the interaction between intra- and extratumoral expression. This hypothesis can be formulated by a qdODE, expressed as

$$\dot{G}(E_i) = Q_S\left(\hat{G}(E_i) : \psi_S\right)$$

$$+ Q_{ST}\left(\hat{Y}(E_i) : \psi_{ST}\right) + Q_{SM}\left(\hat{Z}(E_i) : \psi_S\right) \tag{8.18}$$

$$+ Q_{S(TM)}\left(W(E_i) : \psi_{S(TM)}\right)$$

where the size of a tumor is decomposed into its three components, (1) independent component $Q_S\left(\hat{G}(E_i) : \psi_S\right)$ due to the intrinsic capacity of the tumor, specified as a function of tumor size with parameters ψ_S, (2) dependent components $Q_{ST}\left(\hat{Y}(E_i) : \psi_{ST}\right)$ and $Q_{SM}\left(\hat{Z}(E_i) : \psi_{SM}\right)$ due to the activity of the gene expressed within and outside the tumor, specified as a function of gene expression levels in the tumor and its microenvironment with parameters ψ_{ST} and ψ_{SM}, respectively, and (3) dependent component $Q_{S(TM)}\left(W(E_i) : \psi_{S(TM)}\right)$ due to tumor-TME crosstalk mediated by the gene, specified as a function of the strength of tumor-TME interaction with parameters $\psi_{S(TM)}$. Note that the dependent components quantify how and how much gene expression in each tissue and gene co-expression over different tissues shape tumor growth. All the three components are smoothened by a nonparametric approach with the corresponding parameters.

Although cell-cell interactions occur as a common biological phenomenon, their quantitative definition has not been very clear. Biological interactions can be classified into four broad types, i.e., mutualism (where two entities benefit from each other), antagonism (where each entity benefits at the expense of the other), altruism (where one entity benefits the other, at a cost to itself), and aggression (where one entity is more aggressive to exploit the resource than the other). By integrating game theory and ecological behavior theory, Jiang et al. (2019) proposed a mathematical descriptor for each interaction type, regarded as the first quantitative measurement of interactions. The biological justification of these descriptors was appreciated by rearing pairs of microbes in monoculture and co-culture and comparing their relative growth of each microbe between the two cultural experiments (Jiang et al. 2019; Wu et al. 2021). These descriptors can be used to measure tumor-TME interactions, which are expressed as

$$W(E_i) = \begin{cases} \dfrac{\hat{Y}(E_i)\hat{Z}(E_i)}{\left|\hat{Y}(E_i) - \hat{Z}(E_i)\right|}, & \text{for mutualism} \\[3ex] \dfrac{1}{\hat{Y}(E_i)\hat{Z}(E_i)\left|\hat{Z}(E_i) - \hat{Z}(E_i)\right|}, & \text{for antagonism} \\[3ex] \dfrac{\hat{Y}(E_i)}{\hat{Z}(E_i)}, & \hat{Y}(E_i) > \hat{Z}(E_i), \text{altruism} \\[3ex] \dfrac{\hat{Y}(E_i) - \hat{Z}(E_i)}{\hat{Y}(E_i)}, & \hat{Y}(E_i) > \hat{Z}(E_i), \text{aggression} \end{cases} . \tag{8.19}$$

By incorporating the mathematical expression of $W(E_i)$ into the qdODE of equation (8.18c), we can characterize how tumor-TME crosstalk affects tumor growth through mutualism, antagonism, altruism, or aggression. We implement a likelihood approach for estimating these qdODEs parameters in equation (8.18).

Next, we need to test whether tumor-TME crosstalk significantly influence tumor growth. This can be done by formulating two hypotheses:

$$H_0 : Q_{TM}\left(W(E_i) : \psi_{TM}\right) = 0$$

$$H_1 : Q_{TM}\left(W(E_i) : \psi_{TM}\right) \neq 0$$

where the null hypothesis states that tumor-TME crosstalk has no impact on tumor growth and the alternative hypothesis states that tumor-TME crosstalk has an impact on tumor growth. The likelihood under the null hypothesis (L_0) is calculated using equation (8.17), whereas the likelihood under the alternative hypothesis (L_1) is calculated using equation (8.18). The log-LR is then calculated as

$$LR = 2\left(\log L_0 - \log L_1\right) \tag{8.20}$$

which is assumed to follow a chi-square distribution with the degree of freedom equal to the difference of the number of unknown qdODE parameters between the alternative and null hypotheses. Another approach for determining the critical threshold is based on computer simulation. Using the estimated model parameters under the null hypothesis, we simulate tumor size, gene expression in the tumor, and gene expression in the TME and then calculate the LR for the simulated data. This procedure is repeated at least 1,000 times. The 5th percentile of the 1,000 LR values is used as the critical threshold at the 5% significance level.

8.5.4 An Atlas Charting the Impact of Tumor-TME Crosstalk on Liver Size: An Example

We apply the causal qdODE of equation (8.18) to analyze Losic et al.'s (2020) data, aimed to reveal the influence of gene-induced cell-cell crosstalk on tumor size across the tumor and its microenvironment. The data include tumor diameters (in cm) and transcriptional profiles of 28,051 genes from intra- and extratumoral regions for ten patients (Figure 8.2). As the proof of concept, we only consider mutualism and antagonism as two types of tumor-TME crosstalk to investigate its impact on tumor growth. We expand equation (8.18) to include two additional terms that specify how genes are co-expressed across the tumor and TME. The expanded qdODEs are rewritten as

$$\dot{G}(E_i) = Q_S\left(\hat{G}(E_i):\psi_S\right) + Q_{ST}\left(\hat{Y}(E_i):\psi_{ST}\right) + Q_{SM}\left(\hat{Z}(E_i):\psi_{SM}\right)$$
$$+ Q_{S(TM)}\left(W(E_i):\psi_{S(TM)}\right)$$

$$\dot{Y}(E_i) = Q_T\left(\hat{Y}(E_i):\psi_T\right) + Q_{TM}\left(\hat{Z}(E_i):\psi_{TM}\right) \qquad (8.21)$$

$$\dot{Z}(E_i) = Q_M\left(\hat{Z}(E_i):\psi_M\right) + Q_{MT}\left(\hat{Y}(E_i):\psi_{MT}\right)$$

where the notation of the first equation is given as above, $Q_T\left(\hat{Y}(E_i):\psi_T\right)$ and $Q_M\left(\hat{Z}(E_i):\psi_M\right)$ are the independent components of gene expression in the tumor and TME, specified as a function of the corresponding expression levels with parameters ψ_T and ψ_M, respectively, and   is the dependent component of gene expression in the tumor, affected by gene expression in TME (specified by parameter ψ_{TM}) and $Q_{MT}\left(\hat{Y}(E_i):\psi_{MT}\right)$ is the dependent component of gene expression in TME, affected by gene expression in the tumor (specified by parameter ψ_{MT}. Term $Q_{S(TM)}\left(W(E_i):\psi_{S(TM)}\right)$ describes the influence of tumor-TME crosstalk on tumor growth, including its strength and sign.

Based on the impact pattern of tumor-TME crosstalk, we classify all genes into four categories: (1) promotion through intra- and extratumoral cooperation,

(2) inhibition through intra- and extratumoral cooperation, (3) promotion through intra- and extratumoral competition, and (4) inhibition through intra- and extratumoral competition. Figure 8.15 illustrates the examples of these four categories. The expression of gene ENSG00000048052.23 becomes less cooperative with increasing EI between the tumor and its microenvironment, but the across-tissue cooperation induced by this gene substantially promotes tumor growth (Figure 8.15a). Gene ENSG00000048052.23 affects tumor growth differently, depending on where it is expressed; i.e., its expression in TME is favorable to tumor growth but its expression in the tumor

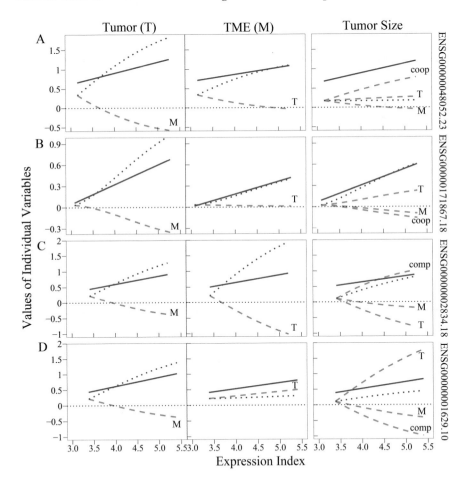

FIGURE 8.15
Dynamic curves of net values of individual variables (tumor size, gene expression in the tumor, and gene expression in TME) (solid line) decomposed into their independent component curves (dotted line) and dependent component curves (broken line) at four representative genes (with names given at the right *y*-axis). The dependent components of tumor size include those due to the expression of the gene in the tumor and TME and its inducing tumor-TME cooperation or competition.

is much less favorable to tumor growth. Considerable promotion of tumor growth by the expression of gene ENSG00000048052.23 in the tumor and its inducing cooperation with expression in the tumor leads to the pronounced amplification of the tumor from its intrinsic capacity. In practice, tumor growth can be prevented and controlled by silencing ENSG00000048052.23's expression in the tumor and uncoupling its inducing tumor-TME cross-talk. The expression of gene ENSG00000171867.18 in the tumor is inhibited by its expression in TME, whereas the latter is less affected by the former (Figure 8.15b). However, the tumor-TME cooperation induced by this gene can substantially inhibit tumor growth. Yet, this inhibition is canceled by promotion from this gene's expression in TME, making the net size of the tumor similar to its independent component.

Gene ENSG00000002834.18 induces an antagonistic relationship between the tumor and TME (Figure 8.15c). It is interesting to see that the expression of this gene in both tissues, especially the tumor, inhibits tumor growth, but its inducing antagonism substantially promotes tumor growth. Stronger promotion, relative to the strength of inhibition, makes the net growth of the tumor larger than its independent component (Figure 8.14c). This finding suggests that by activating the expression of ENSG00000002834.18 in both tissues and also destroying its inducing antagonism, tumor growth can well be controlled. Gene ENSG00000001629.10 expressed in TME inhibits its expression in the tumor, whereas its expression in the tumor promotes its expression in TME (Figure 8.15d). The antagonism induced by this gene substantially inhibits tumor growth, although its expression in different tissues has different signs of influence on tumor growth. By silencing the expression of ENSG00000001629.10 in the tumor and maintaining its inducing tumor-TME competition, tumor growth can well be controlled.

Cooperation and competition are two incompatible, antagonistic phenomena, often regarded as two extremes on a continuum, but they can coexist and even enable each other. Cooperation and competition are intertwined to shape biological evolution, i.e., cooperation is involved in competition whereas competition is also included in cooperation (Pinotti et al. 2020). Because of this, the same gene may induce tumor-TME cooperation or competition. We find that both tumor-TME cooperation and competition induced by the same gene may affect tumor growth, but with different strengths and signs. Among a total of 28,051 genes studied, the whelming majority (28,042) promote tumor growth by inducing tumor-TME cooperation, 16,492 promote tumor growth by inducing tumor-TME competition, 11,559 inhibit tumor growth by inducing tumor-TME competition, and only 9 inhibit tumor growth by inducing tumor-TME cooperation (Figure 8.16). There is considerable overlap for the same genes to affect tumor growth through inducing tumor-TME cooperation or competition. For example, of these 28,042 genes, 16,486 (59%) also promote tumor growth by inducing tumor-TME competition and 11,556 (41%) inhibit tumor growth by inducing tumor-TME competition.

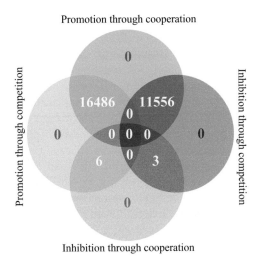

FIGURE 8.16
Venn diagram of the number of genes that promote or inhibit tumor growth through their inducing tumor-TME cooperation or competition.

Since the degrees of promoting tumor growth by tumor-TME cooperation and competition induced by the same gene are likely to differ, oncologists can choose that type of tumor-TME interaction that can better reduce control growth as a strategy for cancer control.

8.6 Concluding Remarks

Despite the success of collective efforts to characterize genetic variants for drug response, the genetic machineries of body-drug interactions remain elusive. It has been recognized that drug response is the consequence of complex interactions between genetic factors and other regulatory mechanisms involved in human cells (Majchrzak-Celinska and Baer-Dubowska 2017; Parca et al. 2019; Peedicayil 2019; Malki and Pearson 2020; Li et al. 2021). Mounting evidence shows that variation in drug response may also be due to cellular heterogeneity (Wu et al. 2020; Zhao et al. 2021). Different cell types of a disease, such as cancer, respond differently to a drug through their diverse transcriptional machineries. Cell-cell communications and temporal-spatial distributions are critical to the contribution of cell heterogeneity to drug response (Wang et al. 2022). Thus, the flow of information linking cell-cell interactions and communication has been streamlined into pharmacogenomic studies, which can promote a paradigm shift of drug discovery in the way targetable mechanisms of drug action can be pieced together for precision medicine (Chambliss and Chan 2016; Farzan et al. 2018; da Silva et al. 2018; Chen et al. 2020; Selevsek et al. 2020; Nassar et al. 2021).

The key to understand the influence of cell-cell interactions on drug response is the application of powerful tools for characterizing cell crosstalk across different tissues. There is a growing body of literature that reports algorithmic tools for inferring cell-cell interactions and cell-cell communication from gene expression (Arnol et al. 2019; Armingol et al. 2021; Brückner et al. 2021). These tools have illustrated how cell-cell interactions shape cellular functions fundamental to biological processes. Each approach has its own assumptions and limitations. Overall, they can characterize the links of different cells induced by genes, proteins, or metabolites, but they cannot capture the full properties of cell-cell interactions including their strength, causality, and sign of causality. Existing approaches infer pairwise interactions between a pair of cells, but lack a capacity to model joint interactions involving multiple cells, especially when the number of cells is large. The limitations of current approaches affect the meaningful application of cell-cell communication and interactions to orchestrate and reconstruct organismal development and pharmacological response.

In this chapter, we describe a versatile theory – functional graph theory to infer cellular interactions from any data domains. It overcomes conceptual, methodological, and technical challenges by integrating different elements of multiple distinct disciplines. The fundamental principle of this theory is to consider interactive cells as a whole (system) guided by game theory. It introduces allometric scaling theory to explain how the function of individual cells changes with system dynamics and integrates it with evolutionary game theory through the Lotka-Volterra predator-prey formulization. By deriving a system of generalized qdODEs, functional graph theory decomposes the function of a cell into two components, one (independent) derived from its own capacity and the other (dependent) from the regulation of other cells. Graph theory enables us to encapsulate the independent components as nodes and the dependent components as edges into mathematical networks. The strength, causality, and sign of cell-cell interactions are coded by the dependent components estimated from qdODEs. Specifically, incredible advantages of functional graph theory can be summarized as follows:

From correlation to causality: Cell-cell interactions and communication inferred by existing approaches actually represent the correlation of function between two cells or the co-expression of genes in two cells. Functional graph theory can characterize the directionality, the causal direction of an interaction, and the sign of the causality. It can also identify two-way interactions or bi-directional interactions; i.e., while one cell regulates the other, the second may simultaneously regulate the first at the same or different strengths and in the same or different signs. In other words, functional graph theory can capture all qualitative and quantitative properties of cell-cell communication or interactions and leverage this concept to a level at which the fundamental role of cells within communities can be best elucidated and translated into practical biomedicine and biotherapeutics.

From linear interactions to nonlinear interactions: Most current approaches analyze cell-cell communication based on a linear relationship. However, linear interactions may only represent a small part of cellular processes, and the majority of cell-cell interactions is virtually the form nonlinearity resulting from substantial uncertainties and random effects across timescales (Gottlieb 2007). Cells use such a nonlinearity to better maintain their robustness to perturbations in environmental exposures (Felix and Barkoulas 2015). In modeling how a cell affects the other cell, functional graph theory implements a nonlinear function to smoothen dynamic changes of the dependent components. Thus, nonlinear cell-cell interactions in any form can be characterized.

From pairwise to joint modeling: By identifying ligand-receptor pairs, current approaches are powerful for analyzing pairwise cell-cell interactions. However, cells often co-exist in communities and co-act to govern community behavior. Thus, pairwise interaction modeling cannot unveil a rock-paper-scissors rule that shapes cell communities as a whole. This issue has been resolved by formulating a system of qdODEs in which the interactions among multiple variables are estimated simultaneously.

Functional graph theory has been applied to analyze real cancer data, showing its biological relevance and statistical robustness. In a commonly used study design, Losic et al. (2020) collected gene expression data from multiple locations within and outside a tumor for multiple patients. Functional graph theory estimates the role of each gene in mediating cell-cell crosstalk across the tumor and its microenvironment. We find that while some genes promote tumor-microenvironment cooperation, some initiate tumor-microenvironment competition. Functional graph theory can specifically infer the direction and sign of tumor-microenvironment interaction induced by each gene. Functional graph theory can predict how gene expression in individual tissues and gene co-expression across different tissues determine tumor growth, providing a complete encyclopedia of the pattern and magnitude of influences of all genes on cancer progression through their differentiated expression over the tumor and its surrounding environment. Taken together, all the above information provides downstream researchers to design precision cancer therapies for obstructing tumor progression by controlling and altering cell-cell communication and interaction using gene-editing strategies.

In studying gene-induced cell-cell interactions, we are often encountered by tens of thousands of genes. How to reconstruct GRNs from such a high-dimensional data is computationally challenging. Functional graph theory integrates developmental modularity theory to split a latent large-scale network into its distinct network communities so that inferring a genetic network for a size-reduced module can be made possible. This treatment enables us to reconstruct a multilayer and multiplex network. By comparing cell type-dependent multilayer networks, we can determine the key topological architecture that distinguishes one cell type from the next. For example, this idea is used to detect why tumor cells perform differently from their microenvironment cells. In Losic et al.'s (2020) data analysis, such key differences are identified between the liver tumor and its microenvironment.

The omics data can be used as biomarkers to differentiate disease from healthy controls, differentiate disease stages and identify subgroups of patients exhibiting different biological signatures (Sun et al. 2020; Wang et al. 2022). Now, functional graph theory promotes the phenomenological application of the omics data to a mechanistic level at which the question of how each omics entity mediates a biological process can be revealed and elucidated. In pharmacological research, by characterizing how cell-cell interactions drive drug response through the transcriptome and proteome, we can glean better insights into molecular mechanisms of drug's action and the prediction of treatment response. The integration of pharmacogenomics and pharmacoproteomics into cell-cell interaction modeling uncovers a whole new direction for diagnostic biomarkers, therapeutic biomarkers, and drug targets. This integration may be a promising avenue in overcoming some of the current limitations in treatment response prediction context.

9

A Graph Model of Personalized Drug–Drug Interactions

9.1 Introduction

Modern biopharmaceutical innovation is shifting its paradigm from the classic monotherapy strategy to a combination therapy modality (Bayat-Mokhtari et al. 2017; Rationalizing combination therapies 2017; Tyers and Wright 2019; Palmer et al. 2019; Deshaies 2020). An increasing body of therapeutical evidence shows that drug combination can achieve cure rates superior to monotherapies that use a single drug to treat a disease or condition (Bayat-Mokhtari et al. 2017; Weinstein et al. 2018). Many ongoing clinical trials have begun to implement combination therapies for cancer, infectious diseases, and metabolic, cardiovascular, autoimmune, and neurological disorders (Perry et al. 2015; Lai et al. 2018; Ciccolini et al. 2019; Joshi and Durden 2019; Coosemans et al. 2019; Asadzadeh et al. 2020; Kholodenko et al. 2021), showing a great promise to increase therapeutic efficacy and decrease drug resistance. When a patient takes multiple medications simultaneously for one or more conditions, drug-drug interactions (DDIs) may occur by which the pharmacological effect of one drug is altered by that of another drug in a combination regimen (Venkatakrishnan and Rostami-Hodjegan 2019; Bain 2019; Meyer et al. 2020). DDIs can be qualitatively classified as synergistic, additive, or antagonistic when the observed effect of the drug combination is greater, equal to, or lesser than the effects of individual drugs, respectively (Weinstein et al. 2018; Niu et al. 2019; Schafer et al. 2020). For this reason, much effort has been devoted to identity synergistic combinations by culturing cell lines (Lehár et al. 2004, 2008) or computational methods (Jansen et al. 2009; Cokol et al. 2017; Yilancioglu et al. 2014; Weinstein et al. 2018).

However, the complexity of DDIs is considerably larger than can be predicted by existing approaches. First, current approaches may only identify the pattern of drug interactions, but fail to estimate their strength and causality. There is little methodology to capture the full properties of DDIs, including bidirectionality, sign, and strength. Second, many approaches infer an overall pattern of drug interaction based on a number of patients,

DOI: 10.1201/9780429171512-11

but they have no power to characterize the patient- and context-specific change of DDIs. Third, while many approaches identify combination synergies based on a pairwise screening, a systematic characterization of how and how strongly different drugs interact as a whole to modulate drug effects is lacking. Although the importance of mathematical models in understanding drug regimens has been recognized (Barbolosi et al. 2016; Shebley and Einolf 2019; Varma et al. 2019), a computational model that can overcome the above limitations has not been developed yet, thereby limiting the capacity of drug combinations to maximize drug efficacy and minimize drug resistance for individual patients (Niu et al. 2019; Zhang et al. 2019; Tran and Grillo 2019).

In this chapter, we propose that functional graph theory can be used to quantify and coalesce multi-drug interactions into mathematical graphs. We expand Sang et al.'s (2022) formulation to provide a more detailed procedure for characterizing clinically meaningful DDI networks. The central tenet of inferring a multi-drug network is to treat it as a game-driven system, in which each drug attempts to maximize its (efficacious or toxic) effect both based on its own strategy and by using the strategies of other drugs through the host's metabolic response. We derive a computational framework that encapsulates bidirectional, signed, and weighted DDIs in quantitative networks and characterizes how each drug interacts antagonistically or synergistically with other drugs to determine pharmacological response. Functioning within the pharmacokinetic (PK) and pharmacodynamic (PD) context, DDI networks are likely patient-dependent. We reconstruct the personalized networks that interrogate and impact PK-PD processes, providing essential information for the precise design and discovery of combination therapies.

9.2 Inferring DDI Networks

9.2.1 Combination of Ecosystem Theory and Evolutionary Game Theory

Drugs produce therapeutic effects through their interactions with the body, including how drugs move throughout the body (PK) and how the body responds to drugs (PD). Administered together to the body, multiple drugs constitute a complex system in which DDIs intertwine with PK and PD processes (Corrie and Hardman 2011; Palleria et al. 2013). This system behaves like an ecosystem in nature where different species (drugs) compete for the access to space and resources (receptors or signaling pathways) or cooperate for common, mutual, or some underlying benefit by sharing space or resources. We argue that such inter-drug interactions can be interpreted through the lens of game theory. Since its inception in economic research in the 1940s (von Neumann and Morgenstern 1944; Nash 1950), game theory has been extensively expanded to a broad range of scientific disciplines, even thought to be more readily applied to biology than to the field of where it is originated (Maynard Smith 1982).

To accommodate the dynamic feature of a game, the dynamic generalization of the Nash equilibrium – evolutionarily stable strategy (Maynard Smith and Price 1973) has been proposed to characterize how a player changes its strategy in response to its counterparts over a regime (Bomze and Pötscher 1989; Ray-Mukherjee and Mukherjee 2016). Under the framework of such evolutionary game theory, all of the standard stability concepts can be assembled through dynamic modeling of temporal changes (Cressman and Tao 2014), without relying the rationality assumption. As the combination of game theory with evolutionary biology, evolutionary game theory is as readily applied to economic research as the field of biology for which it was originally proposed (Alexander 2021).

Evolutionary game theory has been integrated with predator-prey theory and graph theory to form functional graph theory, a new theory that holds great promise to disentangle ecological and genetic complexities (Sun et al. 2021; Wu and Jiang 2021). This theory has been successfully used to study interspecific interactions in ecology (Zhu et al. 2016; Jiang et al. 2018a, b), gene regulatory networks (Chen et al. 2019; Sun et al. 2020; Wang et al. 2022), genetic interactions in quantitative genetics (Wang et al. 2021; Yang et al. 2021), intratumoral cell interactions in cancer etiology (Sang et al. 2019a), and maternal-offspring interaction in reproductive biology (Wang et al. 2017a, b). According to game theory, a player strives to maximize its advantage by rationally designing an optimal strategy based on the strategies of its counterparts, and this pursuit continues until the Nash equilibrium is reached (Nash 1950). Based on this notation, functional graph theory uses predator-prey equations to decompose the overall effect of an entity in a game system into the *independent* component derived from its own strategy and accumulative *dependent* components from its interactions with other entities. Network theory allows us to coalesce the independent effect components of different entities as nodes and the dependent effect components of different entity pairs as edges into a mathematical graph, in which the direct or indirect roadmap of each entity toward system outcome can be charted.

9.2.2 A Procedure of DDI Network Reconstruction

In the PK process of interaction with body, drugs are absorbed, distributed, metabolized, and excreted, leading their concentration to decrease with time. Through their metabolism in the body, drugs produce PD effects on molecular, biochemical, and physiological processes, with the extent depending on the concentration of drugs. In combination therapies, PK and PD processes of each drug are not only determined by its intrinsic interaction with the body but also influenced by its extrinsic interactions with other drugs. The relative contributions of intrinsic vs. extrinsic interactions can provide precise guidance in designing optimal drug combinations, but this information is hidden in observed PK-PD data, which cannot be separated without a powerful computational approach. We address this issue by modeling PK as a function of time and PD as a function of drug concentration through evolutionary game theory.

Suppose there is a multi-drug PK-PD study that tests the pharmacological effect of simultaneously using m drugs on the treatment of a disease for n patients in Phase I and II. We collect blood samples for each patient at a series of (say T) time points before and after dosing and determine the plasma levels of each drug at each time point. Also, we measure physiological parameters that describe drug response at these time points. The PK describes how drug concentration changes as a function of time, whereas the PD specifies how physiological responses change with plasma drug concentration.

PK-based inter-drug network: Let $C_j(t)$ denote the concentration of a drug j ($j=1, \ldots, m$) for a given patient at time t ($t=1, \ldots, T$). Considering all m drugs that constitute a functional system in the body, the ordinary differential equation (ODE) model of functional graph theory is expressed as

$$\dot{C}_j(t) = Q_j\left(C_j(t); \phi_j\right) + \sum_{j'=1, j' \neq j}^{m} Q_{jj'}\left(C_{j'}(t); \phi_{jj'}\right) \tag{9.1}$$

where the concentration of drug j at time t is decomposed into its independent component $Q_j\left(C_j(t); \phi_j\right)$ and aggregate dependent component $\sum_{j'=1, j' \neq j}^{m} Q_{jj'}\left(C_{j'}(t); \phi_{jj'}\right)$. The independent concentration of a drug is only determined by the drug intrinsic capacity to interact with the body, which occurs when it is assumed to be in a socially isolated condition. Thus, the independent concentration of drug j is expressed as a function of its own concentration $C_j(t)$, specified by parameters ϕ_j. The dependent concentration of a drug results from the influence of the other co-existing drugs on this drug. The dependent concentration of drug j due to the effect of drug j' is expressed as a function of the concentration $C_{j'}(t)$ of drug j', specified by $\phi_{jj'}$.

There are no explicit forms for the time-varying functions of independent and dependent components. As such, we implement a nonparametric approach, such as the Legendre Orthogonal Polynomials (LOPs), to smoothen these functions. There have been a number of mathematical equations at different levels of sophistication developed to describe PK (Simeoni et al. 2004; Ahn et al. 2010; Wang et al. 2015a; McKenna et al. 2019). Among a toolkit of these equations, we choose an optimal one for a given PK data and implement it to model $Q_j\left(C_j(t); \phi_j\right)$ and $Q_{jj'}\left(C_{j'}(t); \phi_{jj'}\right)$ based on the LOP approach.

We formulate a maximum likelihood approach based on the PK data, implemented with the m-dimensional ODEs of equation (9.1) and the first-order structured antedependence (SAD(1)) model. We implement a hybrid of the fourth-order Runge-Kutta algorithm and the simplex algorithm to estimate the ODE parameters of equation (1) and SAD(1) parameters structuring

TABLE 9.1

Qualitative and Quantitative Classification of DDI by Functional Graph Theory

		Quantitative Description		
Type	Qualitative Definition	$Q_{jj'}(\cdot)$	Compare	$Q_{jj'}(\cdot)$
1	Symmetric synergism	+	=	+
2	Asymmetric synergism	+	≠	+
3	Directional synergism toward j	+		0
4	Directional synergism toward j'	0		+
5	Altruism toward j or exploitation by j	+		−
6	Altruism toward j' or exploitation by j'	−		+
7	Symmetric antagonism	−	=	−
8	Asymmetric antagonism		≠	−
9	Directional antagonism toward j	−		0
10	Directional antagonism toward j'	0		0
11	Coexistence	0		0

Note: $Q_{j'j}(\cdot)$ and $Q_{jj'}(\cdot)$ may take positive (+), negative (−), or zero (0) values

the residual covariance matrix. The maximum likelihood estimates (MLEs) of the ODE parameters are used to reconstruct a DDI interaction network at the PK space. Based on the comparison of reciprocal dependent components for a pair of drugs $Q_{jj'}\left(C_{j'}(t);\phi_{jj'}\right)$ and $Q_{j'j}\left(C_{j}(t);\phi_{j'j}\right)$, we can qualitatively classify DDIs into different types and quantitatively define the strength, bi-causality, and sign of each inter-drug interaction. The qualitative classifications of different DDI types and their quantitative measures are illustrated in Table 9.1.

PD-based inter-drug network: The above procedure described is based on the PK process, aimed to characterize how the concentration of each drug is affected by those of every other drug across a time scale. The dissection of concentration change for each drug is of critical importance to a better understanding of dose-response relationship in drug efficacy and drug toxicity. Next, we expand functional graph theory to reveal how DDIs shape pharmacological effects on disease treatment. Let $R(C_j)$ denote the response value of drug j ($j=1, ..., m$) at its concentration C_j for a given patient. A new system of ODEs that characterize dose-response changes of m drugs is formulated as

$$\dot{R}(C) = W_j\left(R(C_j);\psi_j\right) + \sum_{j'=1,j'\neq j}^{m} W_{jj'}\left(R(C_{j'});\psi_{jj'}\right) \tag{9.2}$$

where the observed effect of drug j contains two components, the independent component $W_j\left(R(C_j);\psi_j\right)$ that explains that part of drug response due to this drug's intrinsic capacity in isolation and the dependent component $W_{jj'}\left(R\left(C_{j'}\right);\psi_{jj'}\right)$ that explains the rest of drug response resulting from the influence of another drug on this drug. These two components are smoothened by LOP, specified by parameters ψ_j and $\psi_{jj'}$, respectively. As one of the most popular PD models for characterizing dose-response curves (Giraldo 2003; Lin et al. 2005a), the Hill equation can be implemented into ODEs of equation (9.2) to fit the component functions. This equation is expressed as

$$R\left(C_j\right) = E_{0j} + \frac{E_{\max j}C_j^{H_j}}{EC_{50}^{H_j} + C_j^{H_j}} \tag{9.3}$$

where E_{0j} is the baseline, $E_{\max j}$ is the maximal effect that can be evoked by drug j, EC_{50j} is the drug concentration that produces a 50% maximal response, and H_j is the Hill coefficient, the slope of the dose-response curve at the midpoint. We first fit the Hill equation to the PD data for each drug and implemented the predictive values of drug response at different drug concentrations to model the independent and dependent effect components in the ODEs of equation (9.3). As described above, the ODEs are solved by a maximum likelihood approach. The MLEs of independent and dependent effect values are coalesced into graphs, called PD-based DDI networks filled by bidirectional, signed, and weighted inter-drug interactions.

9.2.3 Reconstructing Personalized DDI Networks

Ample evidence shows that considerable variation occurs in the type, pattern, and strength of DDIs among individuals (Coosemans et al. 2019). Functional graph theory can assemble and analyze all PK-PD data from different patients in a clinical trial to reconstruct subject-specific DDI networks. Consider n patients participating in the therapeutic study. Let $\mathbf{y}_i = \left(\mathbf{y}_{i1};...;\mathbf{y}_{im}\right) = \left(\left(y_{i1}\left(t_{i11}\right),...,y_{i1}\left(t_{i1T_i}\right);...;y_{im}\left(t_{im1}\right),...,y_{im}\left(t_{imT_i}\right)\right)\right)$ denote the observed drug-specific concentration values of m drugs at T_i times after administration for patient i ($i=1$, ..., n) and let $\mathbf{z}_i = \left(\mathbf{z}_{i1};...;\mathbf{z}_{im}\right) = \left(z_{i1}\left(C_{i11}\right),...,z_{i1}\left(C_{i1D_i}\right);...;z_{im}\left(C_{im1}\right),...,z_{im}\left(C_{imD_i}\right)\right)$ denote the drug-specific response values of patient i at D_i concentrations for m drugs. Assuming that m patients are independent, the likelihood functions of the PK and PD data for all patients are formulated as

$$L_K\left(\mathbf{y}\right) = \prod_{i=1}^{n} f_i\left(\mathbf{y}_i : \boldsymbol{\mu}_{Ki}, \boldsymbol{\Sigma}_{Ki}\right) \tag{9.4}$$

$$L_D\left(\mathbf{y}\right) = \prod_{i=1}^{n} f_i\left(\mathbf{y}_i : \boldsymbol{\mu}_{Di}, \boldsymbol{\Sigma}_{Di}\right) \tag{9.5}$$

where $f_i(\bullet)$ is an m-variate longitudinal normal density function for patient i characterized by mean vectors and covariance matrices as shown in the equations. We have the mean vectors for patient i,

$$\mu_{Ki} = \left(\mu_{Ki1}; \ldots; \mu_{Kim}\right)$$

$$= \left(\left(\mu_{Ki1}(t_{i11}), \ldots, \mu_{Ki1}(t_{i1T_i}); \ldots; \mu_{Kim}(t_{im1}), \ldots, \mu_{Kim}(t_{imT_i})\right)\right) \quad (9.6)$$

for equation (9.4), and

$$\mu_{Di} = \left(\mu_{Di1}; \ldots; \mu_{Dim}\right)$$

$$= \left(\left(\mu_{Di1}(C_{i11}), \ldots, \mu_{Di1}(C_{i1D_i}); \ldots; \mu_{Dim}(C_{im1}), \ldots, \mu_{Dim}(C_{imD_i})\right)\right) \quad (9.7)$$

for equation (9.5).

We implement individualized PK-based ODEs (i.e., all terms are subscripted by i) with the form of equation (9.1) to model the PK mean vector in equation (9.6) and individualized PD-based ODEs (i.e., all terms are subscripted by i) with the form of equation (9.2) to model the PD mean vector in equation (9.7). Also, we implement SAD(1) to model covariance matrices Σ_{Ki} and Σ_{Di}. A hybrid of the fourth-order Runge-Kutta algorithm and simplex algorithm is implemented to solve the likelihood functions of equations (9.4) and (9.5) under the maximization condition. The MLEs of the independent and dependent components for PK and PD models can be obtained and used to reconstruct personalize PK-based and PD-based DDI networks. Using these personalized networks, we can compare and test inter-individual variability in DDIs, which provides important information for individualized therapies. Specifically, for two patients i and i', we can test how network topology differs from each other by comparing the difference between $Q_{ij}\left(y_{ij}(t); \phi_{ij}\right)$ vs. $Q_{i'j}\left(y_{i'j}(t); \phi_{i'j}\right)$ for nodes and the difference between $Q_{ijj'}\left(y_{ijj'}(t); \phi_{ijj'}\right)$ vs. $Q_{i'jj'}\left(y_{i'jj'}(t); \phi_{i'jj'}\right)$ for edges in the PK network and $W_{ij}\left(z_{ij}(C); \psi_{ij}\right)$ vs. $W_{i'j}\left(z_{i'j}(C); \psi_{i'j}\right)$ for nodes and $W_{ijj'}\left(z_{ijj'}(C); \psi_{ijj'}\right)$ vs. $W_{i'jj'}\left(z_{i'jj'}(C); \psi_{i'jj'}\right)$ for edges in the PD network ($i, i' = 1, \ldots, n$; $j, j' = 1, \ldots, m$). For example, if $W_{ijj'}\left(z_{ij'}(C); \psi_{ijj'}\right) \neq W_{i'jj'}\left(z_{i'jj'}(C); \psi_{i'jj'}\right)$, this means that depending on the genetic context, the therapeutic response of patient i caused by the interaction between drug j and j' is different from that of patient i'.

In summary, personalized DDI networks can depict interpersonal difference in how individual drugs act and interact to determine therapeutic response. For example, one drug exerts many outgoing impacts on other drugs in one patient, but it turns to receive incoming influences by other drugs in the other patient. If patients involved in the PK-PD study receive different treatments or are classified into different groups, such as genders and ages, we can convert personalized networks into context-specific networks. By comparing the topological structure of average networks among different groups, we can extract general rules and mechanisms that distinguish one group from the other. Linking personalized and context-specific networks to the host's genetic blueprints can build more precise predictive models for pharmacological response in combination therapies, understand drug-environment interactions, and, ultimately, facilitate the translation of pharmacological information into the clinic.

9.2.4 Unveiling the Mechanisms behind Drug Interactions

DDI networks inferred from functional graph theory can reveal the mechanisms of inter-drug interactions across two geometrically linked PK and PD spaces (see a diagram in Figure 1.5). The five hypothesized drugs are linked in PK- and PD-initiated networks, from which we can trace the roadmap of how each drug interacts with every other drug to mediate pharmacological effects for individual patients. Different from traditional approaches for DDI network inference, functional graph theory can decompose the concentration change of a drug into its independent component due to its intrinsic interaction with the body and dependent component from its extrinsic interactions with other drugs (Figure 9.1a). The overall concentration of drug D1 is higher than its independent concentration because there is a positive dependent concentration due to the influence of drug D5. This suggests that if D1 does not co-occur with D5, its time-varying concentration decrease will be more dramatic; i.e., D1 will be more quickly excreted from the body. The interaction of D5 with D1 activates the pharmacological effect of D1 (Figure 9.1b). An inverse pattern was found for D2 whose pharmacological effect is inhibited by D5. Figure 9.1 illustrates how the pharmacological effects of drugs D3–D5 are affected by other drugs, providing a detailed atlas of DDIs in the body.

9.3 Inferring Dynamic DDI Networks from Static Data

9.3.1 Theoretical Foundation

To reconstruct a DDI network at PK or PD spaces, one needs to collect data at a number of time points and a number of concentration levels for sufficient dynamic fitting. However, in practice, PK-PD data may be sparse, irregular in time and concentration, and heterogeneous among patients. Chen et al. (2019) implemented allometric scaling theory, a widely used eco-physiological concept (Brown et al. 2004), to contextualize all patients into a unified framework. The central tenet of this theory is that the component trait of a system

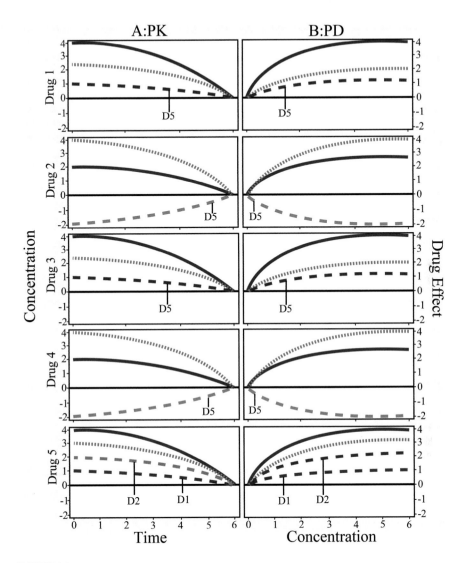

FIGURE 9.1
The decomposition of the overall time-varying concentrations and concentration-varying effects (solid line) of individual drugs into their respective independent (dotted line) and dependent components (broken line) due to regulation by other drugs (with names shown) at PK and PD spaces. The red and blue lines denote the direction by which one drug activates and inhibits the other drug, respectively.

allometrically scales with the whole system in the power law (Shingleton 2010; Findlay and Thagard 2012). Considering all drugs as a functional system, a power relationship occurs between the effects of individual drugs (part) and the total effect of all drugs (whole) across patients. This part-whole relationship projects sparse, irregular, and discrete data on a dense, continuous space, founding a basis for dynamic modeling of evolutionary game theory.

The integration of game theory and allometric scaling theory allows us to derive a system of quasi-dynamic ODEs (qdODEs) that characterize how the concentration of a drug changes during PK-PD processes (Sang et al. 2022). Different from traditionally defined time-derived ODEs, qdODEs are based on the derivative of part-whole relationship, and they are constituted by two components, the independent component that occurs when a drug is assumed to be in isolation and the dependent component that is caused by the interactions of other drugs with this drug. The qdODE-based graph model is founded on the quantitative connection of discrete patients by allometric scaling law, equipped with a capacity to reconstruct DDI networks for individual patients, i.e., personalized networks.

9.3.2 Procedure for Network Inference from Static or Semi-Static Data

Assume a PD-based clinical trial involving n patients who participate in testing the therapeutic response of multiple (say m) drugs for the treatment of a disease. All patients are measured for a drug response variable at multiple concentrations of a drug, but the schedule of the measurement is patient-dependent; i.e., some patients receive drug administration at more densely spaced concentration levels than others and for individual patients, concentration levels are unevenly spaced. Also, because the number of concentration levels may be insufficient for each patient, the fitting of the Hill equation to this data is impossible. We call such longitudinally less informative data static or semi-static data.

Let C_{ijd} denote the concentration value of drug j ($j=1, ..., m$) measured at its concentration level d ($d=1, ..., D_i$) for patient i ($i=1, ..., n$) and $z_{ij}(C_{ijd})$ denote the response value of patient i at concentration C_{ijd}. Note that despite the use of drug-dependent concentration values, concentration level d at which m drugs are administrated simultaneously is consistent for all drugs. To clearly describe the data structure of such a trial, we use a toy example illustrated in Table 9.2. We show how to reconstruct personalized DDI networks from this data.

We assume that m drugs constitute a PD system in the body. In this system, each drug functions individually and also co-functions jointly with other drugs to shape therapeutic response. We define the sum of the observed response values at concentration level d over all drugs for patient i, i.e.,

$$R_{id} = \sum_{j=1}^{m} z_{ij}(C_{ijd})$$ as response index (RI) at this concentration level for this

patient. Thus, $z_{ij}(C_{ijd})$ and R_{id} establish a part-whole relationship that is thought to follow allometric scaling law. We view a concentration level of a drug for a

patient as a sample, thus, R_{id} is generally expressed as R_l ($l = 1, ..., \sum_{i=1}^{n} D_i$) and

TABLE 9.2

Data Structure from a Toy Example for PD-Based Clinical Trial

	Patient							
	1			**2**		**3**	**4**	
Drug	C_{1j1}	C_{1j2}	C_{1j3}	C_{2j1}	C_{2j2}	C_{3j1}	C_{4j1}	C_{4j2}
D_1	$z_{11}(C_{111})$	$z_{11}(C_{112})$	$z_{11}(C_{113})$	$z_{21}(C_{211})$	$z_{21}(C_{212})$	$z_{31}(C_{311})$	$z_{41}(C_{411})$	$z_{41}(C_{412})$
D_2	$z_{12}(C_{121})$	$z_{12}(C_{122})$	$z_{12}(C_{123})$	$z_{22}(C_{221})$	$z_{22}(C_{222})$	$z_{32}(C_{321})$	$z_{42}(C_{421})$	$z_{42}(C_{422})$
D_3	$z_{13}(C_{131})$	$z_{13}(C_{132})$	$z_{13}(C_{133})$	$z_{23}(C_{231})$	$z_{23}(C_{232})$	$z_{33}(C_{331})$	$z_{43}(C_{431})$	$z_{43}(C_{432})$
D_4	$z_{14}(C_{141})$	$z_{14}(C_{142})$	$z_{14}(C_{143})$	$z_{24}(C_{241})$	$z_{24}(C_{242})$	$z_{34}(C_{341})$	$z_{44}(C_{441})$	$z_{44}(C_{442})$
Response Index	R_1	R_2	R_3	R_4	R_5	R_6	R_7	R_8

Note: Each patients receives a different and limited number of drug concentrations

$z_{ij}\left(C_{ijd}\right)$ is generally expressed as $z_j\left(R_l\right)$. We use the power equation to specify the part-whole relationship expressed as

$$z_j\left(R_l\right) = \alpha_j R_l^{\beta_j} \tag{9.8}$$

where α_j and β_j are the proportionality coefficient and allometric exponent of the power equation for drug j, respectively. This power equation provides a key step to describe how the response of a drug changes with RI across samples. Its integration with evolutionary game theory allows us to derive a system of ODEs as

$$\dot{z}_j\left(R_l\right) = W_j\left(z_j\left(R_l\right); \psi_j\right) + \sum_{j'=1, j' \neq j}^{m} W_{jj'}\left(z_{j'}\left(R_l\right); \psi_{jj'}\right) \tag{9.9}$$

where the observed response value to drug j in sample l is decomposed into the independent component $W_j\left(z_j\left(R_l\right); \psi_j\right)$ and the aggregate dependent component $\sum_{j'=1, j' \neq j}^{m} W_{jj'}\left(z_{j'}\left(R_l\right); \psi_{jj'}\right)$ due to the interaction of other drugs with it. Equation (9.4) is called qdODEs because their time derivative is replaced by the RI derivative. Mathematical properties of the qdODEs were discussed in Griffin et al. (2020). Parameters ψ_j specifies how the overall response to drug j changes with RI when this drug is assumed to be independent from other drugs, whereas $\psi_{jj'}$ specifies how drug j' influences the overall response of a patient to drug j through physical or chemical bindings. Nonparametric LOP approaches are used to fit the RI-varying independent and dependent components, where $z_j\left(R_l\right)$ and $z_{j'}\left(R_l\right)$ are the fitted values of the PD data (see Table 9.2) by the power equation.

Under the likelihood of the observed PD data, we implement the fourth-order Runge-Kutta algorithm to estimate the qdODE parameters and SAD(1) to model the structure of the covariance matrix. The covariance matrix is sparse because it is assumed that residuals are independent among patients. Covariances are considered to only occur among different concentration levels for the same patient, whose structure can be fitted by SAD(1). The MLEs of the independent and dependent components are used to reconstruct DDI networks.

The qdODE model of equation (9.4) unifies the static and semi-static information from multiple patients. After qdODE parameters are estimated, we take integrals of the independent and dependent components of qdODEs over the RI range of each patient. Using these integrals, we can reconstruct patient- and context-specific DDI networks. Such personalized inter-drug networks can help to systematically characterize inter-personal variability in the impact of DDIs on therapeutic efficacy.

9.3.3 A Proof of Concept: Analyzing a Real Data Set

Currently, we have no multi-drug clinical data to demonstrate the utility of the DDI network model derived from functional graph theory. However, the model can be tested by analyzing a metal mixture data because the impact of metals on organismic processes complies to a similar rule applying to the body-drug interactions. Versieren et al. (2016) conducted a well-designed study aimed to investigate how Cu, Ni, Cd, and Zn impair barley root elongation. Their experimental design allowed mixture toxicity and interactions in binary and ternary mixture to be assessed across multiple treatments. Versieren et al. found that the toxicity of quaternary mixture was larger than the summed effect of individual metals at single metal concentrations, suggesting the existence of metal-metal interactions in the mixture. This finding suits the validation of the DDI network reconstruction model. We assemble the data from their two toxicity experiments, each including the concentrations of each metal in the mixture and their total toxic effects on root elongation. Let t_{ij} denote the overall toxicity of a metal j to an organism growing in treatment i ($i=1, ..., s$). We define the overall toxicity of a metal as the ratio of the total toxicity to the concentration of this metal. To reflect the part-whole relationship of the systems, we use the sum of the overall toxicity of individual metals, expressed as $T_i = \sum_{j=1}^{m} t_{ij}$, as a proxy to measure the total toxicity of metal mixture in environment i. We call T_i a toxicity index. We illustrate the allometric relationship of the overall toxicity of individual metals with toxicity index by the power equation.

As can be seen, Zn and Ni increase their toxicity dramatically (with a large slope) with toxicity index, whereas the toxicity of Cd and Cn increases slightly (with a smaller slope but with a larger intercept) (Figure 9.2). These differences imply the dynamic existence of complex metal-metal interactions

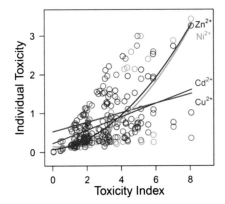

FIGURE 9.2
The allometric relationship of the overall toxicity of individual metals (Zn, blue; Ni, green; Cd, purple; Cu, red) with the total toxicity of metal mixture (toxicity index) to root length growth for barley (*Hordeum vulgare*). The circles represent the position of a metal in this relationship and curves stand for the fitting of overall toxicity data by the power equation. Data from Versieren et al. (2016).

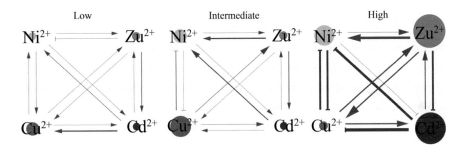

FIGURE 9.3
Metal networks whose varying strengths of metal-metal interactions may cause different levels of toxicity. The size of circles is proportional to the magnitude of the independent toxicity of a metal. The arrowed and T-shaped lines indicate the promotion or inhibition of one metal to the next, respectively, with the thickness proportional to the strength of influence.

(MMIs). We use the qdODE model of equation (9.4) to reconstruct four-node MMI networks that can interpret the toxicity of metal mixture to barley root elongation (Figure 9.3). In the networks, we can identify hub metals that have more links with other metals than average. Hub metals are thought to play a pivotal role in mediating the overall behavior of metal mixtures. We can further identify the direction of the role of a hub. An outgoing or incoming role implies that the hub affects, or is affected by, other metals, respectively. Based on the values of toxicity index, we classify the treatments into three categories, low toxicity, intermediate toxicity, and high toxicity, and infer an MMI networks for each category (Figure 9.3). These toxicity-specific networks provide much useful information for interpreting how MMIs mediate metal toxicity to plant growth.

We find that the contribution of the independent toxicity of individual metals to the total toxicity differs strikingly among metals (Figure 9.3). Ni contributes to the total toxicity in a graduate manner from low to intermediate to high, whereas both Zu and Cd and Cu make the largest considerable contribution to the high- and intermediate-level total toxicity, respectively. It is interesting to find that the strength and complexity of metal interactions are strikingly higher at high-level than low- and intermediate-level total toxicity, implying that the high toxic effect of metal mixture on barley root length growth results from specific metal interactions. These interactions include the predation of Cd toward Cu, the predation of Zu toward Cd, asymmetrical synergism between Ni and Zu, symmetric antagonism between Ni and Cu, symmetric synergism between Cu and Zu, and directional antagonism of Cd toward Ni. A detailed characterization of these interactions, as described above, can help increase the precision of risk assessment and prediction for metal mixture in natural environments.

9.4 Coalescing High-Order DDIs into Hypernetworks

In biology, the complexity of interactions may be largely beyond pairwise networks (Levine et al. 2017). DDIs in combination therapies are not an exception. Mounting evidence shows the pervasion of high-order interactions among drugs in the body, where other drugs modulate the interactions between drug pairs (Cokol et al. 2017; Tekin et al. 2017; Katzir et al. 2019). While the paradigm of pairwise interactions can capture the effect of a drug devoured by other drugs (Figure 9.4a), it misses multilateral relationships and interactions among multispecific drugs. For example, while drug D1 activates a protein that inhibits the expression of a nucleic acid targeted by drug D2, this pairwise inhibitory effect can be attenuated by drug D4 that targets an enzyme that degrades the protein (Figure 9.4b). D4 thus modifies the interaction between the proteins targeted by D1 and D2, without having a direct effect on any of them. The expression or activity of the protein-degrading enzyme may in turn be inhibited by the protein targeted by D3 (Figure 9.3c), thereby generating a four-way interaction. Such interaction processes can quickly lead to interactions at an even higher order.

Functional graph theory can be expanded to detect and coalesce high-order DDIs into quantitative hypernetworks. Different from a pairwise network with edges including two nodes, a hypernetwork is characteristic of hyperedges, i.e., edges containing more than two nodes (Klamt et al. 2009; Kong and Yu 2019). The hypernetworks reconstructed from functional graph theory can characterize DDIs at any order, providing a more complete

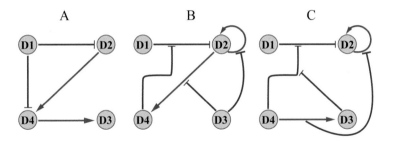

FIGURE 9.4

Pairwise and high-order DDI networks among four drugs D1–D4. (a) Pairwise interactions in a multi-drug community: Drugs affect each other directly. For instance, D1 could be targeting a protein that inhibits the expression of a gene targeted by D2. (b) Three-way interactions in the community: one drug can modulate the interactions between two others. For instance, D3 might degrade a certain protein targeted by D1, thereby attenuating the inhibitory effect of the gene by D2. (c) Four-way interactions in the community. For example, D4 might be a compound that inhibits the protein-degrading enzyme produced by D3-targetted gene. The arrowed and T-shaped lines represent the direction by which one drug activates and inhibits the next drug, respectively, with the strength proportional to the thickness of the lines.

picture of the structure and organization of drug co-regulation communities. These hypernetworks are powerful for understanding, dissecting, and predicting the joint pharmacological response of multiple drugs. The hypernetworks identified are filled by bidirectional, signed, and weighted interactions and such detailed information can facilitate our understanding of the mechanistical basis for combination therapies. Furthermore, since all nodes, edges, and hyperedges of different orders change with allometric scaling relationships across subjects, we can monitor how the topology of hypernetworks varies from subject to subject. In other words, we can reconstruct personalized DDI hypernetworks and convert them into context-specific hypernetworks.

9.5 Learning Large-Scale DDI Networks

To predict potential interactions that were previously unknown, assure that certain interactions should be avoided, and explore how DDIs link to pharmaceutical properties, DDI screening needs to include a large number of drugs in vitro clinical trials (Udrescu et al. 2016). This requires the reconstruction of a large-scale DDI network. The number of interactions increases exponentially with the number of drugs, making it challenging to capture fully interconnected relationships. In living systems, networks are usually sparse; i.e., not all drugs are linked to each other, given that the sparsity of networks is less vulnerable to stochastic disturbances (May 1972; Gross et al.

2009; Allesina and Tang 2012). There are two approaches for inferring sparse DDI networks. First, we implement variable selection to choose a small set of the most significant links for each drug. This can be done by formulating a multiple regression model of a drug on all other drugs built on the ODEs of equations (9.1), (9.2), or (9.9). Some popularly used regularization-based variable selection approaches, such as LASSO (Tibshirani 1996; Zou and Hastie 2005), group LASSO (Yuan and Lin 2006), or adaptive group LASSO (Wang and Leng 2008) can be implemented. Note that this procedure reduces the density of the network, but does not reduce the dimension of the network.

For a large-scale network, it is likely that the network is divided into distinct communities in which genes are more tightly interconnected with each other than with those from other communities. Such modularity theory has been approved to be universal in living systems (Melo et al. 2016; Clune et al. 2013; Kashtan and Alon 2005). This theory allows us to split a whole big network into different communities or called subnetworks. To do so, we implement a functional clustering algorithm, proposed by Kim et al. (2008) and Wang et al. (2012), to classify all drugs into distinct modules based on the similarity of therapeutic response. For high-density PK and PD data, the mathematical models of PK and PD are incorporated into the clustering algorithm. For static or semi-static data, we show that the response level of a drug allometrically scales with the response index across samples in a way following the power law. Thus, the pattern of how one drug functions differently from other drugs can be characterized by differences in power equation coefficients. We formulate a likelihood function based on the drug response data, whose solution can address the questions of how many modules are detected among all drugs (according to information criteria) and which module to which a drug belongs (determined on the basis of posterior probabilities).

The number of drug modules corresponds to the number of DDI network communities. Based on the mean values of communities, we use the same procedure as described above to reconstruct an inter-community connection network. For each module, the number of drugs reduces to a level at which variable selection can work properly. Thus, we reconstruct DDI networks for each module in which the interactions of each drug with other drugs can be charted. In the end, we have a two-layer tridimensional DDI network, composed of the inter-community network at the top and multiple inter-drug networks under each community at the bottom.

9.6 Concluding Remarks

Congruous combinations among multispecific drugs provide a powerful strategy of therapy in the 21st century (Tyers and Wright 2019). The successful deployment of combination strategies as new medicines critically relies upon an understanding of how drugs interact with each other to determine pharmacological response (Levy and Ragueneau-Majlessi 2019; Derendorf et al. 2019). Given the complexities of drug-drug and drug-body interactions, a sophisticated computational approach is sorely needed to extract and excavate the principal mechanisms behind these interactions. Functional graph theory – the integration of graph theory and game theory through PK-PD processes – represents an unprecedented capacity to contextualize all possibly occurring drug interactions into a quantitative network by which one can trace the direct and indirect roadmap of each drug to contribute to the overall therapeutic effects.

As an interdisciplinary framework, functional graph theory has been introduced to the broader community of combination therapies (Sang et al. 2022). It can not only characterize a detailed atlas of drug interactions but also can monitor and trace how drug networks vary among individual patients and change across spatiotemporal gradients. Several network properties are of importance for understanding the role of each drug in mediating therapeutic response. By estimating network density, one can determine the proportion of potential drug-drug links in the network that are actual connections. Network density and sparsity are associated with the pharmacological balance of body-drug interactions. The degree of centrality, referring to the number of connections a drug has, helps to determine hub drugs that are most frequently involved in drug interactions.

There has been a rich body of literature on computational approaches for network inference (Zou and Conzen 2005; Vijesh et al. 2013; Wang and Huang 2014; Han et al. 2016; Chen et al. 2017; Huynh-Thu and Sanguinetti 2019), but most existing approaches can only provide partial information about network topologies (Chen et al. 2019). For example, some approaches can estimate the strength of interactions but fail to identify their causality (Huynh-Thu and Sanguinetti 2019). Some can identify causality but cannot characterize the sign of interactions (Marbach et al. 2012). Functional graph theory can reconstruct fully informative networks, encapsulated by bi-causal, signed, and weighted DDIs, which can address fundamental pharmacological questions that cannot be answered by traditional approaches.

Functional graph theory is extended to reconstruct hypernetworks (Wu and Jiang 2021) because we believe that higher-order interactions of three or more drugs are omnipresent at the sites of drug action. Drug interaction hypernetworks can precisely characterize the inherent complexity of inter-drug interactions and, therefore, better reveal the pharmacological machineries of drug response. There is still much room to modify functional graph theory in terms of how to jointly model drug efficacy vs. drug toxicity (Chhibber et al. 2014), drug sensitivity vs. drug resistance, and drug generality vs. drug specificity. We are in the era of genomic revolution when omics data at the multiorganizational levels can be collected and monitored for the host. By marrying these data and DDI interaction networks and hypernetworks, functional graph theory can be developed into a critical tool for checking and identifying drug synergism that maximizes efficacy but minimizes toxicity in practical clinics.

Networks are fundamental to the functionality of complex systems (Newman 2003). The quantitative reconstruction of DDI networks can help to trace the mechanistic roadmaps of how each drug acts and interacts with every other drug within the PK-PD context. Conventionally, drug discovery has obeyed the well-accepted paradigm of one drug – one target – one disease, aimed to identify the most specific drugs that act against a specific target for a specific disease (Hopkins 2008; Galan-Vasquez and Perez-Rueda 2021). However, diseases are caused by complex biological processes, which can be resistant to the activity of any single drug. Functional graph theory can help to make a paradigm shift from monotherapies to the polypharmacy of multi-drugs-multi-targets-multi-diseases (Bansal et al. 2014).

10

Pharmacogenomics as a Cornerstone of Precision Medicine: Methodological Leveraging

10.1 Introduction

While precision medicine, aimed to tailor medical treatments to individual subjects or to a group of subjects, is becoming the cornerstone of modern medicine, there is no doubt that its own cornerstone is pharmacogenomics (Primorac et al. 2020). Pharmacogenomics plays a pivotal role in making a paradigm shift from a traditional "one-size-fits-all" prescribing approach to individualized medicine. It investigates how patients' DNA variants affect the way they respond to drugs and, more specifically, determine whether a drug helps the patient remove disease or whether the patient has an adverse reaction to the drug or has no influence. As such, pharmacogenomics can be used to improve human health by discovering, designing, and delivering the most appropriate medicine for specific patients.

The successful translation of pharmacogenomics into clinical practices critically relies on a profound understanding of how a person's unique molecular and genetic profile affects his/her susceptibility to certain diseases and predicts which medical treatments can be safe and effective and which ones may cause side-effects (Zhang and Nebert 2017). To achieve these scientific breakthroughs, big data collected from multifaceted aspects of human health and drug response and statistical algorithms for extracting useful information from these data have been widely thought to be sorely needed. Unfortunately, although data collection and acquirement have become less and less difficult, statistical modeling and analysis of these data represent a significant challenge. Much current analysis of genetic and pharmacogenomic data simply, and even indiscriminately, uses existing statistical models, without taking into account the mechanistic details of data formation. Furthermore, beyond statistical methods for the genetic dissection of complex diseases, those for mapping drug response require integrating body-drug interactions, presenting an additional dimension of consideration for data analysis.

The central theme of this book is to introduce several fundamental quantitative mechanistically based approaches for pharmacogenomic studies, which can better inform precision medicine of useful medical curriculums. The key component of these approaches includes the integration of pharmacokinetic (PK) and pharmacodynamic (PD) reactions into functional mapping and network mapping models, allowing us to characterize not only key individual genetic variants for drug response but also chart a comprehensive picture of how different variants work together to determine drug response. While the conventional framework of drug development focuses on the "average" of the population, precision medicine emphasizes the uniqueness of individual patients. The approaches introduced in this book can particularly disentangle the genetic control of drug response specifically occurring in individual patients. It is expected that the application of these approaches will promote a better understanding of the heterogeneity in processes that contribute to how a patient reacts to a specific drug at a specific time and dose. All this allows prescribers to tailor medicines to the nuanced but often unique features possessed by individual patients (Schork 2019; Primorac et al. 2020).

In this chapter, we first review the biochemical principle of how pharmacogenomics works to impact drug response on which the quantitative approaches introduced in this book were developed. We then discuss several issues that may impair the effective applications of these approaches as well as the way these issues can be resolved. We pinpoint how the application of these approaches can be augmented by incorporating omics data that have become increasingly available in pharmacogenomic studies.

10.2 How Drug Works

The strength and pattern of drug effects depend on how drugs interact with patients' body through their unique PK and PD processes. After a drug is administered, the body will first break it down and then transport it to the intended area. This process contains multiple steps of body-drug interactions, each determined by patients' DNA variants. Specifically, these steps are characterized in the following subsections.

10.2.1 Drug–Receptor Interaction

Generally, drugs work by interacting with receptors on the surface of cells or enzymes within cells (Lambert 2014). A specific three-dimensional structure, characterized by receptor and enzyme molecules, allows only substances (drugs) that fit precisely to attach to it, forming a lock-key relationship. In

A Drug-Receptor Interactions

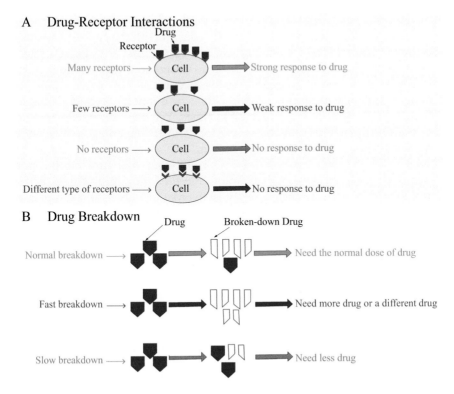

FIGURE 10.1
Diagram of pharmacological processes underlying drug-body interactions. (a) Drug-receptor interactions by which activated receptors by a drug (ligand) directly or indirectly regulate cellular biochemical processes, depending on the degree of drug-receptor match affected by the host's genes. (b) The breakdown of a drug is an important step for drug efficacy, with the degree of drug breakdown being affected by the host's genes.

order to work properly, a drug needs to attach to specific receptors. The types and number of receptors are patient-dependent and, thus, patients' DNA variants directly affect how and how strongly the patients respond to the drug. If a patient has rich receptors that fit precisely the drug, then he or she would have a strong response to the drug (Figure 10.1a). If a patient has fewer such receptors, he or she needs a higher amount of the drug to make it effective. Some patients may have no such receptors or different types of receptors and, then, no response is detected. It is expected that receptors as proteins, coded by genes, are under cis- or trans-genetic control.

In most cases, drugs work through either blocking the physiological function of the protein or mimicking its effect while binding to the target receptor site. A drug is called an agonist if it causes the protein receptor to respond in the same way as the naturally occurring substance. Examples of agonists include morphine (μ-opioid receptor), clonidine (α_2-adrenoceptor), nicotine, phenylephrine, and isoproterenol. The ability to produce a response is termed efficacy (or intrinsic activity), which varies with the type of response measured (Lambert 2004). A drug is called an antagonist if it interacts selectively with receptors but does not lead to an observed effect. An antagonist may reduce the action of an agonist at the receptor site involved. Examples of antagonist drugs are beta-blockers, such as propranolol. Receptor antagonists include reversible and irreversible types. Whereas reversible antagonists readily dissociate from their receptor, irreversible antagonists form a stable chemical bond with their receptor (e.g., in alkylation).

Instead of receptors, some drugs target enzymes that regulate the rate of chemical reactions. Drugs that target enzymes may inhibit their activity (inhibitors) or activate their activity (activators or inducers). Examples of drugs that target enzymes are aspirin, cox-2 inhibitors, and HIV protease inhibitors.

10.2.2 Drug Metabolism

Through specialized enzymatic systems of patients, drugs are broken down into compounds that are more easily excreted from the body. This process, called drug metabolism, is highly variable, which can be influenced by a number of factors. There are specific enzymes responsible for the metabolic breakdown of drugs. For example, the breakdown of the antidepressant drug amitriptyline is determined by CYP enzymes (including CYP2D6 and CYP2CI9), encoded by two genes called *CYP2D6* and *CYP2C19.* The amount of drug-metabolizing enzymes affects how quickly a patient's body breaks down a drug (Figure 10.1b). If one patient breaks the drug down more quickly than others, this implies that his or her body gets rid of the drug faster so that a higher amount of the drug is needed or a different drug should be used. In practice, by genetic texting for the *CYP2D6* and *CYP2C19* genes, doctors can better decide what dose of the drug a specific patient needs.

10.2.3 Targeted Drug Development

Effective drugs can be developed by targeting underlying drug receptor sites or enzymes. However, until recently design of new drugs was very difficult because it is difficult to know what the drug binding sites of the proteins look like and where they are. Modern molecular modeling makes it possible to view the 3-D structure of proteins and their binding sites using data from X-ray crystallography and NMR spectroscopy. For example, the synthesis of several recent drugs, such as HIV protease inhibitors for the treatment of AIDS, has been made using the 3-D structure of proteins. This tool can be benefitted by precisely detecting these proteins. Quantitative and network pharmacogenomics plays a critical role in the systematical characterization of drug receptors and relevant enzymes through gene mapping

10.3 Correcting for Relatedness in Pharmacogenomics Genome-wide Association Studies (GWAS)

10.3.1 Population Structure and Kinship

GWAS have widely been used as a powerful tool to seek to identify genetic variants that contribute to drug receptors, drug metabolism, and drug effects (Motsinger-Reif et al. 2013; Dolgin 2014; Giacomini et al. 2017; Barrett 2019; Koromina et al. 2020; McInnes and Altman 2021; McInnes et al. 2020; Wolking et al. 2021). GWAS discover these genetic factors by correlating a subject's genotype at each SNP with a drug response phenotype. An SNP is considered as being significant if its specific variant is correlated with drug response. In order for GWAS data to be analyzed appropriately, all subjects that comprise the GWAS panel should meet the assumption of independence, implying that these subjects should be sampled under the condition of uniform relatedness.

In recent years, sophisticated technologies have emerged that allow us to sample and assemble any subjects with known or unknown founders into GWAS. Such a broad collection of genetic variants is not only powerful for identifying a complete set of alleles affecting drug response but also provides an unprecedented resource to study the genetic architecture of how pharmacogenes diversify and evolve with environmental change to form pharmacogenetic variation. Violating the independence assumption, however, genetic inference from these heterogeneous GWAS cohorts is impaired by two types of relatedness, population structure, and kinship. The former is formed when subjects sharing ancestry are more closely related than those from different ancestries, whereas the latter exists when some subjects are closely related, but this shared ancestry is unknown. Both types of relatedness may produce high rates of false positive associations; i.e., significant associations detected are driven by the GWAS cohort's relatedness rather than true variants that affect the phenotype.

In the past two decades, numerous statistical and computational methods have been developed to effectively test for associations through correcting for population structure and kinship (Hoffman 2013; Li and Zhu 2013; Sul et al. 2018). Among these methods, genomic control (Evlin and Roeder 1999; Pritchard and Rosenberg 1999), structured association (Pritchard et al. 2000; Rosenberg et al. 2002), principal components analysis (Patterson et al. 2006; Novembre and Stephens 2008; Price et al. 2006), and multidimensional scaling (Purcell et al. 2007; Lee et al. 2010) can correct the population stratification by detecting and visualizing subpopulations contained in the GWAS cohorts (Li and Zhu 2013). These are powerful for controlling population structure but fail to account for the complete genealogy of the subjects. Because of its capacity to account for non-independent samples, linear mixed models (LMMs), originally in animal breeding (Henderson 1975), have emerged as a major tool to correct any relatedness existing among individuals (Yu et al. 2006; Kang et al. 2010; Segura et al. 2012; Listgarten et al. 2012; Zhou and Stephens 2012; Widmer et al. 2014; Wen et al. 2018; Runcie and Crawford 2019). The application of these approaches can well mitigate the inflated effects of both population structure and relatedness in association studies. Below, we describe LMM-based methods for relatedness correction and trace their development to accommodate various purposes of GWAS. We discuss the issue of population correction, typical of pharmacological GWAS incorporating PK and PD principles.

10.3.2 A General LMM Framework

Suppose there is a panel of genotyped subjects involved in pharmacogenetic GWAS. Subjects vary in genetic background, demographic factors, lifestyle, etc. Each subject is measured for a phenotypic trait that reflects its response to a particular drug. Let y_i denote the trait value of subject i. Consider an SNP with three genotypes AA, Aa, and aa. A full LMM model that specifies all genetic and non-genetic effects for this SNP is expressed as

$$y_i = \sum_{r=1}^{R} x_{ir} u_r + \sum_{s=1}^{S} \sum_{l=1}^{L_s} z_{isl} v_{sl} + \xi_i a + \varsigma_i d + g_i + e_i, \tag{10.1}$$

at the right side of which the first two terms are the effect of continuous and discrete covariates, the third term is the genetic effect of the SNP, the fourth term is the random polygenic background effect, and the last term is the error effect. Notation includes, x_{ir}, value of subject i for continuous covariate r ($r=1, ..., R$); u_r, effect of covariate r; z_{isl}, indicator variable of subject i which receives level l ($l=1, ..., L_s$) of discrete covariate s ($s=1, ..., S$); v_{sl}, effect of level l for covariate s, with $\sum_{l=1}^{L_s} v_{sl} = 0$; ξ_i, indicator variable that is defined as 1 for genotype is AA, 0 for genotype Aa, and 0 for genotype aa; a, the additive genetic effect of the SNP; ς_i, indicator variable that is defined as 1 for genotype is Aa, 0 for genotypes AA and aa; d, the dominant genetic effect of the SNP; g_i, polygenic effect of subject i; and e_i, the random residual effect assumed to be normally distributed with mean zero and variance $\sigma^2 \mathbf{I}$ where σ^2 is the residual variance.

Of the discrete covariates, one can be population structure that occurs in GWAS cohorts. Whether a GWAS population has subpopulations and how many subpopulations occur can be determined by package Structure (Pritchard and Rosenberg 1999; Pritchard et al. 2000). The polygenic effects are assumed to follow a normal distribution with mean zero and variance-covariance matrix $\sigma_g^2 \mathbf{G}$, where σ_g^2 is the polygenic variance of the trait and $\mathbf{G}$ is the kinship coefficient matrix between subjects. Restricted maximum likelihood approaches have been developed to solve unknown parameters that specify LMM in equation (10.1).

The genetic part of equation (10.1), denoted as G, includes the fixed additive effect (A) and fixed dominant effect (D) of the SNP, fixed subpopulation effect (Q), and random kinship effect (K), representing a general strategy for GWAS data analysis. A full genetic model is expressed as

$$G = A + D + Q + K \tag{10.2a}$$

In practice, this model may be overfit. To find the most parsimonious model, the following reduced models are considered:

$$G = A + D \tag{10.2b}$$

$$G = A + D + Q \tag{10.2c}$$

$$G = A + D + K \tag{10.2d}$$

The choice of an optimal model that interprets a given GWAS data can be made empirically by comparing Q-Q plots. A Q-Q plot is a graphical representation of the deviation of the observed P values for each SNP from the null hypothesis (Ehret 2010). We sort the observed P values from largest to smallest and then plot them against expected values from a theoretical χ^2-distribution across all SNPs, producing scatter points. If all points are on or near the diagonal line between the x-axis and the y-axis, this suggests that the observed values correspond to the expected values. If points move toward the y-axis, this suggests that some observed P values are more significant than expected under the null hypothesis. An early separation of the expected from the observed implies that many moderately significant P values are more significant than expected under the null hypothesis. This result is likely to be due to genetic relatedness, i.e., systematic differences in allele frequencies between subpopulations of the GWAS cohort, leading to a large number of P values to be smaller than expected by chance alone.

An optimal model can be statistically chosen by likelihood ratio tests. By comparing the reduced Q model of equation (10.2c) or the reduced K model of equation (10.2d) to the full model of equation (10.2a), one can determine whether population structure and kinships should be considered. Both reduced Q and K models are rejected, this means that the full model should be chosen. If the full model is rejected, we can further compare the reduced Q model or K model to the A+D model of equation (10.2b) to determine whether population structure or kinships should be involved in the final GWAS analysis model.

10.3.3 Dynamic Issue in PGx GWAS

The simplest design of a GWAS is to test the association between each SNP and a single trait. However, a sophisticated design that can better characterize the complexity of genetic studies may include multiple traits and multiple environments. To correct population stratification, several modifications to LMM have been made. In particular, Zhou and Stephens (2012) extended LMM to multivariate LMM (mvLMM) for simultaneously analyzing multiple traits, displaying increased power of association detection. More recently, Moore et al. (2019) proposed a structured LMM (StructLMM) model to test and estimate multivariate gene-environment interactions when the dimension of environmental variables is extremely high (>400).

Different from traditional GWAS, pharmacogenomic GWAS may repeatedly measure drug response at a series of time points and drug concentrations, forming dynamically varying traits. To consider the dynamic feature of a complex trait, Ning et al. (2019) implemented a longitudinal LMM (longLMM) to correct population structure and genetic relatedness. However, longLMM expresses dynamic changes using a nonparametric function, and, thereby, its application to PGx GWAS may be limited given the nonlinear PK and PD change of drug response. A nonlinear mixed-effect model (Hou et al. 2008) integrating pharmacologically meaningful equations should be developed to correct any type of relatedness among subjects in PGx GWAS. This integration is likely to strengthen our capacity to reveal the genetic control of drug response that is a function of time and drug concentration and gain new insight into pharmacogenetic architecture.

10.4 Family-Based Designs for PGx Studies

10.4.1 Advantages of Family-Based Designs

Large-scale studies of genetic variation and next-generation sequencing assays revealed that roughly 30%–40% of the variability in pharmacogenes is attributed to rare genetic variants and in some gene families, rare variants even comprise >90% of the pharmacogenetic variation (Fujikura et al. 2015; Kozyra et al. 2017; Bush et al. 2016; Ingelman-Sundberg et al. 2018; Caspar et al. 2021). To detect rare variants, an extremely large sample size is required to assure those genotypes composed of rare alleles to be observed, but such a condition is rarely met for a PGx GWAS. Family-based designs, in which all alleles (including rare ones) are transmitted from parents to their offspring in a Mendelian ratio, can overcome this issue.

Required sample sizes for the identification of rare variants can be much smaller than those for designs composed of unrelated subjects (Wijsman 2016; Ott et al. 2011).

The additional advantage of family-based designs lies in their capacity to control for heterogeneity and population stratification (Ott et al. 2011; Li et al. 2011b). The subjects used for association studies are necessary of the same ethnic origin and, therefore, are genetically uniform, with no existence of population stratification, as opposed to population-based cohorts. In addition, by making use of the transmission information from parents to offspring, family-based designs allow investigation of parent-of-origin effects, thereby better charting the genetic architecture of drug response than designs based on unrelated subjects (Haghighi and Hodge 2002; Li et al. 2011b, 2014b; Sui et al. 2014).

The parent-of-origin effect, or called genetic imprinting, is an epigenetic phenomenon in which an allele from one parent will be expressed while the same allele from the other parent remains inactive. The expression of imprinted genes from only one parental allele results from differential epigenetic marks that are established during gametogenesis. Since its first discovery in the early 1980s, genetic imprinting has been thought to play an important role in embryonic growth and development and disease pathogenesis in a variety of organisms. Several dozen genes in the mouse were detected to express from only one of the two parental chromosomes (Barton et al. 1984; Cattanach and Kirk 1985; Lawson et al. 2013), some of which have been tested in other mammals (Morison et al. 2005) including humans. Family-based designs can facilitate the systematical investigation of the role played by imprinting effects in mediating pharmacogenetic variation.

10.4.2 Genetic Modeling

Consider a panel of families sampled for a PGx GWAS trial. Each family is composed of the maternal parent (M), paternal parent (P), and one or more offspring. Both parents and offspring are genotyped for genome-wide SNPs. The offspring are subject to drug interventions, whose drug response is measured at a series of time points or concentrations. Consider an SNP with three genotypes AA, Aa, and aa, which, as M and P parents, form nine mating types (Table 10.1). Each mating type produces offspring with genotypes segregating in a Mendelian ratio. For example, type $AA \times AA$ only produces offspring genotype AA, type $AA \times Aa$ produces offspring genotypes AA and Aa with the same proportion, so on and so forth. Offspring heterozygote Aa derived from types $AA \times Aa$, $AA \times aa$, and $Aa \times aa$ has its allele A that must come from the M parent and that derived from $Aa \times AA$, $aa \times AA$, and $aa \times Aa$ has its allele A from the P parent. Thus, based on these mating types, we can distinguish two configurations of the offspring heterozygote, expressed as $A|a$ and $a|A$, where the vertical line separates the alleles' origin of parent.

TABLE 10.1

Offspring Genotypes and Their Values Derived from Different Combinations of Maternal (M) and Paternal (P) Genotypes

	Family			Offspring Genotype		
	Genotype		AA	$A\|a$	$a\|A$	aa
No	M×F	Size	$\mu_2=\mu+a$	$\mu_{1+}=\mu+d-i$	$\mu_{1-}=\mu+d-i$	$\mu_0=\mu$
1	$AA\times AA$	n_{22}	1	0	0	0
2	$AA\times Aa$	n_{21}	½	½	0	0
3	$AA\times aa$	n_{20}	0	1	0	0
4	$Aa\times AA$	n_{12}	½	0	½	0
5	$Aa\times Aa$	n_{11}	¼	¼	¼	¼
6	$Aa\times aa$	n_{10}	0	½	0	½
7	$aa\times AA$	n_{02}	0	0	1	0
8	$aa\times Aa$	n_{01}	0	0	½	½
9	$aa\times aa$	n_{00}	0	0	0	1

These two configurations produced from type $Aa\times Aa$ cannot be separated from each other. Taken together, all nine mating types produce four configurations, whose genotypic values can be formulated as

$$AA: \mu_2 = \mu + a$$
$$A\,|\,a: \mu_{1+} = \mu + d + h$$
$$a\,|\,A: \mu_{1-} = \mu + d - h$$
$$aa: \mu_0 = \mu - a$$

(10.3)

where μ is the overall mean, a is the additive genetic effect, d is the dominant genetic effect, and h is the genetic imprinting effect due to the alleles' origin of parent. If there is no effect due to the origin of parent, i should be equal to zero. Thus, by estimating the magnitude of h and testing its significance, we can characterize whether and how imprinting effect affects drug response.

10.4.3 Statistical Modeling

Assume there are n families sampled, which are allotted into different mating types, with size denoted in Table 10.1. Let $n_{2|i}$, $n_{1+|i}$, $n_{1-|i}$ and $n_{0|i}$ denote the observations of offspring configurations AA, $A|a$, $a|A$, and aa derived from family i. For type $Aa\times Aa$, the observation of its offspring heterozygote is denoted as $n_{1|i}$. Let $\mathbf{y}_j|_i=(y_j|_i(t_{j1}), ..., y_j|_i(t_{jT_j}))$ denote the drug concentrations of offspring j from family i measured at time points $(t_{j1}, ..., t_{jT_j})$. The likelihood of phenotypic values at an SNP is formulated as

$$L(\mathbf{y}) = \prod_{i=1}^{n_{22}+n_{21}+n_{12}+n_{11}} \prod_{j=1}^{n_{2|i}} f_2\left(\mathbf{y}_{j|i};\boldsymbol{\mu}_2,\Sigma\right)$$

$$\prod_{i=1}^{n_{21}+n_{20}+n_{10}} \prod_{j=1}^{n_{1+|i}} f_{1+}\left(\mathbf{y}_{j|i};\boldsymbol{\mu}_{1+},\Sigma\right)$$

$$\prod_{i=1}^{n_{12}+n_{02}+n_{01}} \prod_{j=1}^{n_{1-|i}} f_{1-}\left(\mathbf{y}_{j|i};\boldsymbol{\mu}_{1-},\Sigma\right) \qquad (10.4)$$

$$\prod_{i=1}^{n_{11}+n_{10}+n_{01}+n_{00}} \prod_{j=1}^{n_{0|i}} f_0\left(\mathbf{y}_{j|i};\boldsymbol{\mu}_2,\Sigma\right)$$

$$\prod_{i=1}^{n_{11}} \prod_{j=1}^{n_{1|i}} \left(\frac{1}{2} f_{1+}\left(\mathbf{y}_{j|i};\boldsymbol{\mu}_{1+},\Sigma\right) + \frac{1}{2} f_{1-}\left(\mathbf{y}_{j|i};\boldsymbol{\mu}_{1-},\Sigma\right)\right)$$

where $f_2(.)$, $f_{1+}(.)$, $f_{1+}(.)$, and $f_0(.)$ are multivariate normal density functions of offspring j carrying configurations AA, $A|a$, $a|A$, and aa, respectively, with the corresponding mean vectors $\boldsymbol{\mu}_2$, $\boldsymbol{\mu}_{1+}$, $\boldsymbol{\mu}_{1-}$, $\boldsymbol{\mu}_0$, and covariance matrix Σ. Functional mapping integrates a PD equation, e.g., the Hill equation, to model the mean vectors and SAD(1) to model the covariance structure.

Since there are two mixture components for the offspring heterozygote derived from $Aa \times Aa$, we implement the EM algorithm, coupled with the simplex algorithm, to solve the likelihood (10.4). After the maximum likelihood estimates (MLEs) of the PD parameters contained in the mean vectors, we chart configuration-dependent concentration-drug effect curves, from which the additive, dominant and imprinting effect curves can be calculated and tested. Here, we show how to test the significance of imprinting effect. Based on equation (10.3), we formulate the following hypotheses:

$$H_0 : \boldsymbol{\mu}_{1+} = \boldsymbol{\mu}_{1-}$$

$$H_1 : \boldsymbol{\mu}_{1+} \neq \boldsymbol{\mu}_{1-}$$

where the null hypothesis states that there is no imprinting effect and the alternative hypothesis states that there is an imprinting effect. The parameter estimation under the alternative hypothesis has been described as above. To estimate the parameters under the null hypothesis, we rewrite the likelihood of equation (10.4) as

$$
L_0(\mathbf{y}) = \prod_{i=1}^{n_{22}+n_{21}+n_{12}+n_{11}} \prod_{j=1}^{n_{2|i}} f_2\left(\mathbf{y}_{j|i}; \boldsymbol{\mu}_2, \Sigma\right)
$$

$$
\prod_{i=1}^{n_{21}+n_{20}+n_{12}+n_{11}+n_{10}+n_{02}+n_{01}} \prod_{j=1}^{n_{1|i}} f_1\left(\mathbf{y}_{j|i}; \boldsymbol{\mu}_1, \Sigma\right) \tag{10.5}
$$

$$
\prod_{i=1}^{n_{11}+n_{10}+n_{01}+n_{00}} \prod_{j=1}^{n_{0|i}} f_0\left(\mathbf{y}_{j|i}; \boldsymbol{\mu}_2, \Sigma\right)
$$

where the mean vectors of three offspring genotypes in the multivariate normal density probability function are fitted by the PD equation and covariance matrix fitted by the SAD(1) model. The likelihood is solved by implementing the simplex algorithm.

By plugging in the MLEs of model parameters into the likelihoods of equations (8.4) and (8.5), we calculate the log-likelihood ratio under the null and alternative hypotheses as

$$
LR = -2\left(\log L_0 - \log L\right) \tag{10.6}
$$

which is supposed to follow a chi-square distribution with one degree of freedom. Alternatively, we can simulate studies to determine the critical threshold. It is interesting to interpret imprinting causes based on the sign of imprinting effect. According to Table 10.1's formulation, we can say that the *A* allele of the maternal parent exerts a positive imprinting effect or the *a* allele of the paternal parent exerts a positive imprinting effect if *h* is positive. Likewise, the *a* allele of the maternal parent exerts a positive imprinting effect or the *A* allele of the paternal parent exerts a positive imprinting effect if *h* is negative.

Genetic imprinting effects are generally detected through the molecular characterization of mutants (Lawson et al. 2013; Li et al. 2019). This molecular approach can facilitate the mechanistic understanding of how alleles with different parental origins are expressed differently, but is less powerful for a genome-wide characterization of imprinting effects. The statistical model proposed above helps pursue a systematic search for the genome-wide occurrence of imprinting effects and, therefore, gain unique insight into the genomic signature and evolution of the role of this important phenomenon in mediating variation in drug response.

10.5 Intertwined Epistatic and Epistatic Networks

10.5.1 Pleiotropic Networks

Five blood pressure-related variables reflect different aspects of cardiovascular state and disorder but share some common developmental and hemodynamic basis. Thus, it is possible that these variables are controlled by the same genes. A similar principle derived from evolutionary game theory can be used to analyze the pleiotropic control of a trait. If a gene encodes products that can be used to produce different phenotypes, then this gene is said to be pleiotropic. Because of the occurrence of pleiotropic effects, the net genetic variance of a trait may contain its genetic covariance with other traits, which cause inter-trait correlations. Thus, according to evolutionary game theory, we decompose $g_{sk}(d)$ of trait k due to a specific SNP into two components, socially isolated genetic variance (SIGV) and socialized genetic variance (SGV). The SIGV represents how the SNP affects trait k when this trait is assumed to be in isolation, whereas the SGV specifies how and how strongly other traits affect trait k through this SNP. Based on these arguments, we formulate a system of ODEs to quantify these two underlying components, expressed as

$$g'_{sk}(d) = R_{sk}\left(g_{sk}(d) : \Phi_{sk}\right) + \sum_{k'=1, k' \neq k}^{5} R_{skk'}\left(g_{sk'}(d) : \Phi_{skk'}\right), \quad k = 1, \ldots, 5 \quad (10.7)$$

where SIGV $R_{sk}\left(g_{sk}(d) : \Phi_{sk}\right)$ and SDV $R_{skk'}\left(g_{sk'}(d) : \Phi_{skk'}\right)$ are both fitted by a nonparametric function specified by parameters Φ_{sk} and $\Phi_{skk'}$, respectively. We encapsulate $R_{sk}\left(g_{sk}(d) : \Phi_{sk}\right)$ as nodes and $R_{skk'}\left(g_{sk'}(d) : \Phi_{skk'}\right)$ as edges into mathematical networks filled by bidirectional, signed, and weight trait-trait interactions. These networks are called pleiotropic networks in terms of their capacity to characterize how the same gene affects different traits simultaneously. From the pleiotropic networks, one can determine whether, how, and how much one trait is correlated with any other traits due to a given gene.

10.5.2 Epistatic Networks of Pleiotropic Networks

Equation (10.5) characterizes the epistatic network underlying each trait exerted by multiple SNPs, whereas equation (6) illustrates the pleiotropic network underlying multiple traits triggered by each SNP. The combination of the ideas described in these two equations establishes a unified framework for unveiling the epistatic network underlying the pleiotropic network, which is closer to the intrinsic complexity of systems biology and systems medicine. We interpret the effect of SNP s on trait k in terms of three different scenarios. In scenario 1, SNP s only affects trait k but not any other traits, in a way that is independent from other SNPs. In scenario 2, SNP s receives epistatic interactions in a way its effect on trait k is influenced by other SNPs. In scenario 3, SNP s pleiotropically affects multiple traits so that its effect on trait k is regulated by other SNPs. The value of $g_{sk}(d)$ that contributes to genetic architecture is the net consequence of these three scenarios. Based on evolutionary game theory, we decompose $g_{sk}(d)$ using the following replicator equations:

$$g'_{sk}(d) = Q_{sk}\left(g_{sk}(d):\Psi_{sk}\right) + \sum_{s'=1,s'\neq s}^{p} Q_{ss'k}\left(g_{s'k}(d):\Psi_{ss'k}\right)$$

$$+ \sum_{k'=1,k'\neq k}^{5} R_{skk'}\left(g_{sk'}(d):\Psi_{skk'}\right) \tag{10.8}$$

$$s = 1, \dots, p; k = 1, \dots, 5$$

where $Q_{sk}\left(g_{sk}(d):\Psi_{sk}\right)$ is the independent genetic variance of trait k due to SNP s that is expected to occur when both SNP s and trait k are assumed to be in isolation, $\sum Q_{ss'k}\left(g_{s'k}(d):\Psi_{ss'k}\right)$ is the *epistatic dependent genetic variance* of trait k due to interactions of other $p-1$ SNPs with SNP s, and $\sum R_{skk'}\left(g_{sk'}(d):\Psi_{skk'}\right)$ the *pleiotropic dependent variance* of trait k due to influences of other four traits under the control of SNP s. Nonparametric models are used to smoothen the independent genetic variance, the epistatic dependent genetic variance, and pleiotropic dependent variance, with ODE parameters Ψ_{sk}, $\Psi_{ss'k}$, and $\Psi_{skk'}$, respectively. The above three types of genetic variance are contextualized into a tridimensional network that characterizes the epistatic network of the pleiotropic network.

10.6 Pharmacosystems Biology: From Pharmacogenomics to Pharmaco-Omics

10.6.1 Integrating Pharmaco-Omics into Pharmacogenomics

PGx GWAS have proven to be a successful approach for identifying significant SNPs associated with pharmacological response (Auwerx et al. 2022). However, like those detected in disease-oriented GWAS, the majority of statistically significant PGx signals are located in non-coding regions of the human genome (Maurano et al. 2012; Li and Ritchie 2021). The detection of these significant signals is due to linkage disequilibrium between SNPs and causal variants driving the association. Obviously, the gap between non-coding PGx GWAS signals and the causal genes makes it impossible to translate GWAS discoveries into clinical settings. Many bioinformatics approaches integrating functional genomics knowledge have been developed to identify genetically regulated genes from GWAS discoveries.

Driving a genomic walk from GWAS signals to downstream causal genes, these bioinformatics approaches can be broadly classified into two categories, fine mapping and gene prioritization (Li and Ritchie 2021). As one common option for post-GWAS analyses, the fine-mapping approach seeks to identify causal variants or genes for complex diseases or traits through building LD structures and haplotype blocks (Schaid et al. 2018; Broekema et al. 2020). It is known that non-coding DNA of the human genome, located in intergenic and intronic regions, can act as enhancers, promoters, transcription factors, and CCCTC-binding factors, which regulate transcriptional or translational activities of genes. Various genetic variants, like expression quantitative trait loci (eQTLs), splicing QTL, and protein QTL, may be harbored in these regulatory elements (Andersson et al. 2014; ENCODE Project Consortium et al. 2020; GTEx Consortium 2020; Rohde et al. 2019). Thus, genetic variants modulate the expression of causal genes under the regulatory mechanisms shaped by the functional elements. The gene-prioritization approach takes advantage of intermediate molecular traits, such as gene expression, protein expression, and metabolite abundance, to deduct possible molecular mechanisms underpinning complex diseases or traits. It has three types, colocalization, Mendelian Randomization (MR), and transcriptome-wide association study (TWAS).

The colocalization method reveals the co-occurring patterns between eQTLs and GWAS signals and tests the biological hypothesis of whether and how a causal locus or a genetic variant shapes both the intermediate molecular changes and the complex trait of interest (Hukku et al. 2021). A GWAS signal is likely to be functional if it is colocalized within an eQTL. MR is a causal inference approach, striving to explore the causal relationship between a modifiable exposure and complex disease trait (Holmes et al. 2017). For example, blood concentrations of low-density lipoprotein cholesterol (LDL-c) can serve as a modifiable exposure for coronary heart disease (CHD). MR uses LDL-c-related genetic variants as instrumental variables to estimate the causal effects of LDL-c on CHD risk (Li and Ritchie 2021).

10.6.2 TWAS as a Gene-Based Association Approach

TWAS was first developed by Gamazon et al. (2013), which integrates GWAS data with eQTL information to identify transcriptionally regulated genes involved in variation in complex traits. TWAS is characterized by three steps (Figure 10.2), (1) training a predictive model of expression from genotype on a reference panel, such as GTEx, GEUVADIS, DGN, etc., (2) using this model to predict expression for individuals in the GWAS cohort, and (3) associating this predicted expression with the trait (Wainberg et al. 2019). TWAS has two

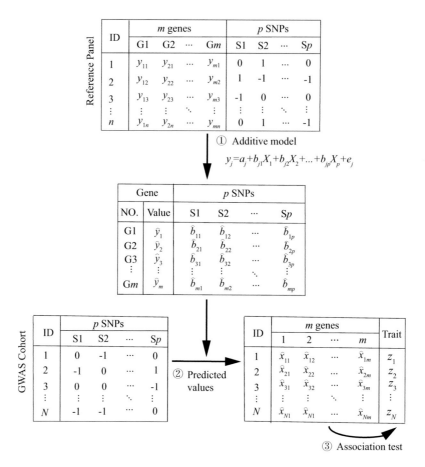

FIGURE 10.2
Data structure for a TWAS analysis. The top panel is the data from the reference transcriptome studies, such as GTEx, including genotype and expression levels, for a sample of n subjects. The total numbers of SNP and genes are m and p, respectively. The middle panel is the additive model of gene expression as a function of SNP genotypes, established with the data from the reference panel. The bottom panel is the predicted expression values of m genes for N subjects from a GWAS cohort based on the subjects' SNP genotypes using the predictive model. The workflow of the TWAS data analysis includes three steps: (1) establish an additive predictive model by regressing the expression values of each gene on SNP data across reference samples, (2) impute the predicted values of gene expression for each subject in the GWAS cohort using the established predictive model, and (3) undertake the (casual) association analysis of the imputed gene expression profiles and trait or disease outcome.

significant advantages: first, it is less relied on GWAS discoveries. Unless a large sample size is used, however, a GWAS can hardly detect small-effect variants (McCarthy et al. 2008; Manolio et al. 2009); second, it mitigates a burden due to multiple comparisons by performing gene-level tests in comparison with variant-based analyses.

Below is a statistical procedure for undertaking TWAS including predicting gene expression levels for individuals based on polygenic risk scores and association analysis of predicted genes and traits. Consider a data structure illustrated in Figure 10.2. The reference panel comes from the reference transcriptome studies (including genotype and expression levels). The reference panel includes n subjects sampled, m genes profiled, and p SNPs genotyped. It is possible that the m genes are measured from multiple tissues. We formulate an additive regression model of gene j ($j=1, ..., m$) on all SNPs across samples, expressed as

$$y_j = a_j + b_{j1}X_1 + b_{j2}X_2 + ... + b_{jp}X_p + e_j \tag{10.9}$$

where y_j is the expression level of gene j (dependent variable ort response), a_j is the intercept, $(b_{j1}, b_{j2}, ..., b_{jp})$ are the regression (effect) coefficients of p SNPs (independent variables or predictors), respectively, $(X_1, X_2, ..., X_p)$ are the genotype design vector of p SNPs, and e_j is the residual error.

Equation (10.9) is a predictive model involving a full set of SNPs, presenting a curse of dimensionality ($p \gg n$) issue. Also, the aggregation of SNP effects across the genome is complicated by the linkage disequilibria among SNPs. As a result, a joint analysis of all SNPs is needed, implemented with the shrinkage of the effect estimates via standard or tailored statistical techniques, such as LASSO or ridge regression (Mak et al. 2017), or Bayesian approaches that perform shrinkage via prior distribution specification (Ge et al. 2019). Different degrees of shrinkage can be achieved; some force most effect estimates to zero or close to zero, some mostly shrink small effects, while others shrink the largest effects (Choi et al. 2020). The other category of computational algorithms for solving equation (10.9) is the best linear unbiased prediction method (Speed and Balding 2014).

The predictive model means that the expression value of any gene can be predicted based on SNP information. Thus, the predictive model built from the reference data (Figure 10.2) can be used to estimate the expression values of each gene in the GWAS cohort. Because each subject carries a genotype at each SNP that has been genotyped in the reference panel, we can estimate polygenic risk scores for individual subjects using the predictive model (Figure 10.2), expressed as

$$\hat{y}_{ij} = \hat{a}_j + \hat{b}_{j1}X_{i1} + \hat{b}_{j2}X_{i2} + ... + \hat{b}_{jp}X_{ip} \tag{10.10}$$

where the hats denote the estimated values from equation (10.9).

Next, with the estimated gene expression values as independent variables and complex traits or diseases as dependent variables, we formulate a linear regression model to estimate the effect of each gene on trait or disease outcomes. Significant genes can explain the molecular mechanisms underlying genotype-phenotype relationship.

10.6.3 A Network Consideration

The predictive model of equation (10.9) is an additive model that assumes the linear combination of the effects of all SNPs. However, as evidenced in a wide body of literature, genetic interactions that occur in a complicated manner are one important determinant of the genetic architecture underlying complex traits and drug response. There is a sore need to take into account SNP-SNP interactions in the predictive model. This issue can be overcome by integrating functional graph theory.

Functional mapping: For a reference panel like GTEx involving n subjects, transcriptional profiles of m genes are measured across multiple tissues (say T) to study the relationship between genetic variation and gene expression in the cell context (GTEx Consortium 2020). Let $y_{ij}(t)$ denote the expression level of gene j ($j=1, ..., m$) in tissue t ($t=1, ..., T$) from subject i ($i=1, ..., n$). We define $E_{it} = \sum_{j=1}^{m} y_{ij}(t)$ as the expression index (EI) of tissue t from subject i. The expression level of individual genes allometrically scales with the EI across tissues, which obeys the power law, mathematically expressed as

$$y_{ij}(E_{it}) = \alpha_{ij} E_{it}^{\beta_{ij}} \tag{10.11}$$

where $y_{ij}(E_{it})$ is the same as $y_{ij}(t)$ and α_{ij} and β_{ij} are the coefficients of the power equation. The GTEx study has genotype data at p SNPs for n subjects. We integrate the power equation into functional mapping to estimate EI-varying expression values of each genotype at individual SNPs, from which the EI-varying additive and dominant expression values of gene j at an SNP s ($s=1, ..., p$), denoted as $a_{js}(E_t)$ and $d_{js}(E_t)$, are estimated. Note that E_t is a generalized, continuous EI.

Bivariate functional clustering: There are p SNPs, thus with p sets of ($a_j(t)$, $d_j(t)$). We implement bivariate functional clustering to classify p SNPs into distinct modules based on their similarity of EI-varying additive and dominant change pattern. If the number of SNPs in a module does not reduce to a level that meets Dunbar's law (Dunbar 1992), we further classify this module into its distinct submodules and, if needed, classify a submodule into its distinct sub-submodules. This process repeats until the number of SNPs within a unit reaches Durbar's number. With this number, we can properly identify and estimate SNP-SNP interactions (Wu and Jiang 2021).

Functional graph theory: Consider a community with the number of SNPs being consistent to Durbar's number. In this community, it is unlikely that all SNPs have complete interconnections to each other. We implement variable selection to choose a small set of the most significant SNPs (say d_s) with which each SNP (s) is linked. Wu and Jiang (2021) integrated evolutionary game theory and predator-prey theory to develop functional graph theory for interaction network modeling. This theory can be used to characterize how each SNP interacts with other SNPs through additive and dominant effects to mediate the expression of a gene. Functional graph theory is formulated by a system of quasi-dynamic ordinary differential equations (qdODEs), expressed as

$$
\left\{
\begin{aligned}
\dot{a}_{js}(E_t) &= Q_{ajs}\left(a_{js}(E_t);\Phi_{ajs}\right) \\
&+ \sum_{s'=1}^{d_s} Q_{aajs'}\left(a_{js'}(E_t);\Phi_{aajs'}\right) + \sum_{s'=1}^{d_s} Q_{adjs'}\left(d_{js'}(E_t);\Phi_{adjs'}\right) \\
\dot{d}_{js}(E_t) &= Q_{djs}\left(d_{js}(E_t);\Phi_{djs}\right) \\
&+ \sum_{s'=1}^{d_s} Q_{dajs'}\left(a_{js'}(E_t);\Phi_{dajs'}\right) + \sum_{s'=1}^{d_s} Q_{ddjs'}\left(d_{js'}(E_t);\Phi_{ddjs'}\right)
\end{aligned}
\right.
\tag{10.12}
$$

where the additive effect of gene j at SNP s is decomposed into this SNP's independent value due to its intrinsic capacity $Q_{ajs}\left(a_{js}(E_t);\Phi_{ajs}\right)$, its dependent values $Q_{aajs'}\left(a_{js'}(E_t);\Phi_{aajs'}\right)$ due to its additive×additive epistasis with SNP s', and its dependent values $Q_{adjs'}\left(d_{js'}(E_t);\Phi_{adjs'}\right)$ due to its additive×dominant epistasis with SNP s'; and the dominant effect of gene j at SNP s is decomposed into this SNP's independent value due to its intrinsic capacity $Q_{djs}\left(d_{js}(E_t);\Phi_{djs}\right)$, its dependent values $Q_{dajs'}\left(a_{js'}(E_t);\Phi_{dajs'}\right)$ due to its dominant×additive epistasis with SNP s', and its dependent values $Q_{ddjs'}\left(d_{js'}(E_t);\Phi_{ddjs'}\right)$ due to its dominant×dominant epistasis with SNP s'. We implement a nonparametric Legendre Orthogonal Polynomial (LOP) approach to smoothen EI-varying independent and dependent values, specified by qdODE parameters Φ_{ajs} and Φ_{djs} and $\Phi_{aajs'}$, $\Phi_{adjs'}$, $\Phi_{dajs'}$ and $\Phi_{ddjs'}$.

We implement the fourth-order Runge-Kutta algorithm to solve the qdODEs in equation (10.12). After the qdODE parameters are estimated, we plug them into the qdODEs to estimate the additive and dominant effects of each SNP in gene j by taking the integrals of the ODEs. These estimated values contain the independent effect of an SNP and its epistatic interaction effects with all other possible SNPs, which can be used as a predictive effect value of a subject at the same SNP in the GWAS cohort.

Association tests: Under the additive assumption, the aggregated genetic effect value of all SNPs in the expression of a gene for each subject from the GWAS cohort is the sum of additive or dominant effects at each SNP. These values represent EI-varying expression levels of m genes for N subjects. Association analysis of these values with trait or disease outcomes measured in the GWAS cohort can characterize the molecular mechanisms behind the trait or disease formation.

In modern biology and biomedicine, much effort has been devoted to integrate data from "omics" disciplines, i.e., transcriptomics, epigenomics,

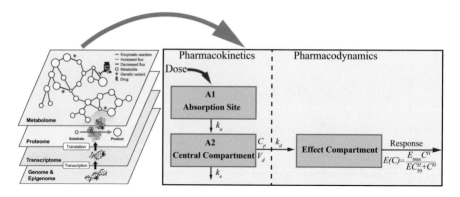

FIGURE 10.3

Pharmacosystems biology of body-drug interactions. When a drug is administered to the body, it produces PK and PD interactions with the body (illustrated on the right). This interactive process stimulates the activity of genetic (and epigenetic) variants (denoted by stars) that propagate their information through several intermediate molecular layers (e.g., transcriptome and proteome) to guide the metabolic interaction network composed of metabolites (nodes) connected by enzymatic reactions (edges). (Adapted from Auwerx et al. 2022.)

proteomics, and metabolomics, into the genomic context (Figure 10.3). Wu (2021) proposed a tridimensional model for flowing and propagating genetic information into the end-point phenotype space through multilayer, multiplex, multiscale, and multifunctional networks across gene, protein, metabolic, and microbiome spaces. By moving beyond pharmacogenomics to what might be called "pharmaco-omics," this model may provide a computational tool to study pharmacosystems biology, further gaining unique insight into the pharmacogenomic architecture of drug response and thus helping to accelerate an attempt to optimize and individualize drug therapy.

10.7 Concluding Remarks

The application of genomics to pharmacological variation leads to pharmacogenomics. As an ever-growing discipline, pharmacogenomics strikes to use genomic – and other "omic" information – to help inform, design, and deliver optimal drug therapy for specific individuals, which has become the cornerstone of precision medicine. The importance and significance of pharmacogenomics result from its capacity to help maximize drug efficacy and minimize the occurrence of adverse drug reactions. The demonstration of this capacity critically relies on how useful genetic information can be modeled, excavated, and extracted from various data at different levels streaming from high-throughput experiments and biobanks. For this reason, the progress of pharmacogenomic research has occurred in parallel with the striking advances that have occurred in methodological and computational development for data modeling and analysis during the past decades.

Although many statistical methods for pharmacogenomic GWAS have been developed to map pharmacogenes, their capacity is limited to identify individual genes associated with end-point drug response phenotypes, without consideration of biochemical processes and principles behind drug-body interactions. Wu and Lin (2008) summarized and outlined a set of computational models for pharmacogenetic and pharmacogenomic mapping. The properties of these models lie in their seamless integration with PK and PD processes that capture how a drug is absorbed, distributed, metabolized, and excreted throughout the body and how the drug targets molecular receptors and enzymes for cellular function. Although Wu and Lin's functional mapping models are advantageous in terms of revealing the molecular mechanisms of drug-body interactions, their philosophical theme was still based on a reductionist thinking, assuming that drug response is controlled by individual genes and proteins.

The past more than one decade has witnessed the enormous paradigm shift of genomic research from a more conventional reductionist thinking to a holistic, systems-oriented consideration (Ozdemir et al. 2018; Wu 2021). All pharmacological mechanisms are far more complex than previously appreciated a decade ago (Hendrickx et al. 2020). Thus, molecular reductionist views of highly complex therapeutic drug efficacy are largely oversimplifications. A new omnigenic theory has emerged to explain the genetic architecture of complex diseases from a complete set of genes the organism may carry (Boyle et al. 2017). Ample evidence shows that all these genes do not only act individually but also interact with each other to form an intricated but well-orchestrated interaction network. More recently, a new theory – functional graph theory – combines Wu and Lin's previous functional mapping models and evolutionary game theory through predator-prey theory to infer and interrogate omnigenic interactome networks. In the preceding chapters, we describe and assess the application of functional graph theory to pharmacogenomically based precision medicine.

In this chapter, we outline and discuss several strategies and methods by which functional graph theory can be leveraged to make more substantial contributions to the mechanistic understanding go pharmacogenomic architecture. With the advent of advanced technologies that produce large volumes of high-dimensionality data streams from transcriptomic, proteomic, metabolomics, or epigenomic pipelines, there is an imperative need to develop effective tools for analyzing linking and these highly invaluable high-dimensionality across different spaces data and extract more nuanced, intuitive, and useful information from them. Network modeling that aims at dissecting complex biological systems (Wu 2021) is at the core of systems pharmacology to reveal how perturbations of genetic variants propagate through the metabolic network into high-order phenotypes of drug efficacy

(Figure 10.3). Information flux through multilayer, multispacer, multiplex, and multifunctional networks provide molecular pharmacologists and other healthcare team members with a blueprint to make more reasonable and more highly individualized therapeutic decisions with effectively engineered efficacy profiles.

Bibliography

Abrams PA (2000) The evolution of predator-prey interactions: Theory and evidence. *Annu Rev Ecol Syst* 31(1): 79–105.

Agoram BM, Martin SW, van der Graaf PH (2007) The role of mechanism-based pharmacokinetic-pharmacodynamic (PK-PD) modelling in translational research of biologics. *Drug Discov Today* 12: 1018–1024.

Ahn K, Luo JT, Berg A, Keefe D, Wu RL (2010) Functional mapping of drug response with pharmacodynamic-pharmcokinetic principles. *Trends Pharmacol Sci* 31: 306–311.

Akinola AT, Adigun MO, Mudali P (2019) Network stability based on the amount of available bandwidth in a software defined networking. *IEEE Africon* 2019: 1–6.

Alaoui-Jamali MA, Dupré I, Qiang H (2004) Prediction of drug sensitivity and drug resistance in cancer by transcriptional and proteomic profiling. *Drug Resist Updat* 7(4–5): 245–255.

Alarcon-Barrera JC, Kostidis S, Ondo-Mendez A, Giera M (2022) Recent advances in metabolomics analysis for early drug development. *Drug Discov Today* 27: 1763–1773.

Alcalá-Corona SA, Sandoval-Motta S, Espinal-Enríquez J, Hernández-Lemus E (2021) Modularity in biological networks. *Front Genet* 12: 701331.

Alexander JM (2021) Evolutionary game theory. In: Edward NZ (ed) *The Stanford Encyclopedia of Philosophy*. http://www.plato.stanford.edu/archives/fall2009/entries/game-evolutionary/.

Allesina S, Tang S (2012) Stability criteria for complex ecosystems. *Nature* 483: 205–208.

Andersson R, Gebhard C, Miguel-Escalada I, Hoof I, Bornholdt J, Boyd M, Chen Y, Zhao X, Schmidl C, Suzuki T, et al. (2014) An atlas of active enhancers across human cell types and tissues. *Nature* 507: 455–461.

Archetti M, Ferraro DA, Christofori G (2015) Heterogeneity for IGF-II production maintained by public goods dynamics in neuroendocrine pancreatic cancer. *Proc Natl Acad Sci U S A* 112: 1833–1838.

Armingol E, Officer A, Harismendy O, Lewis NE (2021) Deciphering cell-cell interactions and communication from gene expression. *Nat Rev Genet* 22(2): 71–88.

Arnol D, Schapiro D, Bodenmiller B, Saez-Rodriguez J, Stegle O (2019) Modeling cell-cell interactions from spatial molecular data with spatial variance component analysis. *Cell Rep* 29(1): 202–211.e6.

Asadzadeh Z, Safarzadeh E, Safaei S, Baradaran A, Mohammadi A, Hajiasgharzadeh K, Derakhshani A, Argentiero A, Silvestris N, Baradaran B (2020) Current approaches for combination therapy of cancer: The role of immunogenic cell death. *Cancers (Basel)* 12(4): e1047.

Auwerx C, Sadler MC, Reymond A, Kutalik Z (2022) From pharmacogenetics to pharmaco-omics: Milestones and future directions. *HGG Adv* 3(2): 100100.

Babb de Villiers C, Kroese M, Moorthie S (2020) Understanding polygenic models, their development and the potential application of polygenic scores in healthcare. *J Med Genet* 57(11): 725–732.

Bailey KR, Cheng C (2010) Genome-wide association studies in pharmacogenetics research debate. *Pharmacogenomics* 11(3): 305–308.

Bain KT (2019) Precision medication: An illustrative case series guiding the clinical application of multi-drug interactions and pharmacogenomics. *Clin Case Rep* 8(2): 305–312.

Baker RL, Leong WF, Brock MT, Markelz RJ, Covington MF, Devisetty UK, Edwards CE, Maloof J, Welch S, Weinig C (2015) Modeling development and quantitative trait mapping reveal independent genetic modules for leaf size and shape. *New Phytol* 208(1): 257–268.

Ballesta A, Innominato PF, Dallmann R, Rand DA, Lévi FA (2017) Systems chrono-therapeutics. *Pharmacol Rev* 69: 161–199.

Banerjee BD, Kumar R, Thamineni KL, Shah H, Thakur GK, Sharma T (2019) Effect of environmental exposure and pharmacogenomics on drug metabolism. *Curr Drug Metab* 20(14): 1103–1113.

Bansal M, Belcastro V, Ambesi-Impiombato A, di Bernardo D (2007) How to infer gene networks from expression profiles. *Mol Syst Biol* 3: 78.

Bansal M, Yang J, Karan C, Menden MP, Costello JC, Tang H, Xiao G, Li Y, Allen J, Zhong R, et al. (2014) A community computational challenge to predict the activity of pairs of compounds. *Nat Biotechnol* 32(12): 1213–1222.

Barbolosi D, Ciccolini J, Lacarelle B, Barlési F, André N (2016) Computational oncology–mathematical modelling of drug regimens for precision medicine. *Nat Rev Clin Oncol* 13: 242–254.

Barrett JH (2019) Genome-wide association studies of therapeutic response: Addressing the complexities. *Pharmacogenomics* 20(4): 213–216.

Barton SC, Surani MA, Norris ML (1984) Role of paternal and maternal genomes in mouse development. *Nature* 311(5984): 374–376.

Basanta D, Anderson AR (2013) Exploiting ecological principles to better understand cancer progression and treatment. *Interface Focus* 3: 20130020.

Basanta D, Scott JG, Fishman MN, Ayala G, Hayward SW, Anderson AR (2011) Investigating prostate cancer tumour-stroma interactions – Clinical and biological insights from an evolutionary game. *Br J Cancer* 106: 174–181.

Bateson W (1907) The progress of genetics since the rediscovery of Mendel's paper. *Progressus Rei Botanicae* 1: 368–382.

Bayat-Mokhtari R, Homayouni TS, Baluch N, Morgatskaya E, Kumar S, Das B, Yeger H (2017) Combination therapy in combating cancer. *Oncotarget* 8(23): 38022–38043.

Baye TM, Wilke RA (2010) Mapping genes that predict treatment outcome in admixed populations. *Pharmacogenomics J* 10: 465–477.

Ben-David U, Siranosian B, Ha G, Tang H, Oren Y, Hinohara K, Strathdee CA, Dempster J, Lyons NJ, Burns R, et al. (2018) Genetic and transcriptional evolution alters cancer cell line drug response. *Nature* 560(7718): 325–330.

Berryman AA (1992) The origins and evolution of predator-prey theory. *Ecology* 73: 1530–1535.

Bhullar BA, Marugán-Lobón J, Racimo F, Bever GS, Rowe TB, Norell MA, Abzhanov A (2012) Birds have paedomorphic dinosaur skulls. *Nature* 487(7406): 223–226.

Biswas A, Haldane A, Arnold E, Levy RM (2019) Epistasis and entrenchment of drug resistance in HIV-1 subtype B. *eLife* 8: e50524.

Boger E, Wigström O (2018) A partial differential equation approach to inhalation physiologically based pharmacokinetic modeling. *CPT Pharmacometrics Syst Pharmacol* 7(10): 638–646.

Bomze IM, Pötscher BM (1989) *Game Theoretical Foundations of Evolutionary Stability.* Springer, Berlin.

Bonnans C, Chou J, Werb Z (2014) Remodelling the extracellular matrix in development and disease. *Nat Rev Mol Cell Biol* 15: 786–801.

Boyle EA, Li YI, Pritchard JK (2017) An expanded view of complex traits: From polygenic to omnigenic. *Cell* 169(7): 1177–1186.

Broekema RV, Bakker OB, Jonkers IH (2020) A practical view of fine-mapping and gene prioritization in the post-genome-wide association era. *Open Biol* 10: 190221.

Browaeys R, Saelens W, Saeys Y (2020) NicheNet: Modeling intercellular communication by linking ligands to target genes. *Nat Methods* 17(2): 159–162.

Brown JH, Gillooly JF, Allen AP, Savage VM, West GB (2004) Toward a metabolic theory of ecology. *Ecology* 85(7): 1771–1789.

Brückner DB, Arlt N, Fink A, Ronceray P, Rädler JO, Broedersz CP (2021) Learning the dynamics of cell-cell interactions in confined cell migration. *Proc Natl Acad Sci U S A* 118(7): e2016602118.

Brunton LL, Lazo JS, Parker KL (eds) (2006) *The Pharmacologic Basis of Therapeutics,* 11th edition. McGraw Hill, New York.

Busby BP, Niktab E, Roberts CA, Sheridan JP, Coorey NV, Senanayake DS, Connor LM, Munkacsi AB, Atkinson PH (2019) Genetic interaction networks mediate individual statin drug response in saccharomyces cerevisiae. *NPJ Syst Biol Appl* 5: 35.

Bush WS, Crosslin DR, Owusu-Obeng A, Wallace J, Almoguera B, Basford MA, Bielinski SJ, Carrell DS, Connolly JJ, Crawford D, et al. (2016) Genetic variation among 82 pharmacogenes: The PGRNseq data from the eMERGE network. *Clin Pharmacol Ther* 100(2): 160–169.

Busiello DM, Suweis S, Hidalgo J, Maritan A (2017) Explorability and the origin of network sparsity in living systems. *Sci Rep* 7: 12323.

Button-Simons KA, Kumar S, Carmago N, Haile MT, Jett C, Checkley LA, Kennedy SY, Pinapati RS, Shoue DA, McDew-White M, et al. (2021) The power and promise of genetic mapping from Plasmodium falciparum crosses utilizing human liver-chimeric mice. *Commun Biol* 4: 734.

Cabello-Aguilar S, Alame M, Kon-Sun-Tack F, Fau C, Lacroix M, Colinge J (2020) SingleCellSignalR: Inference of intercellular networks from single-cell transcriptomics. *Nucleic Acids Res* 48: e55.

Callebaut W, Rasskin-Gutman D (eds) (2005) *Modularity: Understanding the Development and Evolution of Natural Complex Systems.* MIT Press, Cambridge, MA.

Cang Z, Nie Q (2020) Inferring spatial and signaling relationships between cells from single cell transcriptomic data. *Nat Commun* 11: 2084.

Cano-Gamez E, Trynka G (2020) From GWAS to function: Using functional genomics to identify the mechanisms underlying complex diseases. *Front Genet* 11: 424.

Cao JG, Wang LL, Huang ZW, Gai JY, Wu RL (2017) Functional mapping of multiple dynamic traits. *J Agri Biol Environ Stat* 22: 60–75.

Carlsten C, Brauer M, Brinkman F, Brook J, Daley D, McNagny K, Pui M, Royce D, Takaro T, Denburg J (2014) Genes, the environment and personalized medicine: We need to harness both environmental and genetic data to maximize personal and population health. *EMBO reports* 15: 76–79.

Caspar SM, Schneider T, Stoll P, Meienberg J, Matyas G (2021) Potential of whole-genome sequencing-based pharmacogenetic profiling. *Pharmacogenomics* 22(3): 177–190.

Cattanach BM, Kirk M (1985) Differential activity of maternally and paternally derived chromosome regions in mice. *Nature* 315(6019): 496–498.

Cecil C, Walton E, Smith R, et al. (2016) DNA methylation and substance-use risk: A prospective, genome-wide study spanning gestation to adolescence. *Transl Psychiatry* 6: e976.

Chambliss AB, Chan DW (2016) Precision medicine: From pharmacogenomics to pharmacoproteomics. *Clin Proteom* 13: 25.

Chang AY, Hsu E, Patel J, Li YQ, Zhang M, Iguchi H, Rogoff HA (2019) Evaluation of tumor cell-tumor microenvironment component interactions as potential predictors of patient response to napabucasin. *Mol Cancer Res* 17(7): 1429–1434.

Chauvet C, Crespo K, Ménard A, Roy J, Deng AY (2013) Modularization and epistatic hierarchy determine homeostatic actions of multiple blood pressure quantitative trait loci. *Hum Mol Genet* 22: 4451–4459.

Chen B, Garmire L, Calvisi DF, Chua MS, Kelley RK, Chen X (2020) Harnessing big 'omics' data and AI for drug discovery in hepatocellular carcinoma. *Nat Rev Gastroenterol Hepatol* 17: 238–251.

Chen C, Jiang L, Fu G, Wang M, Wang Y, Shen B, Liu Z, Wang Z, Hou W, Berceli SA, et al. (2019) An omnidirectional visualization model of personalized gene regulatory networks. *NPJ Syst Biol Appl* 5: 38.

Chen C, Shen B, Ma T, Wang M, Wu RL (2022) A statistical framework for recovering pseudo-dynamic networks from static data. *Bioinformatics* 26: btac038.

Chen CX, Jiang LB, Shen BY, Wang M, Griffin CH, Chinchilli V, Wu RL (2021) A computational atlas of tissue-specific regulatory networks. *Front Syst Biol* 1: 714161.

Chen S, Shojaie A, Witten DM (2017) Network reconstruction from high-dimensional ordinary differential equations. *J Am Stat Assoc* 112(520): 1697–1707.

Chen T, He HL, Church GM (1999) Modeling gene expression with differential equations. *Pac Symp Biocomput* 29–40.

Cheng F, Desai RJ, Handy DE, Wang R, Schneeweiss S, Barabási A-L (2018) Network-based approach to prediction and population-based validation of in silico drug repurposing. *Nat Commun* 9(1): 2691.

Cheng F, Lu W, Liu C, Fang J, Hou Y, Handy DE (2019) A genome-wide positioning systems network algorithm for in silico drug repurposing. *Nat Commun* 10(1): 3476.

Cheverud JM, Routman EJ (1995) Epistasis and its contribution to genetic variance components. *Genetics* 139(3): 1455–1461.

Chhibber A, Kroetz DL, Tantisira KG, McGeachie M, Cheng C, Plenge R, Stahl E, Sadee W, Ritchie MD, Pendergrass SA (2014) Genomic architecture of pharmacological efficacy and adverse events. *Pharmacogenomics* 15(16): 2025–2048.

Choi H, Sheng J, Gao D, Li F, Durrans A, Ryu S, Lee SB, Narula N, Rafii S, Elemento O, Altorki NK, Wong ST, Mittal V (2015) Transcriptome analysis of individual stromal cell populations identifies stroma-tumor crosstalk in mouse lung cancer model. *Cell Rep* 10: 1187–1201.

Choi SW, Mak TS, O'Reilly PF (2020) Tutorial: A guide to performing polygenic risk score analyses. *Nat Protoc* 15(9): 2759–2772.

Choy E, Yelensky R, Bonakdar S, Plenge RM, Saxena R, De Jager PL, Shaw SY, Wolfish CS, Slavik JM, Cotsapas C (2008) Genetic analysis of human traits in vitro: Drug response and gene expression in lymphoblastoid cell lines. *PLoS Genet* 4(11): e1000287.

Ciccolini J, Barbolosi D, André N, Benzekry S, Barlesi F (2019) Combinatorial immunotherapy strategies: Most gods throw dice, but fate plays chess. *Ann Oncol* 30(11): 1690–1691.

Cillo AR, Kürten CHL, Tabib T, Qi Z, Onkar S, Wang T, Liu A, Duvvuri U, Kim S, Soose RJ, et al. (2020) Immune landscape of viral- and carcinogen-driven head and neck cancer. *Immunity.* 52(1): 183–199.e9.

Clairambault J (2007) Modeling oxaliplatin drug delivery to circadian rhythms in drug metabolism and host tolerance. *Adv Drug Deliv Rev* 59(9–10): 1054–1068.

Clayton D, Cuzick J (1985) Multivariate generalizations of the proportional hazards model. *J Roy Stat Soc Ser A (General)* 48: 82–117.

Clayton TA, Lindon JC, Cloarec O, Antti H, Charuel C, Hanton G, Provost JP, Le Net JL, Baker D, Walley RJ, Everett JR, Nicholson JK (2006) Pharmaco-metabonomic phenotyping and personalized drug treatment. *Nature* 440: 1073–1077.

Clune J, Mouret JB, Lipson H (2013) The evolutionary origins of modularity. *Proc Biol Sci* 280(1755): 20122863.

Coelho MTP, Diniz-Filho JA, Rangel TR (2019) A parsimonious view of the parsimony principle in ecology and evolution. *Ecography* 42: 968–976.

Cokol M, Kuru N, Bicak E, Larkins-Ford J, Aldridge BB (2017) Efficient measurement and factorization of high-order drug interactions in mycobacterium tuberculosis. *Sci Adv* 3(10): e1701881.

Collins FS, Varmus H (2015) A new initiative on precision medicine. *N Engl J Med* 372: 793–795.

Contreras MG, Fagiolo G (2014) Propagation of economic shocks in input-output networks: A cross-country analysis. *Phys Rev E Stat Nonlin Soft Matter Phys* 90(6): 062812.

Cooper GM, Johnson JA, Langaee TY, Feng H, Stanaway IB, Schwarz UI, Ritchie MD, Stein CM, Roden DM, Smith JD, et al. (2008) A genome-wide scan for common genetic variants with a large influence on warfarin maintenance dose. *Blood* 112: 1022–1027.

Coosemans A, Vankerckhoven A, Baert T, Boon L, Ruts H, Riva M, Blagden S, Delforge M, Concin N, Mirza MR, Ledermann JA, et al. (2019) Combining conventional therapy with immunotherapy: A risky business? *Eur J Cancer* 113: 41–44.

Corona G, Rizzolio F, Giordano A, Toffoli G (2012) Pharmaco-metabolomics: An emerging "omics" tool for the personalization of anticancer treatments and identification of new valuable therapeutic targets. *J Cell Physiol* 227(7): 2827–2831.

Corrie K, Hardman JG (2011) Mechanisms of drug interactions: Pharmacodynamics and pharmacokinetics. *Anaesth Intensive Care Med* 15: 305–308.

Cortez M, Ellner SP (2010) Understanding rapid evolution in predator-prey interactions using the theory of fast-slow dynamical systems. *Am Nat* 176(5): e109–e127.

Costanzo M, Kuzmin E, van Leeuwen J, Mair B, Moffat J, Boone C, Andrews B (2019) Global genetic networks and the genotype-to-phenotype relationship. *Cell* 177(1): 85–100.

Costanzo M, VanderSluis B, Koch EN, Baryshnikova A, Pons C, Tan G, Wang W, Usaj M, Hanchard J, Lee SD, et al. (2016) A global genetic interaction network maps a wiring diagram of cellular function. *Science* 353(6306): aaf1420.

Cressman R, Tao Y (2014) The replicator equation and other game dynamics. *Proc Natl Acad Sci U S A* 111: 10810–10817.

Crouch DJM, Bodmer WF (2020) Polygenic inheritance, GWAS, polygenic risk scores, and the search for functional variants. *Proc Natl Acad Sci U S A* 117(32): 18924–18933.

Custódio CA, Mano JF (2016) Cell surface engineering to control cellular interactions. *Chem Nano Mat* 2(5): 376–384.

D'Argenio D, Park K (1997) Uncertain pharmacokinetic/pharmacodynamic systems: Design, estimation and control. *Control Eng Pract* 5: 1707–1716.

da Silva A, Bowden M, Zhang S, Masugi Y, Thorner AR, Herbert ZT, Zhou CW, Brais L, Chan JA, Hodi FS, et al. (2018) Characterization of the neuroendocrine tumor immune microenvironment. *Pancreas* 47: 1123–1129.

da Silva BS, Leffa DT, Beys-da-Silva WO, Torres ILS, Rovaris DL, Victor MM, Dallmann R, Okyar A, Lévi F (2016) Dosing-time makes the poison: Circadian regulation and pharmacotherapy. *Trends Mol Med* 22: 430–445.

Daly AK (2009) Pharmacogenomics of anticoagulants: Steps toward personal dosage. *Genome Med* 1: 10.

Daly AK (2010) Genome-wide association studies in pharmacogenomics. *Nat Rev Genet* 11(4): 241–246.

Daly AK, Donaldson PT, Bhatnagar P, Shen Y, Pe'er I, Floratos A, Daly MJ, Goldstein DB, John S, Nelson MR, et al. (2009) HLA-B*5701 genotype is a major determinant of drug-induced liver injury due to flucloxacillin. *Nat Genet* 41: 816–819.

Daniels MJ, Hogan JW (2008) *Missing Data in Longitudinal Studies: Strategies for Bayesian Modeling and Sensitivity Analysis.* Chapman & Hall/CRC, London, pp. 188–189.

Darne B, Girerd X, Safar M, Cambien F, Guize L (1989) Pulsatile versus steady component of blood pressure: A cross-sectional analysis and a prospective analysis on cardiovascular mortality. *Hypertension* 13: 392400.

Dart AM (2017) Should pulse pressure influence prescribing? *Aust Prescr* 40: 26–29.

Darwiche A (2009) *Modeling and Reasoning with Bayesian Networks.* Cambridge University Press, Cambridge.

Das K, Li R, Huang Z, Gai J, Wu RL (2012) A Bayesian framework for functional mapping through joint modeling of longitudinal and time-to-event data. *Int J Plant Genomics* 2012: 680634.

Davidson S (2000) Research suggests importance of haplotypes over SNPs. *Nat Biotechnol* 18: 1134–1135.

Davis JD, Bansal A, Hassman D, Akinlade B, Li M, Li ZY, Swanson B, Hamilton JD, DiCioccio AT (2018) Evaluation of potential disease-mediated drug–drug interaction in patients with moderate-to-severe atopic dermatitis receiving dupilumab. *Clin Pharmacol Ther* 104(6): 1146–1154.

de Lartigue J (2018) Tumor heterogeneity: A central foe in the war on cancer. *JCSO* 16: e167–e174.

de Looff M, de Jong S, Kruyt FAE (2019) Multiple interactions between cancer cells and the Tumor microenvironment modulate TRAIL signaling: Implications for TRAIL receptor targeted therapy. *Front Immunol* 10: 1530.

De Luca M, Aiuti A, Cossu G, Parmar M, Pellegrini G, Robey PG (2019) Advances in stem cell research and therapeutic development. *Nat Cell Biol* 21(7): 801–811.

de Vries Schultink AH, Zwart W, Linn SC, Beijnen JH, Huitema AD (2015) Effects of pharmacogenetics on the pharmacokinetics and pharmacodynamics of tamoxifen. *Clin Pharmacokinet* 54: 797–810.

DeGruttola V, Tu XM (1994) Modelling progression of CD4-lymphocyte count and its relationship to survival time. *Biometrics* 50(4): 1003–1014.

Delgado FM, Gómez-Vela F (2019) Computational methods for gene regulatory networks reconstruction and analysis: A review. *Artif Intell Med* 95: 133–145.

Demichelis S, Ritzberger K (2003) From evolutionary to strategic stability. *J Econ Theory* 113(1): 51–75.

Dempster AP, Laird NM, Rubin DB (1977) Maximum likelihood from incomplete data via the EM algorithm. *J Roy Stat Soc Ser B (Methodological)* 39: 1–38.

Derendorf H, von Richter O, Hermann R, Rostami-Hodjegan A (2019) Drug–drug interactions: Progress over the past decade and looking ahead to the future. *Clin Pharmacol Ther* 105(6): 1289–1291.

Deshaies RJ (2020) Multispecific drugs herald a new era of biopharmaceutical innovation. *Nature* 580: 329–338.

Diggle P, Kenward MG (1994) Informative drop-out in longitudinal data analysis. *Appl Stat* 49–93.

Ditlevsen S, Gaetano AD (2005) Stochastic vs. deterministic uptake of dodecanedioic acid by isolated rat livers. *Bull Math Biol* 67: 547–561.

Ditlevsen S, Yip K, Holstein-Rathlou N (2005) Parameter estimation in a stochastic model of the tubuloglomerular feedback mechanism in a rat nephron. *Math Biosci* 194: 49–69.

Dolgin E (2014) Massive schizophrenia genomics study offers new drug directions. *Nat Rev Drug Discov* 13(9): 641–643.

Domanski MJ, Davis BR, Pfeffer MA, Kastantin M, Mitchell GF (1999) Isolated systolic hypertension: Prognostic information provided by pulse pressure. *Hypertension* 34: 375–380.

Domingo J, Baeza-Centurion P, Lehner B (2019) The causes and consequences of genetic interactions (epistasis). *Annu Rev Genomics Hum Genet* 20: 433–460.

Dong A, Feng L, Yang DC, Wu S, Zhao JS, Wang J, Wu RL (2021) FunGraph: A statistical protocol to reconstruct omnigenic multilayer interactome networks for complex traits. *STAR Protocols* 2: 100985.

Donnet S, Foulley J, Samson A (2010) Bayesian analysis of growth curves using mixed models defined by stochastic differential equations. *Biometrics* 66: 733–741.

Donnet S, Samson A (2013) A review on estimation of stochastic differential equations for pharmacokinetic/pharmacodynamic models. *Adv Drug Deliv Rev* 65(7): 929–939.

Dugger SA, Platt A, Goldstein DB (2018) Drug development in the era of precision medicine. *Nat Rev Drug Discov* 17: 183–196.

Dunbar RIM (1992) Neocortex size as a constraint on group size in primates. *J Hum Evol* 22: 469–493.

Durisová M, Dedík L (2005) New mathematical methods in pharmacokinetic modeling. *Basic Clin Pharmacol Toxicol* 96(5): 335–342.

Dzobo K, Senthebane DA, Thomford NE, Rowe A, Dandara C, Parker MI (2018) Not everyone fits the mold: Intratumor and intertumor heterogeneity and innovative cancer drug design and development. *OMICS* 22(1): 17–34.

Ebert P, Audano PA, Zhu QH, Rodriguez-Martin B, Porubsky D, Bonder MJ, Sulovari A, Ebler J, Zhou WC, Serra Mari R, et al. (2021) Haplotype-resolved diverse human genomes and integrated analysis of structural variation. *Science* 372(6537): eabf7117.

Efremova M, Vento-Tormo M, Teichmann SA, Vento-Tormo R (2020) CellPhoneDB: Inferring cell-cell communication from combined expression of multi-subunit ligand-receptor complexes. *Nat Protoc* 15: 1484–1506.

Ehret GB (2010) Genome-wide association studies: Contribution of genomics to understanding blood pressure and essential hypertension. *Curr Hypertens Rep* 12(1): 17–25.

Eichelbaum M, Ingelman-Sundberg M, Evans WE (2006) Pharmacogenomics and individualized drug therapy. *Annu Rev Med* 57: 119–137.

El-Deiry WS, Taylor B, Neal JW (2017) Tumor evolution, heterogeneity, and therapy for our patients with advanced cancer: How far have we come? *Am Soc Clin Oncol Educ Book* 37: e8–e15.

Elton CS (1958) *Ecology of Invasions by Animals and Plants*. Chapman & Hall/CRC, London.

ENCODE Project Consortium, Moore JE, Purcaro MJ, Pratt HE, Epstein CB, Shoresh N, et al. (2020) Expanded encyclopaedias of DNA elements in the human and mouse genomes. *Nature* 583: 699–710.

Espinosa-Soto C (2018) On the role of sparseness in the evolution of modularity in gene regulatory networks. *PLoS Comput Biol* 14(5): e1006172.

Evans WE, Johnson JA (2001) Pharmacogenomics: The inherited basis for interindividual differences in drug response. *Annu Rev Genomics Hum Genet* 2: 9–39.

Evans WE, McLeod HL (2013) Pharmacogenomics – Drug disposition, drug targets, and side effects. *N Engl J Med* 348(6): 538–549.

Evlin B, Roeder K (1999) Genomic control for association studies. *Biometrics* 55: 997–1004.

Farzan N, Vijverberg SJ, Kabesch M, Sterk PJ, Maitland-van der Zee AH (2018) The use of pharmacogenomics, epigenomics, and transcriptomics to improve childhood asthma management: Where do we stand? *Pediatr Pulmonol* 53(6): 836–845.

Felix MA, Barkoulas M (2015) Pervasive robustness in biological systems. *Nat Rev Genet* 16: 483–496.

Felmlee MA, Morris ME, Mager DE (2012) Mechanism-based pharmacodynamic modeling. *Methods Mol Biol* 929: 583–600.

Feng L, Jiang P, Li CF, Zhao JS, Dong A, Yang DC, Wu RL (2021) Genetic dissection of growth trajectories: From funmap to fungraph. *Forest Res* 1: 19.

Ferrante L, Bompadre S, Leone L, Montanari M (2005) A stochastic formulation of the gompertzian growth model for in vitro bactericidal kinetics: Parameter estimation and extinction probability. *Biom J* 47: 309–318.

Findlay SD, Thagard P (2012) How parts make up wholes. *Front Physiol* 3: 455.

Finlay DB, Duffull SB, Glass M (2020) 100 years of modelling ligand-receptor binding and response: A focus on GPCRs. *Br J Pharmacol* 177(7): 1472–1484.

Fisher RA (1918) The correlation between relatives on the supposition of Mendelian inheritance. *Proc Roy Soc Edinburgh* 52: 399–433.

Fitzmaurice GM, Laird NM (2000) Generalized linear mixture models for handling nonignorable dropouts in longitudinal studies. *Biostatistics* 1(2): 141–156.

Follmann D, Wu M (1995) An approximate generalized linear model with random effects for informative missing data. *Biometrics* 51: 151–168.

Franklin SS, Gustin W IV, Wong ND, Larson MG, Weber MA, Kannel WB, Levy D (1997) Hemodynamic patterns of age-related changes in blood pressure: The framingham heart study. *Circulation* 96: 308–315.

Fu GF, Liu JY, Luo JT, Wang Z, Wang YQ, Wang NT, Wu RL (2013) *Systems mapping for personalized medicine*. In: Vizirianakis I (ed) *Handbook of Personalized Medicine: Advances in Nanotechnology, Drug Delivery and Therapy*. Pan Stanford Publishing, Greece.

Fu GF, Luo J, Berg A, Wang Z, Li JH, Das K, Li R, Wu RL (2010) A dynamic model for functional mapping of biological rhythms. *J Biol Dyn* 4: 1–10.

Fu GF, Wang Z, Li JH, Wu RL (2011) A mathematical framework for functional mapping of complex systems using delay differential equations. *J Theor Biol* 289: 206–216.

Fu LY, Sun LD, Han H, Jiang LB, Zhu S, Ye MX, Tang SZ, Huang MR, Wu RL (2017) How trees allocate carbon for optimal growth: Insight from a game-theoretic model. *Brief Bioinform* 19: 593–602.

Fujikura K, Ingelman-Sundberg M, Lauschke VM (2015) Genetic variation in the human cytochrome P450 supergene family. *Pharmacogenet Genomics* 25(12): 584–594.

Fuselli S (2019) Beyond drugs: The evolution of genes involved in human response to medications. *Proc Biol Sci* 286(1913): 20191716.

Galan-Vasquez E, Perez-Rueda E (2021) A landscape for drug–target interactions based on network analysis. *PLoS ONE* 16(3): e0247018.

Galon J, Bruni D (2020) Tumor immunology and tumor evolution: Intertwined histories. *Immunity* 52(1): 55–81.

Gamazon ER, Wheeler HE, Shah KP, Mozaffari SV, Aquino-Michaels K, Carroll RJ, Eyler AE, Denny JC; GTEx Consortium, Nicolae DL, et al. (2015) A gene-based association method for mapping traits using reference transcriptome data. *Nat Genet* 47: 1091–1098.

Gamfeldt L, Snäll T, Bagchi R, Jonsson M, Gustafsson L, Kjellander P, Ruiz-Jaen MC, Fröberg M, Stendahl J, Philipson CD, et al. (2013) Higher levels of multiple ecosystem services are found in forests with more tree species. *Nat Commun* 4: 1340.

Gan JW (2021) A stochastic differential equation model for systems mapping of complex traits. PhD thesis, Beijing Forestry University, China.

Gardner MR, Ashby WR (1970) Connectance of large dynamic (cybernetic) systems: Critical values for stability. *Nature* 228(5273): 784.

Gardner TS, di Bernardo D, Lorenz D, Collins JJ (2003) Inferring genetic networks and identifying compound mode of action via expression profiling. *Science* 301(5629): 102–105.

Gatenby RA, Gillies RJ (2008) A microenvironmental model of carcinogenesis. *Nat Rev Cancer* 8: 56–61.

Ge D, Fellay J, Thompson AJ, Simon JS, Shianna KV, Urban TJ, Heinzen EL, Qiu P, Bertelsen AH, Muir AJ, et al. (2009) Genetic variation in IL28B predicts hepatitis C treatment-induced viral clearance. *Nature* 461: 399–401.

Ge T, Chen CY, Ni Y, Feng YA, Smoller JW (2019) Polygenic prediction via bayesian regression and continuous shrinkage priors. *Nat Commun* 10: 1–10.

Gesztelyi R, Zsuga J, Kemeny-Beke A, Varga B, Juhasz B, Tosaki A (2012) The hill equation and the origin of quantitative pharmacology. *Arch Hist Exact Sci* 66: 427–438.

Giacomini KM, Yee SW, Mushiroda T, Weinshilboum RM, Ratain MJ, Kubo M (2017) Genome-wide association studies of drug response and toxicity: An opportunity for genome medicine. *Nat Rev Drug Discov* 16: 70.

Giraldo J (2003) Empirical models and hill coefficients. *Trends Pharmacol Sci* 24: 63–65.

Girvan M, Newman ME (2002) Community structure in social and biological networks. *Proc Natl Acad Sci U S A* 99(12): 7821–7826.

Gómez-González S, Paniw M, Blanco-Pastor JL, García-Cervigón AI, Godoy O, Herrera JM, Lara A, Miranda A, Ojeda F, Ochoa-Hueso R (2022) Moving towards the ecological intensification of tree plantations. *Trends Plant Sci* 27(7): 637–645.

Gonzalez-Covarrubias V, Urena-Carrion J, Villegas-Torres B, Cossío-Aranda JE, Gottlieb G (2007) Probabilistic epigenesis. *Dev Sci* 10: 1–11.

Goutelle S, Maurin M, Rougier F, Barbaut X, Bourguignon L, Ducher M, Maire P (2008) The Hill equation: A review of its capabilities in pharmacological modelling. *Fundam Clin Pharmacol* 22(6): 633–648.

Goyal A (2022) How diverse ecosystems remain stable. *Nat Ecol Evol* 6: 667–668. https://doi.org/10.1038/s41559-022-01758-3.

Graham RM, Perez DM, Hwa J, Piascik MT (1996) Alpha 1-adrenergic receptor subtypes: Molecular structure, function, and signaling. *Circ Res* 78: 737–749.

Griffin C, Jiang LB, Wu RL (2020) Analysis of quasi-dynamic ordinary differential equations and the quasi-dynamic replicator. *Physica A: Stat Mech its Appl (Physica A)* 555: 124422.

Grisel JE, Belknap JK, O'Toole LA, Helms ML, Wenger CD, Crabbe JC (1997) Quantitative trait loci affecting methamphetamine responses in BXD recombinant inbred mouse strains. *J Neurosci* 17(2): 745–754.

Gross CG, Rocha-Miranda CE, Bender DB (1972) Visual properties of neurons in inferotemporal cortex of the macaque. *J Neurophysiol*, 35: 96–111.

Gross T, Rudolf L, Levin SA, Dieckmann U (2009) Generalized models reveal stabilizing factors in food webs. *Science* 325(5941): 747–750.

Grzywa TM, Paskal W, Włodarski PK (2017) Intratumor and intertumor heterogeneity in melanoma. *Transl Oncol* 10(6): 956–975.

GTEx Consortium (2020) The GTEx consortium atlas of genetic regulatory effects across human tissues. *Science* 369: 1318–1330.

Guessous I, Gwinn M, Khoury MJ (2009) Genome-wide association studies in pharmacogenomics: Untapped potential for translation. *Genome Med* 1: 46.

Guo W, Ratcliffe SJ, Have TTT (2004) A random pattern-mixture model for longitudinal data with dropouts. *J Am Stat Assoc* 99: 929–937.

Guo YQ, Luo JT, Wang JX, Wu RL (2011) How to compute which genes control drug resistance dynamics. *Drug Discov Today* 16: 339–334.

Haghighi F, Hodge SE (2002) Likelihood formulation of parent-of-origin effects on segregation analysis, including ascertainment. *Am J Hum Genet* 70(1): 142–156.

Han SW, Chen G, Cheon MS, Zhong H (2016) Estimation of directed acyclic graphs through two-stage adaptive lasso for gene network inference. *J Am Stat Assoc* 111(515): 1004–1019.

Hanna J, Hossain GS, Kocerha J (2019) The potential for microRNA therapeutics and clinical research. *Front Genet* 10: 478.

Hanson C, Cairns J, Wang L, Sinha S (2016) Computational discovery of transcription factors associated with drug response. *Pharmacogenomics J* 16: 573–582.

Harré MS, Prokopenko M (2016) The social brain: Scale-invariant layering of Erdős-Rényi networks in small-scale human societies. *J Roy Soc Interface* 13(118): 20160044.

Hayford CE, Tyson DR, Robbins CJ 3rd, Frick PL, Quaranta V, Harris LA (2021) An in vitro model of tumor heterogeneity resolves genetic, epigenetic, and stochastic sources of cell state variability. *PLoS Biol* 19(6): e3000797.

Heeren A, McNally RJ (2016) An integrative network approach to social anxiety disorder: The complex dynamic interplay among attentional bias for threat, attentional control, and symptoms. *J Anxiety Disord* 42: 95–104.

Henderson CR (1975) Best linear unbiased estimation and prediction under a selection model. *Biometrics* 31(2): 423–447.

Henderson R, Diggle P, Dobson A (2000) Joint modelling of longitudinal measurements and event time data. *Biostatistics* 1: 465–480.

Hendrickx JO, van Gastel J, Leysen H, Martin B, Maudsley S (2020) High-dimensionality data analysis of pharmacological systems associated with complex diseases. *Pharmacol Rev* 72(1): 191–217.

Hey SP, Gerlach CV, Dunlap G, Prasad V, Kesselheim AS (2020) The evidence landscape in precision medicine. *Sci Transl Med* 12: eaaw7745.

Hicks JK, Sangkuhl K, Swen JJ, Ellingrod VL, Müller DJ, Shimoda K, Bishop JR, Kharasch ED, Skaar TC, Gaedigk A, et al. (2017) Clinical pharmacogenetics implementation consortium guideline (CPIC) for CYP2D6 and CYP2C19 genotypes and dosing of tricyclic antidepressants. *Clin Pharmacol Ther* 102(1): 37–44. (2016 Update)

Hockings JK, Pasternak AL, Erwin AL, Mason NT, Eng C, Hicks JK (2020) Pharmacogenomics: An evolving clinical tool for precision medicine. *Cleve Clin J Med* 87: 91–99.

Hoffman GE (2013) Correcting for population structure and kinship using the linear mixed model: Theory and extensions. *PLoS ONE* 8(10): e75707.

Hogan JW, Laird NM (1997) Mixture models for the joint distribution of repeated measures and event times. *Stat Med* 16: 239–257.

Holmes MV, Ala-Korpela M, Smith GD (2017) Mendelian randomization in cardiometabolic disease: Challenges in evaluating causality. *Nat Rev Cardiol* 14: 577–590.

Hong KW, Min H, Heo BM, Joo SE, Kim SS, Kim Y (2012) Recapitulation of genome-wide association studies on pulse pressure and mean arterial pressure in the Korean population. *J Hum Genet* 57: 391–393.

Hood L, Perlmutter RM (2004) The impact of systems approaches on biological problems in drug discovery. *Nat Biotechnol* 22: 1215–1217.

Hopkins AL (2008) Network pharmacology: The next paradigm in drug discovery. *Nat Chem Biol* 4(11): 682–690.

Hou W, Garvan CW, Zhao W, Behnke M, Eyler FD, Wu RL (2005) A general model for detecting genetic determinants underlying longitudinal traits with unequally spaced measurements and nonstationary covariance structure. *Biostatistics* 6: 420–433.

Hou W, Garvan CW, Zhao W, Behnke M, Eyler FD, Wu RL (2006) A general likelihood model for characterizing cocaine-induced genetic determinants for developmental trajectories in early childhood. *Stat Med* 25: 4020–4035.

Hou W, Li HY, Zhang B, Huang MR, Wu RL (2008) A nonlinear mixed-effect mixture model for functional mapping of longitudinal traits. *Heredity* 101: 321–328.

Hsieh F, Tseng YK, Wang JL (2006) Joint modeling of survival and longitudinal data: Likelihood approach revisited. *Biometrics* 62: 1037–1043. https://doi.org/10.1038/nm.4426.

Huang J, Niu C, Green CD, Yang L, Mei H, Han J-DJ (2013) Systematic prediction of pharmacodynamic drug–drug interactions through protein-protein-interaction network. *PLoS Comput Biol* 9(3): e1002998.

Hukku A, Pividori M, Luca F, Pique-Regi R, Im HK, Wen X (2021) Probabilistic colocalization of genetic variants from complex and molecular traits: Promise and limitations. *Am J Hum Genet* 108: 25–35.

Huynh-Thu V, Sanguinetti G (2019) Gene regulatory network inference: An introductory survey. *Methods Mol Biol* 1883: 1–23.

Imoto S, Tamada Y, Savoie CJ, Miyano S (2007) Analysis of gene networks for drug target discovery and validation. *Methods Mol Biol* 360: 33–56.

Ingelman-Sundberg M, Mkrtchian S, Zhou Y, Lauschke VM (2018) Integrating rare genetic variants into pharmacogenetic drug response predictions. *Hum Genom* 12: 26.

Irvine DJ, Dane EL (2020) Enhancing cancer immunotherapy with nanomedicine. *Nat Rev Immunol* 20(5): 321–334.

Iyengar R, Zhao S, Chung S-W, Mager DE, Gallo JM (2012) Merging systems biology with pharmacodynamics. *Sci Transl Med* 4: 126ps7.

Jacob F, Salinas RD, Zhang DY, Nguyen PTT, Schnoll JG, Wong SZH, Thokala R, Sheikh S, Saxena D, Prokop S, et al. (2020) A patient-derived glioblastoma organoid model and biobank recapitulates inter- and intra-tumoral heterogeneity. *Cell* 180(1): 188–204.

Jansen G, Lee AY, Epp E, Fredette A, Surprenant J, Harcus D, Scott M, Tan E, Nishimura T, Whiteway M, Hallett M, Thomas DY (2009) Chemogenomic profiling predicts antifungal synergies. *Mol Syst Biol* 5: 338.

Jazwinsky A (1970) *Stochastic Processes and Filtering Theory*. Academic Press, New York.

Jiang L, Clavijo JA, Sun L, Zhu X, Bhakta MS, Gezan SA, Carvalho M, Vallejos CE, Wu RL (2015) Plastic expression of heterochrony quantitative trait loci (*h*QTL) for leaf growth in the common bean (Phaseolus vulgaris L.). *New Phytol* 207: 872–882.

Jiang LB, He XQ, Jin Y, Ye MX, Sang MM, Chen N, Zhu J, Zhang ZR, Li JT, Wu RL (2018a) A mapping framework of collaboration-competition QTLs that drive community dynamics. *Nat Commun* 9(1): 3010. (Chapter 9)

Jiang LB, Shi CZ, Ye MX, Xi FF, Cao YG, Wang L, Zhang MM, Sang MN, Wu RL (2018b) A computational-experimental framework for mapping plant coexistence. *Methods Ecol Evol* 9: 1335–1352.

Jiang LB, Liu J, Zhu X, Ye M, Sun L, Lacaze X, Wu RL (2015) 2HiGWAS: A unifying high-dimensional platform to infer the global genetic architecture of trait development. *Brief Bioinform* 16(6): 905–911.

Jiang LB, Xu J, Zhang Y, Sang MM, Ye MX, Wei K, Xu P, Tai R, Zhao Z, Wu RL, et al. (2019) A drive to driven model of mapping intraspecific interaction networks. *iScience* 22: 109–122.

Jin S, Guerrero-Juarez CF, Zhang L, Chang I, Ramos R, Kuan CH, Myung P, Plikus MV, Nie Q (2021) Inference and analysis of cell-cell communication using CellChat. *Nat Commun* 12(1): 1088.

Johnson D, Wilke MAP, Lyle SM, Kowalec K, Jorgensen A, Wright GEB, Drögemöller BI (2022) A systematic review and analysis of the use of polygenic scores in pharmacogenomics. *Clin Pharmacol Ther* 111(4): 919–930.

Joshi S, Durden DL (2019) Combinatorial approach to improve cancer immunotherapy: Rational drug design strategy to simultaneously hit multiple targets to kill tumor cells and to activate the immune system. *J Oncol* 2019: 1.

Jusko WJ (1995) Pharmacokinetics and receptor-mediated pharmacodynamics of corticosteroids. *Toxicology* 102(1–2): 189–196.

Jusko WJ, Ko HC, Ebling WF (1995) Convergence of direct and indirect pharmacodynamic response models. *J Pharmacokinet Biopharm* 23: 5–8.

Kalman RE (1960) A new approach to linear filtering and prediction problems. *Trans ASME – J Basic Eng* 82(Ser D): 35–45.

Kang HM, Sul JH, Service SK, Zaitlen NA, Kong SY, Freimer NB, et al. (2010) Variance component model to account for sample structure in genome-wide association studies. *Nat Genet* 42(4): 348–354.

Kashtan N, Alon U (2005) Spontaneous evolution of modularity and network motifs. *Proc Natl Acad Sci U S A* 102(39): 13773–13778.

Kashtan N, Noor E, Alon U (2007) Varying environments can speed up evolution. *Proc Natl Acad Sci U S A* 104(34): 13711–13716.

Katzir I, Cokol M, Aldridge BB, Alon U (2019) Prediction of ultra-high-order antibiotic combinations based on pairwise interactions. *PLoS Comput Biol* 15(1): e1006774.

Kaur G, Gan YL, Phillips CL, Wong K, Saini B (2016) Chronotherapy in practice: The perspective of the community pharmacist. *Int J Clin Pharm* 38: 171–182.

Keyte AL, Smith KK (2014) Heterochrony and developmental timing mechanisms: Changing ontogenies in evolution. *Sem Cell Develop Biol* 34: 99–107.

Kholodenko BN, Rauch N, Kolch W, Rukhlenko OS (2021) A systematic analysis of signaling reactivation and drug resistance. *Cell Rep* 35(8): 109157.

Kiessling S, Cermakian N (2017) The tumor circadian clock: A new target for cancer therapy? *Future Oncology* 13: 29.

Kim BR, Zhang L, Berg A, Fan J, Wu RL (2008) A computational approach to the functional clustering of periodic gene-expression profiles. *Genetics* 180(2): 821–834.

Kim HS, Fay JC (2009) A combined-cross analysis reveals genes with drug-specific and background-dependent effects on drug sensitivity in Saccharomyces cerevisiae. *Genetics* 183(3): 1141–1151.

Klamt S, Haus UU, Theis F (2009) Hypergraphs and cellular networks. *PLoS Comput Biol* 5(5): e1000385.

Klein TE, Altman RB, Eriksson N, Gage BF, Kimmel SE, Lee MT, Limdi NA, Page D, Roden DM, Wagner MJ, Caldwell MD, et al. (2009) Estimation of the warfarin dose with clinical and pharmacogenetic data. *N Engl J Med* 360: 753–764.

Klengel T, Binder EB (2013) Gene-environment interactions in major depressive disorder. *Can J Psychiatry* 58(2): 76–83.

Koh-Tan HH, Dashti M, Wang T, Beattie W, Mcclure J, Young B, Dominiczak AF, McBride MW, Graham D (2017) Dissecting the genetic components of a quantitative trait locus for blood pressure and renal pathology on rat chromosome 3. *J Hypertens* 35: 319–329.

Koido M, Kawakami E, Fukumura J, Noguchi Y, Ohori M, Nio Y, Nicoletti P, Aithal GP, Daly AK, Watkins PB, et al. (2020) Polygenic architecture informs potential vulnerability to drug-induced liver injury. *Nat Med* 26: 1541–1548.

Kong YC, Yu TW (2019) A hypergraph-based method for large-scale dynamic correlation study at the transcriptomic scale. *BMC Genomics* 20: 397.

Korolev KS, Xavier JB, Gore J (2014) Turning ecology and evolution against cancer. *Nat Rev Cancer* 14: 371–380.

Koromina M, Koutsilieri S, Patrinos GP (2020) Delineating significant genome-wide associations of variants with antipsychotic and antidepressant treatment response: Implications for clinical pharmacogenomics. *Hum Genom* 14: 4.

Kozyra M, Ingelman-Sundberg M, Lauschke VM (2017) Rare genetic variants in cellular transporters, metabolic enzymes, and nuclear receptors can be important determinants of interindividual differences in drug response. *Genet Med* 19(1): 20–29.

Kraft K, Hoffmann W (2012) Challenge of evidence in individualized medicine. *Person Med* 9: 65–71.

Kristensen N, Madsen H (2010) Continuous time stochastic modeling. CTSM 2.3. *Math Guide.*

Kristensen NR, Madsen H, Ingwersen SH (2005) Using stochastic differential equations for PK/PD model development. *J Pharmacokinet Pharmacodyn* 32(1): 109–141.

Kuhlman SJ, Mackey SR, Duffy JF (2017) Biological rhythms workshop I: Introduction to chronobiology. *Cold Spring Harb Symp Quant Biol* 72: 1–6.

Lai X, Stiff A, Duggan M, Wesolowski R, Carson WE, Friedman A (2018) Modeling combination therapy for breast cancer with BET and immune checkpoint inhibitors. *Proc Natl Acad Sci U S A* 115(21): 5534–5539.

Laird NM (2006) Missing data in longitudinal studies. *Stat Med* 7: 305–315.

Lambert DG (2014) Drugs and receptors. *BJA CEPD Rev* 4: 181–184.

Lander ES, Botstein D (1989) Mapping mendelian factors underlying quantitative traits using RFLP linkage maps. *Genetics* 121(1): 185–199.

Landi P, Minoarivelo HO, Brännström Å, Hui C, Dieckmann U (2018) Complexity and stability of ecological networks: A review of the theory. *Popul Ecol* 60: 319–345.

Lange K (1997) An approximate model of polygenic inheritance. *Genetics* 147(3): 1423–1430.

Lankelma J, Fernández Luque R, Dekker H, van den Berg J, Kooi B (2013) A new mathematical pharmacodynamic model of clonogenic cancer cell death by doxorubicin. *J Pharmacokinet Pharmacodyn* 40: 513–525.

Larstorp AC, Ariansen I, Gjesdal K, Olsen MH, Ibsen H, Devereux RB, Okin PM, Dahlöf B, Kjeldsen SE, Wachtell K (2012) Association of pulse pressure with new-onset atrial fibrillation in patients with hypertension and left ventricular hypertrophy: The Losartan Intervention For Endpoint (LIFE) reduction in hypertension study. *Hypertension* 60: 347–353.

Lawson DA, Kessenbrock K, Davis RT, Pervolarakis N, Werb Z (2018) Tumour heterogeneity and metastasis at single-cell resolution. *Nat Cell Biol* 20(12): 1349–1360.

Lawson HA, Cheverud JM, Wolf JB (2013) Genomic imprinting and parent-of-origin effects on complex traits. *Nat Rev Genet* 14(9): 608–617.

Leander J, Lundh T, Jirstrand M (2014) Stochastic differential equations as a tool to regularize the parameter estimation problem for continuous time dynamical systems given discrete time measurements. *Math Biosci* 251: 54–62.

Lee AB, Luca D, Klei L, Devlin B, Roeder K (2010) Discovering genetic ancestry using spectral graph theory. *Genet Epidemiol* 34: 51–59.

Lee D, Zhang J, Liu J, Gerstein M (2020a) Epigenome-based splicing prediction using a recurrent neural network. *PLoS Comput Biol* 16: e1008006.

Lee JH, Park YR, Jung M, Lim SG (2020b) Gene regulatory network analysis with drug sensitivity reveals synergistic effects of combinatory chemotherapy in gastric cancer. *Sci Rep* 10: 3932.

Lehár J, Krueger A, Zimmermann G, Borisy A (2008) High-order combination effects and biological robustness. *Mol Syst Biol* 4: 215.

Lehár SM, Dooley J, Farr AG, Bevan MJ (2004) Notch ligands Delta1 and Jagged1 transmit distinct signals to T cell precursor. *Blood* 105: 1440–1447.

Lemmer B (2007) Chronobiology, drug-delivery, and chronotherapeutics. *Adv Drug Deliv Rev* 59: 825–827.

Levine J, Bascompte J, Adler P, et al. (2017) Beyond pairwise mechanisms of species coexistence in complex communities. *Nature* 546: 56–64.

Levy G (1964) Relationship between elimination rate of drugs and rate of decline of their pharmacologic effects. *J Pharm Sci* 53: 342–343.

Levy RH, Ragueneau-Majlessi I (2019) Past, present, and future of drug–drug interactions. *Clin Pharmacol Ther* 105(6): 1286–1288.

Li B, Ritchie MD (2021) From GWAS to gene: Transcriptome-wide association studies and other methods to functionally understand GWAS discoveries. *Front Genet* 12: 713230.

Li G, Zhu H (2013) Genetic studies: The linear mixed models in genome-wide association studies. *Open Bioinform J* 7(1): 27–33.

Li HY, Wu RL (2012) A pattern-mixture model for functional mapping of quantitative trait nucleotides with non-ignorable dropout data. *Stat Sinica* 22: 337–357.

Li J, Li X, Zhang S, Snyder M (2019) Gene-environment interaction in the era of precision medicine. *Cell* 177: 38–44.

Li JH, Das K, Fu GF, Li R, Wu RL (2011a) Bayesian lasso for genome-wide association studies. *Bioinformatics* 27: 516–523.

Li Y, Guo YQ, Hou W, Chang M, Liao DP, Wu RL (2011b) A statistical design for testing transgenerational genomic imprinting in natural human populations. *PLoS ONE* 6(2): e16858.

Li JH, Wang Z, Li R, Wu RL (2015) Bayesian group lasso for nonparametric varying-coefficient models with application to functional genome-wide association studies. *Ann Appl Stat* 9(2): 640–664.

Li JH, Zhong W, Li R, Wu RL (2014a) A fast algorithm for detecting gene-gene interactions in genome-wide association studies. *Ann Appl Stat* 8: 2292–2318. (Chapter 5)

Li X, Sui Y, Liu T, Wang J, Li Y, Lin Z, Hegarty J, Koltun WA, Wang Z, Wu RL (2014b) A model for family-based case-control studies of genetic imprinting and epistasis. *Brief Bioinform* 15(6): 1069–1079.

Li N, McMurry T, Berg A, Wang Z, Berceli SA, Wu RL (2010) Functional clustering of periodic transcriptional profiles through ARMA(p, q). *PLoS ONE* 5(4): e9894.

Li Y, Umbach DM, Krahn JM, et al. (2021) Predicting tumor response to drugs based on gene-expression biomarkers of sensitivity learned from cancer cell lines. *BMC Genomics* 22: 272.

Li YY, Li JS (2019) Technical advances contribute to the study of genomic imprinting. *PLoS Genet* 15(6): e1008151.

Li Z, Sillanpää MJ (2015) Dynamic quantitative trait locus analysis of plant phenomic sata. *Trends Plant Sci* 20(12): 822–833.

Liang J, Crowther TW, Picard N, Wiser S, Zhou M, Alberti G, Schulze ED, McGuire AD, Bozzato F, Pretzsch H, et al. (2016) Positive biodiversity-productivity relationship predominant in global forests. *Science* 354(6309): aaf8957.

Lim AJW, Lim LJ, Ooi BNS, Koh ET, Tan JWL, TTSH RA Study Group, Chong SS, Khor CC, Tucker-Kellogg L, Leong KP, et al. (2022) Functional coding haplotypes and machine-learning feature elimination identifies predictors of methotrexate response in rheumatoid arthritis patients. *EBioMedicine* 75: 103800.

Lim B, Woodward WA, Wang X, Reuben JM, Ueno NT (2018) Inflammatory breast cancer biology: The tumour microenvironment is key. *Nat Rev Cancer* 18(8): 485–499.

Lin L, Chen Q, Hirsch JP, Yoo S, Yeung K, Bumgarner RE, Tu ZD, Schadt EE, Zhu J (2018) Temporal genetic association and temporal genetic causality methods for dissecting complex networks. *Nat Commun* 9(1): 3980.

Lin M, Aqvilonte C, Johnson JA, Wu RL (2005a) Sequencing drug response with HapMap. *Pharmacogenomics J* 5: 149–156.

Lin M, Wu RL, Johnson JA (2005b) A bivariate functional mapping model for gene identification of drug response for systolic and diastolic blood pressures. *Pac Symp Biocomput* 11: 572–583.

Lin M, Berg A, Wu RL (2010) Modeling the genetic etiology of pharmacokinetic-pharmacodynamic links with the ARMA process. *J Biopharm Stat* 20: 351–372.

Lin M, Hou W, Li HY, Johnson JA, Wu RL (2007) Modeling sequence-sequence interactions for drug response. *Bioinformatics* 23: 1251–1257.

Lin M, Wu RL (2005) Theoretical basis for the identification of allelic variants that encode drug efficacy and toxicity. *Genetics* 170: 919–928.

Link E, Parish S, Armitage J, et al. (2008) SLCO1B1 variants and statin-induced myopathy – A genomewide study. *N Engl J Med* 359: 789–799.

Liou YJ, Bai YM, Lin E, Chen JY, Chen TT, Hong CJ, Tsai SJ (2012) Gene-gene interactions of the INSIG1 and INSIG2 in metabolic syndrome in schizophrenic patients treated with atypical antipsychotics. *Pharmacogenomics J* 12: 54–61.

Listgarten J, Lippert C, Kadie CM, Davidson RI, Eskin E, Heckerman D (2012) Improved linear mixed models for genome-wide association studies. *Nat Methods* 9(6): 525–526.

Little RJA (1993) Pattern-mixture models for multivariate incomplete data. *J Am Stat Assoc* 88 125–134.

Little RJA (1995) Modeling the drop-out mechanism in repeated-measures studies. *J Am Stat Assoc* 90: 1112–1121.

Little RJA, Rubin DB (1987) *Statistical Analysis with Missing Data*. Wiley, New York.

Liu E, Zhang ZZ, Cheng X, Liu X, Cheng L (2020) SCNrank spectral clustering for network-based ranking to reveal potential drug targets and its application in pancreatic ductal adenocarcinoma. *BMC Med Genom* 13: 50.

Liu GD, Kong L, Wang Z, Wu RL (2013) Systems mapping of metabolic genes through control theory. *Adv Drug Deliv Rev* 65: 918–928.

Liu J, Dang H, Wang X (2018) The significance of intertumor and intratumor heterogeneity in liver cancer. *Exp Mol Med* 50: e416.

Liu T, Johnson JA, Casella G, Wu RL (2004) Sequencing complex diseases with HapMap. *Genetics* 168: 503–511.

Liu T, Liu XL, Chen YM, Wu RL (2007) A unifying differential equation model for functional genetic mapping of circadian rhythms. *Theor Biol Med Model* 4: 5.

Liu T, Wu RL (2009) A Bayesian algorithm for functional mapping of dynamic complex traits. *Algorithms* 2: 667–691.

Liu YY, Slotine JJ, Barabási AL (2011) Controllability of complex networks. *Nature* 473: 167–173.

Lomonosov A, Sitharam M (2007) Stability, optimality and complexity of network games with pricing and player dropouts. *Scal Comput Pract Exp* 8: 79–86.

Losic B, Craig AJ, Villacorta-Martin C, Martins-Filho SN, Akers N, Chen X, Ahsen ME, von Felden J, Labgaa I, D'Avola D, et al. (2020) Intratumoral heterogeneity and clonal evolution in liver cancer. *Nat Commun* 11: 291.

Lozovsky ER, Daniels RF, Heffernan GD, Jacobus DP, Hartl DL (2021) Relevance of higher-order epistasis in drug resistance. *Mol Biol Evol* 38(1): 142–151.

Lu J, Deng K, Zhang X, Liu G, Guan Y (2021) Neural-ODE for pharmacokinetics modeling and its advantage to alternative machine learning models in predicting new dosing regimens. *iScience* 24(7): 102804.

Lu J, Wang XZ, Wan LL, Fu JL, Huo Y, Zhao YW, Guo C (2020) Gene polymorphisms affecting the pharmacokinetics and pharmacodynamics of donepezil efficacy. *Front Pharmacol* 11: 934.

Luizon MR, Ahituv N (2015) Uncovering drug–responsive regulatory elements. *Pharmacogenomics* 16(16): 1829–1841.

Luo JT, Hager WW, Wu RL (2010) A differential equation model for functional mapping of a virus-cell dynamic system. *J Math Biol* 65: 1–15.

Ma CX, Casella G, Wu RL (2002) Functional mapping of quantitative trait loci underlying the character process: A theoretical framework. *Genetics* 161: 1751–1762.

MacArthur RH (1955) Fluctuations of animal populations and a measure of community stability. *Ecology* 36: 533–536.

Macheras P, Iliadis A (2006) *Modeling in Biopharmacokinetics, and Pharmacodynamics.* Springer, New York.

Mackay TF, Stone EA, Ayroles JF (2009) The genetics of quantitative traits: Challenges and prospects. *Nat Rev Genet* 10: 565–577.

Madadi P, Ross CJD, Hayden MR, Carleton BC, Gaedigk A, Leeder JS (2009) Pharmacogenetics of neonatal opioid toxicity following maternal use of codeine during breastfeeding: A case-control study. *Clin Pharmacol Ther* 85(1): 31–35.

Madian AG, Wheeler HE, Jones RB, Dolan ME (2012) Relating human genetic variation to variation in drug responses. *Trends Genet* 28(10): 487–495.

Magaña J, Contreras MG, Keys KL, Risse-Adams O, Goddard PC, Zeiger AM, Mak ACY, Elhawary JR, Samedy-Bates LA, Lee E, et al. (2020) An epistatic interaction between pre-natal smoke exposure and socioeconomic status has a significant impact on bronchodilator drug response in African American youth with asthma. *BioData Min* 13: 7.

Mager DE (2006) Quantitative structure-pharmacokinetic/pharmacodynamic relationships. *Adv Drug Deliv Rev* 58(12–13): 1326–1356.

Mager DE, Mascelli MA, Kleiman NS, Fitzgerald DJ, Abernethy DR (2003) Simultaneous modeling of abciximab plasma concentrations and ex vivo pharmacodynamics in patients undergoing coronary angioplasty. *J Pharmacol Exp Ther* 307(3): 969–976.

Mager DE, Wyska E, Jusko WJ (2003) Diversity of mechanism-based pharmacodynamic models. *Drug Metab Dispos* 31: 510–518.

Majchrzak-Celinska A, Baer-Dubowska W (2017) Pharmacoepigenetics: An element of personalized therapy? *Expert Opin Drug Metab Toxicol* 13(4): 387–398.

Mak TSH, Porsch RM, Choi SW, Zhou X, Sham PC (2017) Polygenic scores via penalized regression on summary statistics. *Genet Epidemiol* 41: 469–480.

Malki MA, Pearson ER (2020) Drug–drug–gene interactions and adverse drug reactions. *Pharmacogenomics J* 20: 355–366.

Mani R, St Onge RP, Hartman JL 4th, Giaever G, Roth FP (2008) Defining genetic interaction. *Proc Natl Acad Sci U S A* 105(9): 3461–3466.

Manolio TA (2010) Genome-wide association studies and assessment of the risk of disease. *N Engl J Med* 363: 166–176.

Manolio TA, Collins FS, Cox NJ, Goldstein DB, Hindorff LA, Hunter DJ, McCarthy MI, Ramos EM, Cardon LR, et al. (2009) Finding the missing heritability of complex diseases. *Nature* 461: 747–753.

Marbach D, Costello JC, Küffner R, Vega NM, Prill RJ, Camacho DM, Allison KR, Kellis M, Collins JJ, Stolovitzky G, et al. (2012) Wisdom of crowds for robust gene network inference. *Nat Methods* 9: 796–804.

Marderstein AR, Davenport ER, Kulm S, Van Hout CV, Elemento O, Clark AG (2021) Leveraging phenotypic variability to identify genetic interactions in human phenotypes. *Am J Hum Genet* 108(1): 49–67.

Marrow P, Dieckmann U, Law R (1996) Evolutionary dynamics of predator-prey systems: An ecological perspective. *J Math Biol* 34(5–6): 556–578.

Maurano MT, Humbert R, Rynes E, Thurman RE, Haugen E, Wang H, Reynolds AP, Sandstrom R, Qu H, Brody J (2012) Systematic localization of common disease-associated variation in regulatory DNA. *Science* 337: 1190–1195.

May RM (1972) Will a large complex system be stable? *Nature* 238: 413–414.

May RM (1973) *Stability and Complexity in Model Ecosystems*. Princeton University Press, Princeton, NJ.

Maynard Smith J (1982) *Evolution and the Theory of Games*. Cambridge University Press, Cambridge.

Maynard Smith J, Price G (1973) The logic of animal conflict. *Nature* 246: 15–18.

McCarthy MI, Abecasis GR, Cardon LR, Goldstein DB, Little J, Ioannidis JP, Hirschhorn JN (2008) Genome-wide association studies for complex traits: Consensus, uncertainty and challenges. *Nat Rev Genet* 9: 356–369.

McGillivray P, Clarke D, Meyerson W, Zhang J, Lee D, Gu M (2018) Network analysis as a grand unifier in biomedical data science. *Ann Rev Biomed Data Sci* 1(1): 153–180.

McInnes G, Altman RB (2021) Drug response pharmacogenetics for 200,000 UK biobank participants. *Pac Symp Biocomput* 26: 184–195.

McInnes G, Dalton R, Sangkuhl K, Whirl-Carrillo M, Lee SB, Tsao PS, Gaedigk A, Altman RB, Woodahl EL (2020) Transfer learning enables prediction of CYP2D6 haplotype function. *PLoS Comput Biol* 16(11): e1008399.

McInnes G, Yee SW, Pershad Y, Altman RB (2021) Genome-wide association studies in pharmacogenomics. *Clin Pharmacol Ther* 110(3): 637–648.

McKenna MT, Weis JA, Quaranta V, Yankeelov TE (2019) Leveraging mathematical modeling to quantify pharmacokinetic and pharmacodynamic pathways: Equivalent dose metric. *Front Physiol* 10: 616.

McKinstry-Wu AR, Wasilczuk AZ, Harrison BA, Bedell VM, Sridharan MJ, Breig JJ, Pack M, Kelz MB, Proekt A (2019) Analysis of stochastic fluctuations in responsiveness is a critical step toward personalized anesthesia. *eLife* 8: e50143.

McNamara KJ (2012) Heterochrony: The evolution of development. *Evo Edu Outreach* 5: 203–218.

Meibohm B, Derendorf H (1997) Basic concepts of pharmacokinetic/pharmacodynamic (PK/PD) modelling. *Int J Clin Pharmacol Ther* 35(10): 401–413.

Melo D, Porto A, Cheverud JM, Marroig G (2016) Modularity: Genes, development and evolution. *Annu Rev Ecol Evol Syst* 47: 463–486.

Melo X, Santos DA, Ornelas R, Fernhall B, Santa-Clara H, Sardinha LB (2018) Pulse pressure tracking from adolescence to young adulthood: Contributions to vascular health. *Blood Pressure* 27: 19–24.

Meyer CT, Wooten DJ, Lopez CF, Quaranta V (2020) Charting the fragmented landscape of drug synergy. *Trends Pharmacol Sci* 41: 266–280.

Meyer CT, Wooten DJ, Paudel BB, Bauer J, Hardeman KN, Westover D, Lovly CM, Harris LA, Tyson DR, Quaranta V (2019) Quantifying drug combination synergy along potency and efficacy axes. *Cell Syst* 8(2): 97–108.e16.

Michailidis G, d'Alché-Buc F (2013) Autoregressive models for gene regulatory network inference: Sparsity, stability and causality issues. *Math Biosci* 246(2): 326–334.

Mini E, Nobili S (2009) Pharmacogenetics: Implementing personalized medicine. *Clin Cases Miner Bone Metab* 6: 17–24.

Moore R, Casale FP, Jan Bonder M, Horta D; BIOS Consortium, Franke L, Barroso I, Stegle O (2019) A linear mixed-model approach to study multivariate gene-environment interactions. *Nat Genet* 51(1): 180–186.

Morison IM, Ramsay JP, Spencer HG (2005) A census of mammalian imprinting. *Trends Genet* 21(8): 457–465.

Motsinger-Reif AA, Jorgenson E, Relling MV, Kroetz DL, Weinshilboum R, Cox NJ, Roden DM (2013) Genome-wide association studies in pharmacogenomics: Successes and lessons. *Pharmacogenet Genomics* 23(8): 383–394.

Muir AJ, Gong L, Johnson SG, Lee MT, Williams MS, Klein TE, Caudle KE, Nelson DR (2014) Clinical pharmacogenetics implementation consortium (CPIC) guidelines for IFNL3 (IL28B) genotype and PEG interferon-α-based regimens. *Clin Pharmacol Ther* 95: 141–146.

Mustavich LF, Miller P, Kidd KK, Zhao H (2010) Using a pharmacokinetic model to relate an individual's susceptibility to alcohol dependence to genotypes. *Hum Hered* 70: 177–193.

Naiki-Ito A (2010) Gap junction dysfunction reduces acetaminophen hepatotoxicity with impact on apoptotic signaling and connexin 43 protein induction in rat. *Toxicol Pathol* 38: 280.

Naiki-Ito A, Kato H, Asamoto M, Naiki T, Shirai T (2012) Age-dependent carcinogenic susceptibility in rat liver is related to potential of gap junctional intercellular communication. *Toxicol Pathol* 40(5): 715–721.

Najafi M, Goradel NH, Farhood B, Salehi E, Solhjoo S, Toolee H, Kharazinejad E, Mortezaee K (2019) Tumor microenvironment: Interactions and therapy. *J Cell Physiol* 234(5): 5700–5721.

Nash JF (1950) Equilibrium points in N-Person games. *Proc Natl Acad Sci U S A* 36(1): 48–49.

Nassar SF, Raddassi K, Wu T (2021) Single-Cell multiomics analysis for drug discovery. *Metabolites* 11(11): 729.

Nawaz S, Yuan Y (2016) Computational pathology: Exploring the spatial dimension of tumor ecology. *Cancer Lett* 380: 296–303.

Nelander S, Wang W, Nilsson B, She QB, Pratilas C, Rosen N, Gennemark P, Sander C (2008) Models from experiments: Combinatorial drug perturbations of cancer cells. *Mol Syst Biol* 4: 216.

Newman ME (2003) The structure and function of complex networks. *SIAM Rev* 45: 167–256.

Nicholson JK, Holmes E, Lindon JC, Wilson LD (2004) The challenges of modeling mammalian biocomplexity. *Nat Biotechnol* 22: 1268–1274.

Ning C, Wang D, Zhou L, Wei J, Liu Y, Kang H, Zhang S, Zhou X, Xu S, Liu JF (2019) Efficient multivariate analysis algorithms for longitudinal genome-wide association studies. *Bioinformatics* 35(23): 4879–4885.

Niu J, Straubinger RM, Mager DE (2019) Pharmacodynamic drug–drug interactions. *Clin Pharmacol Ther* 105(6): 1395–1406.

Nkhoma SC, Ahmed AOA, Zaman S, Porier D, Baker Z, Stedman TT (2021) Dissection of haplotype-specific drug response phenotypes in multiclonal malaria isolates. *Int J Parasitol Drugs Drug Resist* 15: 152–161.

Noël F, Massenet-Regad L, Carmi-Levy I, Cappuccio A, Grandclaudon M, Trichot C, Kieffer Y, Mechta-Grigoriou F, Soumelis V (2021) Dissection of intercellular communication using the transcriptome-based framework ICELLNET. *Nat Commun* 12(1): 1089. (Chapter 8)

Novembre J, Stephens M (2008) Interpreting principal component analyses of spatial population genetic variation. *Nat Genet* 40: 646–649.

Nowell PC (1976) The clonal evolution of tumor cell populations. *Science* 194: 23–28.

Nussinov R, Jang H, Nir G, Tsai CJ, Cheng F (2021) A new precision medicine initiative at the dawn of exascale computing. *Signal Transduct Target Ther* 6(1): 3.

Odum EP (1953) *Fundamentals of Ecology.* Saunders, Philadelphia.

Orlando PA, Gatenby RA, Brown JS (2012) Cancer treatment as a game: Integrating evolutionary game theory into the optimal control of chemotherapy. *Phys Biol* 9: 1–10.

Ott J, Kamatani Y, Lathrop M (2011) Family-based designs for genome-wide association studies. *Nat Rev Genet* 12: 465–474.

Ozdemir T, Fedorec AJH, Danino T, Barnes CP (2018) Synthetic biology and engineered live biotherapeutics: Toward increasing system complexity. *Cell Syst* 7(1): 5–16.

Pacheco JM, Santos FC, Dingli D (2014) The ecology of cancer from an evolutionary game theory perspective. *Interface Focus* 4: 20140019.

Padmanabhan S, Joe B (2017) Towards precision medicine for hypertension: A review of genomic, epigenomic, and microbiomic effects on blood pressure in experimental rat models and humans. *Physiol Rev* 97: 1469–1528.

Palaniappan L, Simons LA, Simons J, Friedlander Y, McCallum J (2002) Comparison of usefulness of systolic, diastolic, and mean blood pressure and pulse pressure as predictors of cardiovascular death in patients ≥60 years of age (the Dubbo study). *Am J Cardiol* 90: 1398–1401.

Palleria C, Di Paolo A, Giofrè C, Caglioti C, Leuzzi G, Siniscalchi A, De Sarro G, Gallelli L (2013) Pharmacokinetic drug–drug interaction and their implication in clinical management. *J Res Med Sci* 18(7): 601–610.

Palmer AC, Chidley C, Sorger PK (2019) A curative combination cancer therapy achieves high fractional cell killing through low cross-resistance and drug additivity. *eLife* 8: e50036.

Panda S (2016) Circadian physiology of metabolism. *Science* 354: 1008–1015.

Panditrao G, Bhowmick R, Meena C, Sarkar RP (2022) Emerging landscape of molecular interaction networks: Opportunities, challenges and prospects. *J Biosci* 47: 24.

Parca L, Pepe G, Pietrosanto M, Galvan G, Galli L, Palmeri A, Sciandrone M, Ferrè F, Ausiello G, Helmer-Citterich M (2019) Modeling cancer drug response through drug-specific informative genes. *Sci Rep* 9: 15222.

Park J, Lee SY, Baik SY, Park CH, Yoon JH, Ryu BY, Kim JH (2020) Gene-Wise burden of coding variants correlates to noncoding pharmacogenetic risk variants. *Int J Mol Sci* 21(9): 3091.

Park JC, Jang SY, Lee D, Lee J, Kang U, Chang H, Kim HJ, Han SH, Seo J, Choi M, et al. (2021) A logical network-based drug-screening platform for Alzheimer's disease representing pathological features of human brain organoids. *Nat Commun* 12(1): 280.

Parter M, Kashtan N, Alon U (2007) Environmental variability and modularity of bacterial metabolic networks. *BMC Evol Biol* 7: 169.

Patel SJ, Milwid JM, King KR, Bohr S, Iracheta-Vellve A, Li M, Vitalo A, Parekkadan B, Jindal R, Yarmush ML (2012) Gap junction inhibition prevents drug-induced liver toxicity and fulminant hepatic failure. *Nat Biotechnol* 30: 179.

Patterson N, Price AL, Reich D (2006) Population structure and eigenanalysis. *PLoS Genet* 2(12): 2074–2093.

Pawitan Y, Self S (1993) Modeling disease marker processes in AIDS. *J Am Stat Assoc* 88: 719–726.

Peedicayil J (2019) Pharmacoepigenetics and pharmacoepigenomics: An overview. *Curr Drug Discov Technol* 16(4): 392–399.

Pemovska T, Bigenzahn JW, Srndic I, Lercher A, Bergthaler A, César-Razquin A, Kartnig F, Kornauth C, Valent P, Staber PB, et al. (2021) Metabolic drug survey highlights cancer cell dependencies and vulnerabilities. *Nat Commun* 12: 7190.

Perry D, Sperling R, Katz R, Berry D, Dilts D, Hanna D, Salloway S, Trojanowski JQ, Bountra C, Krams M, et al. (2015) Building a roadmap for developing combination therapies for Alzheimer's disease. *Expert Rev Neurotherap* 15(3): 327–333.

Picchini U, Ditlevsen S, Gaetano AD (2006) Modeling the euglycemic hyperinsulinemic clamp by stochastic differential equations. *J Math Biol* 53: 771–796.

Pinotti F, Ghanbarnejad F, Hövel P, Poletto C (2020) Interplay between competitive and cooperative interactions in a three-player pathogen system. *R Soc Open Sci* 7(1): 190305.

Pirmohamed M (2014) Personalized pharmacogenomics: Predicting efficacy and adverse drug reactions. *Annu Rev Genomics Hum Genet* 15: 349–370.

Prantil-Baun R, Novak R, Das D, Somayaji MR, Przekwas A, Ingber DE (2018) Physiologically based pharmacokinetic and pharmacodynamic analysis enabled by microfluidically linked Organs-on-Chips. *Annu Rev Pharmacol Toxicol* 58: 37–64.

Price AL, Patterson NJ, Plenge RM, Weinblatt ME, Shadick NA, Reich D (2006) Principal components analysis corrects for stratification in genome-wide association studies. *Nat Genet* 38: 904–909.

Primorac D, Bach-Rojecky L, Vađunec D, Juginović A, Žunić K, Matišić V, Skelin A, Arsov B, Boban L, Erceg D, et al. (2020) Pharmacogenomics at the center of precision medicine: Challenges and perspective in an era of big data. *Pharmacogenomics* 21(2): 141–156.

Pritchard JK, Rosenberg NA (1999) Use of unlinked genetic markers to detect population stratification in association studies. *Am J Hum Genet* 65: 220–228.

Pritchard JK, Stephens M, Donnelly P (2000) Inference of population structure using multilocus genotype data. *Genetics* 155(2): 945–959.

Purcell S, Neale B, Todd-Brown K, Thomas L, Ferreira MAR, Bender D, Maller J, Sklar P, Daly MJ, Sham PC, et al. (2007) Plink: A tool set for whole-genome association and population-based linkage analyses. *Am J Hum Genet* 81: 559–575.

Rajon E, Plotkin JB (2013) The evolution of genetic architectures underlying quantitative traits. *Proc Biol Sci* 280(1769): 20131552.

Ramanathan M (1999a) An application of Ito's lemma in population pharmacokinetics and pharmacodynamics. *Pharm Res* 16: 584–586.

Ramanathan M (1999b) A method for estimating pharmacokinetic risks of concentration dependent drug interactions from preclinical data. *Drug Metab Dispos* 27: 1479–1487.

Ramón Y, Cajal S, Sesé M, Capdevila C, Aasen T, De Mattos-Arruda L, Diaz-Cano SJ, Hernández-Losa J, Castellví J (2020) Clinical implications of intratumor heterogeneity: Challenges and opportunities. *J Mol Med (Berl)* 98(2): 161–177.

Rationalizing combination therapies (2017). *Nat Med* 23: 1113. https://doi.org/10.1038/nm.4426.

Ray-Mukherjee J, Mukherjee S (2016) Evolutionary stable strategy application of Nash equilibrium in biology. *Resonance: J Sci* 21(9): 803–814.

Reay WR, Atkins JR, Carr VJ, Green MJ, Cairns MJ (2020) Pharmacological enrichment of polygenic risk for precision medicine in complex disorders. *Sci Rep* 10: 879.

Reeve R, Turner JR (2013) Pharmacodynamic models: Parameterizing the hill equation, Michaelis-Menten, the logistic curve, and relationships among these models. *J Biopharm Stat* 23(3): 648–661.

Roden DM, Wilke RA, Kroemer HK (2011) Stein CM. Pharmacogenomics: The genetics of variable drug responses. *Circulation* 123(15): 1661–1670.

Rodriguez-Meira A, Buck G, Clark SA, Povinelli BJ, Alcolea V, Louka E, McGowan S, Hamblin A, Sousos N, Barkas N, et al. (2019) Unravelling intratumoral heterogeneity through high-sensitivity single-cell mutational analysis and parallel RNA sequencing. *Mol Cell* 73(6): 1292–1305.

Rohde LA, Mota NR, Oliveira C, Berger M, et al. (2019) Integrative proteomics and pharmacogenomics analysis of methylphenidate treatment response. *Transl Psychiatry* 9(1): 308.

Román-Pérez E, Casbas-Hernández P, Pirone JR, Rein J (2012) Gene expression in extratumoral microenvironment predicts clinical outcome in breast cancer patients. *Breast Cancer Res* 14(2): R51.

Rosenberg NA, Pritchard JK, Weber JL, Cann HM, Kidd KK, Zhivotovsky LA, Feldman MW (2002) Genetic structure of human populations. *Genetics* 298: 2381–2385.

Rothbauer M, Zirath H, Ertl P (2018) Recent advances in microfluidic technologies for cell-to-cell interaction studies. *Lab Chip* 18: 249–270.

Rouault H, Hakim V (2012) Different cell fates from cell-cell interactions: Core architectures of two-cell bistable networks. *Biophys J* 102: 417–426.

Runcie DE, Crawford L (2019) Fast and flexible linear mixed models for genome-wide genetics. *PLoS Genet* 15(2): e1007978.

Sackton TB, Hartl DL (2016) Genotypic context and epistasis in individuals and populations. *Cell* 166(2): 279–287.

Sadée W, Dai ZY (2005) Pharmacogenetics/genomics and personalized medicine. *Hum Mol Genet Spec No* 2: R207–214.

Safar ME (1989) Pulse pressure in essential hypertension: Clinical and therapeutical implications. *J Hypertens* 7: 769–776.

Saito Y, Maekawa K, Ozawa S, Sawada J (2007) Genetic polymorphisms and haplotypes of major drug metabolizing enzymes in east asians and their comparison with other ethnic populations. *Curr Pharmacog* 5(1): 49–78.

Sandholm WH (2009) Evolutionary game theory. In: Meyers R (eds) *Encyclopedia of Complexity and Systems Science*. Springer, New York.

Sang MM, Rice S, Qiu L, Lin X, Gragnoli C, Belani CP, Wu RL (2019a) A rewiring model of intratumoral interaction networks. *Comput Struct Biotechnol J* 18: 45–51.

Sang M, Shi H, Wei K, Ye M, Jiang L, Sun L, Wu RL (2019b) A dissection model for mapping complex traits. *Plant J* 97(6): 1168–1182.

Sang MM, Dong A, Wu S, Feng J, Wang J, Griffin C, Wu RL (2022) A graph model of combination therapies. *Drug Discov Today* 27(5): 1210–1217.

Sangviroon A, Panomvana D, Tassaneeyakul W, Namchaisiri J (2010) Pharmacokinetic and pharmacodynamic variation associated with VKORC1 and CYP2C9 polymorphisms in Thai patients taking warfarin. *Drug Metab Pharmacokinet* 25(6): 531–538.

Schafer J, Lehmann BD, Gonzalez-Ericsson PI, Marshall CB, Beeler JS, Redman LN, Jin H, Sanchez V, Stubbs MC, et al. (2020) Targeting MYCN-expressing triple-negative breast cancer with BET and MEK inhibitors. *Sci Transl Med* 12: eaaw8275.

Schaid DJ, Chen W, Larson NB (2018) From genome-wide associations to candidate causal variants by statistical fine-mapping. *Nat Rev Genet* 19: 491–504.

Schärfe CPI, Tremmel R, Schwab M, et al. (2017) Genetic variation in human drug-related genes. *Genome Med* 9: 117.

Schork NJ (2019) Artificial intelligence and personalized medicine. In: Von Hoff D, Han H (eds) *Precision Medicine in Cancer Therapy. Cancer Treatment and Research.* Springer, Cham, Switzerland.

Scott SA, Sangkuhl K, Stein CM, Hulot JS, Mega JL, Roden DM, Klein TE, Sabatine MS, Johnson JA, Shuldiner AR (2013) Clinical pharmacogenetics implementation consortium guidelines for CYP2C19 genotype and clopidogrel therapy. *Clin Pharmacol Ther* 94: 317–323. (2013 Update)

Segura V, Vilhjálmsson BJ, Platt A, Korte A, Seren Ü, Long Q, Nordborg M (2012) An efficient multi-locus mixed-model approach for genome-wide association studies in structured populations. *Nat Genet* 44(7): 825–830.

Selevsek N, Caiment F, Nudischer R, Gmuender H, Agarkova I, Atkinson FL, Bachmann I, Baier V, Barel G, Bauer C (2020) Network integration and modelling of dynamic drug responses at multi-omics levels. *Commun Biol* 3: 573.

Sesso HD, Stampfer MJ, Rosner B, Hennekens CH, Gaziano JM, Manson JE Glynn RJ (2000) Systolic and diastolic blood pressure, pulse pressure, and mean arterial pressure as predictors of cardiovascular disease risk in men. *Hypertension* 36: 801–817.

Shahrezaei V, Swain PS (2008) Analytical distributions for stochastic gene expression. *Proc Natl Acad Sci U S A* 105: 17256–17261.

Shebley M, Einolf HJ (2019) Practical assessment of clinical drug–drug interactions in drug development using physiologically based pharmacokinetics modeling. *Clin Pharmacol Ther* 105(6): 1326–1328.

Shingleton A (2010) Allometry: The study of biological scaling. *Nat Ed Knowl* 3(10): 2.

Shirali M, Knott SA, Pong-Wong R, Navarro P, Haley CS (2018) Haplotype heritability mapping method uncovers missing heritability of complex traits. *Sci Rep* 8: 4982.

Shuldiner AR, O'Connell JR, Bliden KP, et al. (2009) Association of cytochrome P450 2C19 genotype with the antiplatelet effect and clinical efficacy of clopidogrel therapy. *JAMA* 302: 849–857.

Simeoni M, Magni P, Cammia C, De Nicolao G, Croci V, Pesenti E, Germani M, Poggesi I, Rocchetti M (2004) Predictive pharmacokinetic-pharmacodynamic modeling of tumor growth kinetics in xenograft models after administration of anticancer agents. *Cancer Res* 64: 1094–1101.

Sistonen J, Fuselli S, Palo JU, Chauhan N, Padh H, Sajantila A (2009) Pharmacogenetic variation at CYP2C9, CYP2C19, and CYP2D6 at global and microgeographic scales. *Pharmacogenet Genomics* 19(2): 170–179.

Smith KK (2003) Time's arrow: Heterochrony and the evolution of development. *Int J Dev Biol* 47(7–8): 613–621.

Smolensky MH, Hermida RC, Ayala DE, Portaluppi F (2015) Bedtime hypertension chronotherapy: Concepts and patient outcomes. *Curr Pharm Des* 21: 773–790.

Snyder MW, Adey A, Kitzman JO, Shendure J (2015) Haplotype-resolved genome sequencing: Experimental methods and applications. *Nat Rev Genet* 16: 344–358.

Sontag E, Kiyatkin A, Kholodenko BN (2004) Inferring dynamic architecture of cellular networks using time series of gene expression, protein and metabolite data. *Bioinformatics* 20(12): 1877–1886.

Sørensen H (2004) Parametric inference for diffusion processes observed at discrete points in time: A survey. *Int Stat Rev* 72: 337–354.

Sosnin S, Karlov D, Tetko IV, Fedorov MV (2019) Comparative study of multitask toxicity modeling on a broad chemical space. *J Chem Inf Model* 59: 1062–1072.

Speed D, Balding DJ (2014) MultiBLUP: Improved SNP-based prediction for complex traits. *Genome Res* 24(9): 1550–1557.

Srividhy J, Crampin EJ, McSharry PE, Schnell S (2007) Reconstructing biochemical pathways from time course data. *Proteomics* 7: 828–838.

Steimer W, Zöpf K, von Amelunxen S, Pfeiffer H, Bachofer J, Popp J (2005) Amitriptyline or not, that is the question: Pharmacogenetic testing of CYP2D6 and CYP2C19 identifies patients with low or high risk for side effects in amitriptyline therapy. *Clin Chem* 51(2): 376–385.

Steuer R, Kurths J, Daub CO, Weise J, Selbig J (2002) The mutual information: Detecting and evaluating dependencies between variables. *Bioinformatics* 18: S231–S240.

Suarez-Kurtz G, Parra EJ (2018) Population diversity in pharmacogenetics: A latin american perspective. *Adv Pharmacol* 83: 133–154.

Sui Y, Wu W, Wang Z, Wang J, Wang Z, Wu RL (2014) A case-control design for testing and estimating epigenetic effects on complex diseases. *Brief Bioinform* 15(2): 319–326.

Sul JH, Martin LS, Eskin E (2018) Population structure in genetic studies: Confounding factors and mixed models. *PLoS Genet* 14(12): e1007309.

Sulli G, Lam MTY, Panda S (2019) Interplay between circadian clock and cancer: New frontiers for cancer treatment. *Trends Cancer* 5(8): 475–494.

Sun L, Jiang L, Grant CN, Wang HG, Gragnoli C, Liu Z, Wu RL (2020) Computational identification of gene networks as a biomarker of neuroblastoma risk. *Cancers (Basel)* 12(8): 2086.

Sun LD, Dong A, Griffin C, Wu RL (2021) Statistical mechanics of clock gene networks underlying circadian rhythms. *Appl Phys Rev* 8: 021313.

Sun LD, Sang M, Zheng C, Wang D, Shi H, Liu K, Guo Y, Cheng T, Zhang Q, Wu RL (2018) The genetic architecture of heterochrony as a quantitative trait: Lessons from a computational model. *Brief Bioinform* 19(6): 1430–1439.

Sun LD, Wu RL (2015a) Mapping complex traits as a dynamic system. *Phys Life Rev* 13: 155–185.

Sun LD, Wu R (2015b) Toward the practical utility of systems mapping. *Phys Life Rev* 13: 198–201.

Sun LD, Ye MX, Hao H, Wang N, Wang YQ, Cheng T, Zhang QZ, Wu RL (2014) A model framework for identifying genes that guide the evolution of heterochrony. *Mol Biol Evol* 31: 2238–2247.

Suppiah V, Moldovan M, Ahlenstiel G, Berg T, Weltman M, Abate ML, Bassendine M, Spengler U, Dore GJ, Powell E (2009) IL28B is associated with response to chronic hepatitis C interferon-α and ribavirin therapy. *Nat Genet* 41: 1100–1104.

Suweis S, Simini F, Banavar JR, Maritan A (2013) Emergence of structural and dynamical properties of ecological mutualistic networks. *Nature* 500: 449–452.

Tabassum DP, Polyak K (2015) Tumorigenesis: It takes a village. *Nat Rev Cancer* 15: 473–483.

Takahashi T, Luzum JA, Nicol MR, Jacobson PA (2020) Pharmacogenomics of COVID-19 therapies. *NPJ Genomic Med* 5: 35.

Takeuchi F, McGinnis R, Bourgeois S, Barnes C, Eriksson N, Soranzo N, Whittaker P, Ranganath V, Kumanduri V, McLaren W, et al. (2009) A genome-wide association study confirms VKORC1, CYP2C9, and CYP4F2 as principal genetic determinants of warfarin dose. *PLoS Genet* 5: e1000433.

Tanaka Y, Nishida N, Sugiyama M, Kurosaki M, Matsuura K, Sakamoto N, Nakagawa M, Korenaga M, Hino K, Ito Y, et al. (2009) Genome-wide association of IL28B with response to pegylated interferon-α and ribavirin therapy for chronic hepatitis C. *Nat Genet* 41: 1105–1109.

Taylor JC, Bongartz T, Massey J, Mifsud B, Spiliopoulou A, Scott IC, Wang J, Morgan M, Plant D, Colombo M, et al. (2018) Consortia: Genome-wide association study of response to methotrexate in early rheumatoid arthritis patients. *Pharmacogenomics J* 18(4): 528–538.

Tegner J, Yeung MK, Hasty J, Collins JJ (2003) Reverse engineering gene networks: Integrating genetic perturbations with dynamical modeling. *Proc Natl Acad Sci U S A* 100: 5944–5949.

Teichert M, Eijgelsheim M, Rivadeneira F, Uitterlinden AG, van Schaik RH, Hofman A, De Smet PA, van Gelder T, Visser LE, Stricker BH (2009) A genome-wide association study of acenocoumarol maintenance dosage. *Hum Mol Genet* 18: 3758–3768.

Tekin E, Savage VM, Yeh PJ (2017) Measuring higher-order drug interactions: A review of recent approaches. *Curr Opin Syst Biol* 4: 16–23.

Tibshirani R (1996) Regression shrinkage and selection via the lasso. *J Roy StatiSoc Ser B* 58: 267–288. (Chapter 9)

Tornøe CW, Agersø H, Senderovitz T, Nielsen HA, Madsen H, Karlsson MO, Jonsson EN (2007) Population pharmacokinetic/pharmacodynamic (PK/PD) modelling of the hypothalamic-pituitary-gonadal axis following treatment with GnRH analogues. *Br J Clin Pharmacol* 63(6): 648–664.

Tornøe CW, Jacobsen JL, Madsen H (2004) Grey-box pharmacokinetic/pharmacodynamic modelling of a euglycaemic clamp study. *J Math Biol* 48: 591–604.

Tran MT, Grillo JA (2019) Translation of drug interaction knowledge to actionable labeling. *Clin Pharmacol Ther* 105(6): 1292–1295.

Truong VT, Baverel PG, Lythe GD, Vicini P, Yates JWT, Dubois VFS (2022) Step-by-step comparison of ordinary differential equation and agent-based approaches to pharmacokinetic-pharmacodynamic models. *CPT Pharmacometrics Syst Pharmacol* 11(2): 133–148.

Tse SM, Tantisira K, Weiss ST (2011) The pharmacogenetics and pharmacogenomics of asthma therapy. *Pharmacogenomics J* 11(6): 383–392.

Tsuyuzaki K, Ishii M, Nikaido I (2019) Uncovering hypergraphs of cell-cell interaction from single cell RNA-sequencing data. Preprint at bioRxiv. https://doi.org/10.1101/566182.

Tuntland T, Ethell B, Kosaka T, Blasco F, Zang RX, Jain M, Gould T, Hoffmaster K (2014) Implementation of pharmacokinetic and pharmacodynamic strategies in early research phases of drug discovery and development at Novartis Institute of Biomedical Research. *Front Pharmacol* 5: 174.

Tyers M, Wright GD (2019) Drug combinations: A strategy to extend the life of antibiotics in the 21st century. *Nat Rev Microbiol* 17(3): 141–155.

Tyler SR, Rotti PG, Sun X, Yi Y, Xie W, Winter MC, Flamme-Wiese MJ, Tucker BA, Mullins RF, Norris AW, et al. (2019) PyMINEr finds gene and autocrineparacrine networks from human islet scRNA-Seq. *Cell Rep* 26: 1951–1964.e8.

Uddin MS, Kabir MT, Al MA, Abdel-Daim MM, Barreto GE, Ashraf GM (2019) APOE and Alzheimer's disease: Evidence mounts that targeting APOe4 may combat Alzheimer's pathogenesis. *Mol Neurobiol* 56: 2450–2465.

Udrescu L, Sbârcea L, Topîrceanu A, Iovanovici A, Kurunczi L, Bogdan P, Udrescu M (2016) Clustering drug–drug interaction networks with energy model layouts: Community analysis and drug repurposing. *Sci Rep* 6: 32745.

Uemoto Y, Pong-Wong R, Navarro P, Vitart V, Hayward C, Wilson JF, Rudan I, Campbell H, Hastie ND, Wright AF, Haley CS (2013) The power of regional heritability analysis for rare and common variant detection: Simulations and application to eye biometrical traits. *Front Genet* 4: 232.

van der Wijst MGP, Brugge H, de Vries DH, Deelen P, Swertz MA, LifeLines Cohort Study, BIOS Consortium, Franke L (2018) Single-cell RNA sequencing identifies celltype-specific cis-eQTLs and co-expression QTLs. *Nat Genet* 50(4): 493–497.

van der Wijst MGP, de Vries DH, Brugge H, Westra HJ, Franke L (2018) An integrative approach for building personalized gene regulatory networks for precision medicine. *Genome Med* 10: 96.

van der Wouden CH, Böhringer S, Cecchin E, Cheung KC, Dávila-Fajardo CL, Deneer VHM, Dolžan V, Ingelman-Sundberg M, Jönsson S, Karlsson MO, et al., Ubiquitous Pharmacogenomics Consortium (2020) Generating evidence for precision medicine: Considerations made by the Ubiquitous Pharmacogenomics Consortium when designing and operationalizing the PREPARE study. *Pharmacogenet Genomics* 30(6): 131–144.

Varma MVS, Bi YA, Lazzaro S, West M (2019) Clopidogrel as a perpetrator of drug–drug interactions: A challenge for quantitative predictions? *Clin Pharmacol Ther* 105(6): 1295–1299.

Venkatakrishnan K, Rostami-Hodjegan A (2019) Come dance with me: Transformative changes in the science and practice of drug–drug interactions. *Clin Pharmacol Ther* 105(6): 1272–1278.

Venkatesan S, Swanton C (2016) Tumor evolutionary principles: How intratumor heterogeneity influences cancer treatment and outcome. *Am Soc Clin Oncol Educ Book* 35: e141–e149.

Vennin S, Li Y, Willemet M, Fok H, Gu H, Charlton P, Alastruey J, Chowienczyk P (2017) Identifying hemodynamic determinants of pulse pressure: A combined numerical and physiological approach. *Hypertension* 70(6): 1176–1182.

Vento-Tormo R, Efremova M, Botting RA, Turco MY, Vento-Tormo M, Meyer KB, Park JE, Stephenson E, Polański K, Goncalves A (2018) Single-cell reconstruction of the early maternal-fetal interface in humans. *Nature* 563: 347–353.

Versieren L, Evers S, De Schamphelaere KAC, Blust R, Smolders E (2016) Mixture toxicity and interactions of copper, nickel, cadmium, and zinc to barley at low effect levels: Something from nothing? *Environ Toxicol Chem* 35: 2483–2492.

Viatte C, Strong K, Hannigan J, Nussbaumer E, Emmons LK, Conway S, Paton-Walsh C, Hartley J, Benmergui L, Lin J (2015) Identifying fire plumes in the Arctic with tropospheric FTIR measurements and transport models. *Atmos Chem Phys* 15: 2227–2246.

Vijesh N, Chakrabarti SK, Sreekumar J (2013) Modeling of gene regulatory networks: A review. *J Biomed Sci Eng* 6: 223–231.

Vogel F (1959) Moderne probleme der humangenetik. *Ergebn Inn Med Kinderheilkd* 12: 52–125.

von Neumann J, Morgenstern O (1944) *Theory of Games and Economic Behavior*. Princeton University Press, Princeton, NJ. (Chapter 9).

Wagner GP, Pavlicev M, Cheverud JM (2007) The road to modularity. *Nat Rev Genet* 8(12): 921–931.

Wagner J, Rapsomaniki MA, Chevrier S, Anzeneder T, Langwieder C, Dykgers A, Rees M, Ramaswamy A, Muenst S, Soysal SD, et al. (2019) A single-cell atlas of the tumor and immune ecosystem of human breast cancer. *Cell* 177(5): 1330–1345.

Wain LV, Vaez A, Jansen R, Joehanes R, van der Most PJ, Erzurumluoglu AM, O'Reilly PF, Cabrera CP, et al. (2017) Novel blood pressure locus and gene discovery using genome-wide association study and expression data sets from blood and the kidney. *Hypertension* 70: e4–e19.

Wain LV, Verwoert GC, O'Reilly PF, Shi G, Johnson T, Johnson AD, Bochud M, Rice KM, Henneman P, Smith AV, et al. (2011) Genome-wide association study identifies six new loci influencing pulse pressure and mean arterial pressure. *Nat Genet* 43: 1005–1011.

Wainberg M, Sinnott-Armstrong N, Mancuso N, Barbeira AN, Knowles DA, Golan D, Ermel R, Ruusalepp A, Quertermous T, Hao K, et al. (2019) Opportunities and challenges for transcriptome-wide association studies. *Nat Genet* 51(4): 592–599.

Wang H, Leng C (2008) A note on the adaptive group Lasso. *Comput Stat Data Analy* 52: 5277–5286.

Wang HJ, Ye MX, Fu YR, Dong A, Zhu XL, Bo WH, Jiang LB, Griffin CH, Liang D, Wu RL (2021) Modeling genome-wide by environment interactions through omnigenic interactome networks. *Cell Rep* 35: 109114.

Wang LW, McLeod HL, Weinshilboum RM (2011) Genomics and drug response. *N Engl J Med* 364: 1144–1153.

Wang Q, Dong A, Jiang L, Griffin C, Wu RL (2022) A single-cell omics network model of cell crosstalk during the formation of primordial follicles. *Cell* 11(3): 332.

Wang Q, Gan J, Wei K, Berceli SA, Gragnoli C, Wu RL (2019a) A unifying framework to map multifaceted pharmacodynamic responses to hypertension interventions. *Drug Discov Today* 24: 883–889.

Wang S, Karikomi M, MacLean AL, Nie Q (2019b) Cell lineage and communication network inference via optimization for single-cell transcriptomics. *Nucleic Acids Res* 47: e66.

Wang X, Zhang HY, Chen XZ (2019c) Drug resistance and combating drug resistance in cancer. *Cancer Drug Resist* 2(2): 141–160.

Wang Y, Wang R, Zhnag S, Song S, Jiang C, Han G, Wang M, Ajani J, Futreal A, Wang L (2019d) iTALK: An R package to characterize and illustrate intercellular communication. Preprint at bioRxiv. https://doi.org/10.1101/507871.

Wang Q, Gosik K, Xing SJ, Jiang LB, Sun LD, Chinchilli VM, Wu RL (2017a) Integration of epigenetic game theory and developmental principles. *Phys Life Rev* 20: 166–169.

Wang Q, Gosik K, Xing SJ, Jiang LB, Sun LD, Chinchilli VM, Wu RL (2017b) Epigenetic game theory: How to compute the epigenetic control of maternal-to-zygotic transition. *Phys Life Rev* 20: 126–137.

Wang Y, Eskridge K, Zhang SP, Wang D (2008) Using spline-enhanced ordinary differential equations for PK/PD model development. *J Pharmacokinet Pharmacodyn* 35: 553–571.

Wang Y, Kilic O, Csizmar CM, Ashok S, Hougland JL, Distefano MD, Wagner CR (2020) Engineering reversible cell-cell interactions using enzymatically lipidated chemically self-assembled nanorings. *Chem Sci* 12(1): 331–340.

Wang YQ, Tong C, Wang Z, Wang Z, Mauger D, Tantisira KG, Israel E, Szefler SJ, Chinchilli VM, Boushey HA, et al. (2015a) Pharmacodynamic genome-wide association study identifies new response loci for glucocorticoid intervention in asthma. *Pharmacogenomics J.* 15: 422–429.

Wang ZH, Butner JD, Cristini V, Deisboeck TS (2015b) Integrated PK-PD and agent-based modeling in oncology. *J Pharmacokinet Pharmacodyn* 42: 179–189.

Wang YQ, Wang NT, Wang JX, Wang Z, Wu RL (2013a) Delivering systems pharmacogenomics towards precision medicine through mathematics. *Adv Drug Deliv Rev* 65: 905–911.

Wang Z, Pang XM, Lv YF, Xu F, Zhou T, Li X, Feng SS, Li JH, Li ZK, Wu RL (2013b) A dynamic framework for quantifying the genetic architecture of phenotypic plasticity. *Brief Bioinform* 14: 82–95.

Wang Z, Li HY, Li JH, Wang JX, Wang YQ, Wang NT, Wu RL (2013c) Statistical resolution of missing longitudinal data in clinical pharmacogenomics. *Adv Drug Deliv Rev* 65: 912–917.

Wang ZH, Wang Z, Fu GF, Luo JT, Wu RL (2013d) Stochastic modeling of systems mapping for drug response. *Adv Drug Deliv Rev* 65: 912–917. (Chapter 1)

Wang YQ, Xu M, Wang Z, Tao M, Wang L, Zhu J, Li RZ, Berceli SA, Wu RL (2012) How to cluster gene expression dynamics in response to environmental signals. *Brief Bioinform* 13: 162–174.

Wang YX, Huang H (2014) Review on statistical methods for gene network reconstruction using expression data. *J Theor Biol* 362: 53–61.

Wang YY, Kang HG, Xu TY, Hao LL, Bao YM, Jia PL (2022) CeDR Atlas: A knowledgebase of cellular drug response. *Nucleic Acids Res* 50(D1): D1164–D1171.

Wang Z, Wang Y, Wang N, Wang J, Wang Z, Vallejos CE, Wu RL (2014) Towards a comprehensive picture of the genetic landscape of complex traits. *Brief Bioinform* 15(1): 30–42.

Wang ZH, Hou W, Wu RL (2005) A statistical model to analyze quantitative trait locus interactions for HIV dynamics from the virus and human genomes. *Stat Med* 25: 495–511.

Wang ZH, Li Y, Li Q, Wu RL (2009) Joint functional mapping of quantitative trait loci for HIV-1 and CD4+ dynamics. *Int J Biostat* 5(1): Article 9.

Wang ZH, Wu RL (2004) A statistical model for high-resolution mapping of quantitative trait loci determining human HIV-1 dynamics. *Stat Med* 23: 3033–3051.

Waring JF, Tang Q, Robieson WZ, King DP, Das U, Dubow J, Dutta S, Marek GJ, Gault LM (2015) APOE-varepsilon4 carrier status and donepezil response in patients with Alzheimer's disease. *J Alzheimers Dis* 47: 137–148.

Watters JW, Kraja A, Meucci MA, Province MA, McLeod HL (2004) Genome-wide discovery of loci influencing chemotherapy cytotoxicity. *Proc Natl Acad Sci U S A* 101(32): 11809–11814.

Wei K, Wang J, Sang MM, Zhang SL, Zhou HC, Jiang LB, Michelangeli JAC, Vallejos CE, Wu RL (2018a) An ecophysiologically based model identifies a major pleiotropic QTL for leaf growth trajectories of *Phaseolus vulgaris*. *Plant J* 95: 775–784.

Wei K, Wang Q, Gan JW, Zhang SL, Gragnoli C, Wu RL (2018b) Mapping genes for drug chronotherapy. *Drug Discov Today* 23: 1883–1888.

Weibull JW (1995) *Evolutionary Game Theory*. MIT Press, Cambridge, MA.

Weigelt B, Reis-Filho JS (2014) Epistatic interactions and drug response. *J Pathol* 232(2): 255–263.

Weinshilboum R (2003) Inheritance and drug response. *N Engl J Med* 348(6): 529–537.

Weinshilboum RM, Wang LW (2006) Pharmacogenetics and pharmacogenomics: Development, science, and translation. *Annu Rev Genomics Hum Genet* 7: 223–245.

Weinshilboum RM, Wang LW (2017) Pharmacogenomics: Precision medicine and drug response. *Mayo Clin Proc* 92(11): 1711–1722.

Weinstein ZB, Kuru N, Kiriakov S, Palmer AC, Khalil AS, Clemons PA, Zaman MH, Roth FP, Cokol M (2018) Modeling the impact of drug interactions on therapeutic selectivity. *Nat Commun* 9: 3452.

Weiss S, Silverman E, Palmer L (2001) Case-Control association studies in pharmacogenetics. *Pharmacogenomics J* 1: 157–158.

Wen S, Wang CG, Berg A, Li Y, Chang MM, Fillingim RB, Wallace MR, Staud R, Kaplan L, Wu RL (2009) Modeling genetic imprinting effects of DNA sequences with multilocus polymorphism data. *Algor Mol Biol* 4: 11.

Wen YJ, Zhang H, Ni YL, Huang B, Zhang J, Feng JY, Wang SB, Dunwell JM, Zhang YM, Wu RL (2018) Methodological implementation of mixed linear models in multi-locus genome-wide association studies. *Brief Bioinform* 19(4): 700–712.

West GB, Brown JH, Enquist BJ (2001) A general model for ontogenetic growth. *Nature* 413(6856): 628–631.

Widmer C, Lippert C, Weissbrod O, Fusi N, Kadie C, Davidson R, Listgarten J, Heckerman D (2014) Further improvements to linear mixed models for genome-wide association studies. *Sci Rep* 4: 6874.

Wijsman EM (2016) Family-based approaches: Design, imputation, analysis, and beyond. *BMC Genet* 17: S9.

Witz IP (2008) Tumor-microenvironment interactions: Dangerous liaisons. *Adv Cancer Res* 100: 203–229.

Wolking S, Campbell C, Stapleton C, McCormack M, Delanty N, Depondt C, Johnson MR, Koeleman BPC, Krause R, Kunz WS, et al. (2021) Role of common genetic variants for drug-resistance to specific anti-seizure medications. *Front Pharmacol* 12: 688386.

Woo AY, Song Y, Xiao RP, Zhu W (2015) Biased β_2-adrenoceptor signalling in heart failure: Pathophysiology and drug discovery. *Br J Pharmacol* 172: 5444–5456.

Wu H, Lu T, Xue H, Liang H (2014) Sparse additive ordinary differential equations for dynamic gene regulatory network modeling. *J Am Stat Assoc* 109: 700–716.

Wu MC, Bailey KR (1989) Estimation and comparison of changes in the presence of informative right censoring: Conditional linear model. *Biometrics* 939–955.

Wu MC, Carroll RJ (1988) Estimation and comparison of changes in the presence of informative right censoring by modeling the censoring process. *Biometrics* 175–188.

Wu RL (2021) Systems genetics. *Front Syst Biol* 1: 738155.

Wu RL, Cao JG, Huang ZW, Wang Z, Gai JY, Vallejos CE (2011a) Systems mapping: How to improve the genetic mapping of complex traits through design principles of biological systems. *BMC Syst Biol* 5: 84.

Wu RL, Tong CF, Wang Z, Mauger D, Chinchilli VM, Tantisira K, Szefler SJ, Israel E (2011b) A conceptual framework for integrating pharmacodynamic principles into genome-wide association studies for pharmacogenomics. *Drug Discov Today* 16: 884–890.

Wu RL, Hou W (2006) A hyperspace model to decipher the genetic architecture of developmental processes: Allometry meets ontogeny. *Genetics* 172(1): 627–637.

Wu RL, Hou W, Cui YH, Li HY, Liu T, Wu S, Ma C-X, Zeng YR (2007) Mapping the genetic architecture of complex traits with molecular markers. *Recent Patents Nanotech* 1: 41–49.

Wu RL, Jiang LB (2021) Recovering dynamic networks in big static datasets. *Phys Rep* 812: 1–57.

Wu RL, Lin M (2006) Functional mapping – How to map and study the genetic architecture of dynamic complex traits. *Nat Rev Genet* 7: 229–237.

Wu RL, Lin M (2008) *Statistical and Computational Pharmacogenomics*. Chapman & Hall/CRC, London.

Wu RL, Ma CX, Casella G (2007) *Statistical Genetics of Quantitative Traits: Linkage, Maps, and QTL*. Springer-Verlag, New York.

Wu RL, Ma C-X, Lin M, Casella G (2004a) A general framework for analyzing the genetic architecture of developmental characteristics. *Genetics* 166: 1541–1551.

Wu RL, Ma C-X, M Lin, Wang ZH, Casella G (2004b) Functional mapping of quantitative trait loci underlying growth trajectories using a transform-both-sides logistic model. *Biometrics* 60: 729–738.

Wu RL, Ma CX, Littell RC, Wu SS, Yin T, Huang M, Wang M, Casella G (2002) A logistic mixture model for characterizing genetic determinants causing differentiation in growth trajectories. *Genet Res* 79(3): 235–245.

Wu RL, Zeng Z-B (2001) Joint linkage and linkage disequilibrium mapping in natural populations. *Genetics* 157: 899–909.

Wu Z, Lawrence PJ, Ma A, Zhu J, Xu D, Ma Q (2020) Single-Cell techniques and deep learning in predicting drug response. *Trends Pharmacol Sci* 41(12): 1050–1065.

Wulfsohn MS, Tsiatis AA (1997) A joint model for survival and longitudinal data measured with error. *Biometrics* 330–339.

Xia X (2017) Bioinformatics and drug discovery. *Curr Top Med Chem* 17: 1709–1726.

Xia XH (2020) Drug efficacy and toxicity prediction: An innovative application of transcriptomic data. *Cell Biol Toxicol* 36: 591–602.

Xie XM, Hanson C, Sinha S (2019) Mechanistic interpretation of non-coding variants for discovering transcriptional regulators of drug response. *BMC Biol* 17: 62.

Xu M, Jiang L, Zhu S, Zhou C, Ye M, Mao K, Sun L, Su X, Pan H, Zhang S, et al. (2006) A computational framework for mapping the timing of vegetative phase change. *New Phytol* 211(2): 750–760.

Yaghoobi H, Haghipour S, Hamzeiy H, Asadi-Khiavi M (2012) A review of modeling techniques for genetic regulatory networks. *J Med Signals Sens* 2(1): 61–70.

Yamamoto TN, Kishton RJ, Restifo NP (2019) Developing neoantigen-targeted T cell-based treatments for solid tumors. *Nat Med* 25(10): 1488–1499.

Yamashita F, Hashida M (2013) Pharmacokinetic considerations for targeted drug delivery. *Adv Drug Deliv Rev* 65: 139–147.

Yang DC, Jin Y, Ye MX, He XQ, Wu RL (2021) Inferring multilayer interactome networks shaping phenotypic plasticity and evolution. *Nat Commun* 12: 5304.

Yap JS, Fan J, Wu RL (2009) Nonparametric modeling of longitudinal covariance structure in functional mapping of quantitative trait loci. *Biometrics* 65(4): 1068–1077.

Yap JS, Fan JQ, Wu RL (2009) Nonparametric modeling of covariance structure in functional mapping of quantitative trait loci. *Biometrics* 65: 1068–1077.

Yilancioglu K, Cokol M, Pastirmaci I, Erman B, Cetiner S (2014) Oxidative stress is a mediator for increased lipid accumulation in a newly isolated *Dunaliella salina* strain. *PLoS ONE* 9: e91957.

Yonatan Y, Amit G, Friedman J, Bashan A (2022) Complexity-stability trade-off in empirical microbial ecosystems. *Nat Ecol Evol* https://doi.org/10.1038/s41559-022-01745-8.

You D, Richardson JR, Aleksunes LM (2020) Epigenetic regulation of multidrug resistance protein 1 and breast cancer resistance protein transporters by histone deacetylase inhibition. *Drug Metab Dispos* 48(6): 459–480.

Yu JM, Pressoir G, Briggs WH, Vroh BI, Yamasaki M, Doebley JF, McMullen MD, Gaut BS, Nielsen DM, Holland JB, et al. (2006) A unified mixed-model method for association mapping that accounts for multiple levels of relatedness. *Nat Genet* 38: 203–208.

Yu MG, Law NJ, Taylor JMG, Sandler HM (2004) Joint longitudinal-survival-cure models and their application to prostate cancer. *Stat Sini* 14: 835–862.

Yuan M, Lin Y (2006) Model selection and estimation in regression with grouped variables. *J Roy Stat Sco B* 68: 49–67.

Zeggini E, Gloyn AL, Barton AC, Wain LV (2019) Translational genomics and precision medicine: Moving from the lab to the clinic. *Science* 365: 1409–1413.

Zhang CL, Yu Z, Li X, Liu D (2014) Chronopharmacodynamics and chronopharmacokinetics of pethidine in mice. *PLoS ONE* 9(7): e102054.

Zhang G, Nebert DW (2017) Personalized medicine: Genetic risk prediction of drug response. *Pharmacol Ther* 175: 75–90.

Zhang JD, Sach-Peltason L, Kramer C, Wang K, Ebeling M (2020) Multiscale modelling of drug mechanism and safety. *Drug Discov Today* 25: 519–534.

Zhang M, Bo W, Xu F, Li H, Ye M, Jiang L, Shi C, Fu Y, Zhao G, Huang Y, et al. (2017) The genetic architecture of shoot-root covariation during seedling emergence of a desert tree, Populus euphratica. *Plant J* 90(5): 918–928.

Zhang TH, Dai L, Barton JP, Du Y, Tan Y, Pang W, Chakraborty AK, Lloyd-Smith JO, Sun R (2020) Predominance of positive epistasis among drug resistance-associated mutations in HIV-1 protease. *PLoS Genet* 16(10): e1009009.

Zhang Y, Giacchetti S, Parouchev A, Hadadi E, Li X, Dallmann R, Xandri-Monje H, Portier L, Adam R, Lévi F, et al. (2018) Dosing time dependent in vitro pharmacodynamics of Everolimus despite a defective circadian clock. *Cell Cycle* 17(1): 33–42.

Zhang Y, Huynh JM, Liu GS, Ballweg R, Aryeh KS, Paek AL, Zhang T (2019) Designing combination therapies with modeling chaperoned machine learning. *PLoS Comput Biol* 15(9): e1007158.

Zhao S, Iyengar R (2012) Systems pharmacology: Network analysis to identify multiscale mechanisms of drug action. *Annu Rev Pharmacol Toxicol* 52(1): 505–521.

Zhao W, Chen YQ, Casella G, Cheverud JM, Wu RL (2005a) A non-stationary model for functional mapping of complex traits. *Bioinformatics* 21: 2469–2477.

Zhao W, Hou W, Littell RC, Wu RL (2005b) Structured antedependence models for functional mapping of multiple longitudinal traits. *Stat Appl Genet Mol Biol* 4(1): 26.

Zhao W, Dovas A, Spinazzi EF, Levitin HM, Banu MA, Upadhyayula P, Sudhakar T, Marie T, Otten ML, Sisti MB, et al. (2021) Deconvolution of cell type-specific drug responses in human tumor tissue with single-cell RNA-seq. *Genome Med* 13(1): 82.

Zhao W, Wu RL, Ma CX, Casella G (2004) A fast algorithm for functional mapping of complex traits. *Genetics* 167(4): 2133–2137.

Zhou K, Pearson ER (2013) Insights from genome-wide association studies of drug response. *Annu Rev Pharmacol Toxicol* 53: 299–310.

Zhou X, Franklin RA, Adler M, Jacox JB, Bailis W, Shyer JA, Flavell RA, Mayo A, Alon U, Medzhitov R (2018) Circuit design features of a stable two-cell system. *Cell* 172(4): 744–757.e17.

Zhou X, Stephens M (2012) Genome-wide efficient mixed-model analysis for association studies. *Nat Genet* 44(7): 821–824.

Zhou Y, Lauschke VM (2019) Pharmacogenomic network analysis of the gene-drug interaction landscape underlying drug disposition. *Comput Struct Biotechnol J* 18: 52–58.

Zhu XL, Jiang LB, Ye MX, Sun LD, Gragnoli C, Wu RL (2016) Integrating evolutionary game theory into mechanistic genotype-phenotype mapping. *Trends Genet* 32: 256–268.

Zimmerman DL, Núñez-Antón VA (2001) Parametric modelling of growth curve data: An overview. *Test* 10: 1–73.

Zimmerman DL, Núñez-Antón VA (2009) *Antedependence Models for Longitudinal Data*. CRC Press, Boca Raton, FL.

Zou H, Hastie T (2005) Regularization and variable selection via the elastic net. *J Roy Stat Soc B* 67: 301–320.

Zou HX, Banerjee P, Leung SSY, Yan XY (2020) Application of pharmacokinetic-pharmacodynamic modeling in drug delivery: Development and challenges. *Front Pharmacol* 11: 997.

Zou M, Conzen SD (2005) A new dynamic Bayesian network (DBN) approach for identifying gene regulatory networks from time course microarray data. *Bioinformatics* 21(1): 71–79.

Zwietering MH, Jongenburger I, Rombouts FM, van't Riet K (1990) Modeling of the bacterial growth curve. *Appl Environ Microbiol* 56(6): 1875–1881.

Index

Note: **Bold** page numbers refer to tables and *italic* page numbers refer to figures.

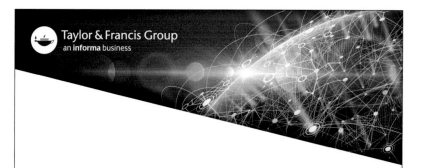